Molecular Analysis of Cancer

METHODS IN MOLECULAR MEDICINE ™

John M. Walker, Series Editor

70. **Cystic Fibrosis Methods and Protocols,** edited by *William R. Skach*, 2002

69. **Gene Therapy Protocols, 2nd ed.**, edited by *Jeffrey R. Morgan*, 2002

68. **Molecular Analysis of Cancer,** edited by *Jacqueline Boultwood and Carrie Fidler*, 2002

67. **Meningococcal Disease:** *Methods and Protocols*, edited by *Andrew J. Pollard and Martin C. J. Maiden*, 2001

66. **Meningococcal Vaccines:** *Methods and Protocols*, edited by *Andrew J. Pollard and Martin C. J. Maiden*, 2001

65. **Nonviral Vectors for Gene Therapy:** *Methods and Protocols*, edited by *Mark A. Findeis*, 2001

64. **Dendritic Cell Protocols,** edited by *Stephen P. Robinson and Andrew J. Stagg*, 2001

63. **Hematopoietic Stem Cell Protocols,** edited by *Christopher A. Klug and Craig T. Jordan*, 2001

62. **Parkinson's Disease:** *Methods and Protocols*, edited by *M. Maral Mouradian*, 2001

61. **Melanoma Techniques and Protocols:** *Molecular Diagnosis, Treatment, and Monitoring*, edited by *Brian J. Nickoloff*, 2001

60. **Interleukin Protocols,** edited by *Luke A. J. O'Neill and Andrew Bowie*, 2001

59. **Molecular Pathology of the Prions,** edited by *Harry F. Baker*, 2001

58. **Metastasis Research Protocols:** *Volume 2, Cell Behavior In Vitro and In Vivo*, edited by *Susan A. Brooks and Udo Schumacher*, 2001

57. **Metastasis Research Protocols:** *Volume 1, Analysis of Cells and Tissues*, edited by *Susan A. Brooks and Udo Schumacher*, 2001

56. **Human Airway Inflammation:** *Sampling Techniques and Analytical Protocols*, edited by *Duncan F. Rogers and Louise E. Donnelly*, 2001

55. **Hematologic Malignancies:** *Methods and Protocols*, edited by *Guy B. Faguet*, 2001

54. *Mycobacterium tuberculosis* **Protocols,** edited by *Tanya Parish and Neil G. Stoker*, 2001

53. **Renal Cancer:** *Methods and Protocols*, edited by *Jack H. Mydlo*, 2001

52. **Atherosclerosis:** *Experimental Methods and Protocols*, edited by *Angela F. Drew*, 2001

51. **Angiotensin Protocols**, edited by *Donna H. Wang*, 2001

50. **Colorectal Cancer:** *Methods and Protocols*, edited by *Steven M. Powell*, 2001

49. **Molecular Pathology Protocols**, edited by *Anthony A. Killeen*, 2001

48. **Antibiotic Resistance Methods and Protocols,** edited by *Stephen H. Gillespie*, 2001

47. **Vision Research Protocols,** edited by *P. Elizabeth Rakoczy*, 2001

46. **Angiogenesis Protocols,** edited by *J. Clifford Murray*, 2001

45. **Hepatocellular Carcinoma:** *Methods and Protocols*, edited by *Nagy A. Habib*, 2000

44. **Asthma:** *Mechanisms and Protocols*, edited by *K. Fan Chung and Ian Adcock*, 2001

43. **Muscular Dystrophy:** *Methods and Protocols*, edited by *Katherine B. Bushby and Louise Anderson*, 2001

42. **Vaccine Adjuvants:** *Preparation Methods and Research Protocols*, edited by *Derek T. O'Hagan*, 2000

41. **Celiac Disease:** *Methods and Protocols*, edited by *Michael N. Marsh*, 2000

40. **Diagnostic and Therapeutic Antibodies,** edited by *Andrew J. T. George and Catherine E. Urch*, 2000

39. **Ovarian Cancer:** *Methods and Protocols*, edited by *John M. S. Bartlett*, 2000

38. **Aging Methods and Protocols,** edited by *Yvonne A. Barnett and Christopher R. Barnett*, 2000

37. **Electrochemotherapy, Electrogenetherapy, and Transdermal Drug Delivery:** *Electrically Mediated Delivery of Molecules to Cells*, edited by *Mark J. Jaroszeski, Richard Heller, and Richard Gilbert*, 2000

36. **Septic Shock Methods and Protocols,** edited by *Thomas J. Evans*, 2000

Methods in Molecular Medicine

Molecular Analysis of Cancer

Edited by

Jacqueline Boultwood

and

Carrie Fidler

*Leukaemia Research Fund Molecular Haematology Unit,
University of Oxford, NDCLS, John Radcliffe Hospital, Oxford, UK*

Humana Press ✳ Totowa, New Jersey

© 2002 Humana Press Inc.
Softcover reprint of the hardcover 1st edition 2002
999 Riverview Drive, Suite 208
Totowa, New Jersey 07512

www.humanapress.com

All rights reserved. No part of this book may be reproduced, stored in a retrieval system, or transmitted in any form or by any means, electronic, mechanical, photocopying, microfilming, recording, or otherwise without written permission from the Publisher. Methods in Molecular Medicine™ is a trademark of The Humana Press Inc.

The content and opinions expressed in this book are the sole work of the authors and editors, who have warranted due diligence in the creation and issuance of their work. The publisher, editors, and authors are not responsible for errors or omissions or for any consequences arising from the information or opinions presented in this book and make no warranty, express or implied, with respect to its contents.

This publication is printed on acid-free paper. ∞
ANSI Z39.48-1984 (American Standards Institute) Permanence of Paper for Printed Library Materials.

Cover Illustration: Fig. 1A from Chapter 3: "Spectral Karyotyping in Cancer Cytogenetics" by E. Hilgenfeld, et al.

Production Editor: Jessica Jannicelli.
Cover design by Patricia F. Cleary.

For additional copies, pricing for bulk purchases, and/or information about other Humana titles, contact Humana at the above address or at any of the following numbers: Tel.: 973-256-1699; Fax: 973-256-8341; E-mail: humana@humanapr.com; Website: humanapress.com

Photocopy Authorization Policy:
Authorization to photocopy items for internal or personal use, or the internal or personal use of specific clients, is granted by Humana Press Inc., provided that the base fee of US $10.00 per copy, plus US $00.25 per page, is paid directly to the Copyright Clearance Center at 222 Rosewood Drive, Danvers, MA 01923. For those organizations that have been granted a photocopy license from the CCC, a separate system of payment has been arranged and is acceptable to Humana Press Inc.

10 9 8 7 6 5 4 3 2 1

Library of Congress Cataloging in Publication Data

Main entry under title:

Methods in molecular medicine™.

Molecular analysis of cancer/edited by Jacqueline Boultwood and Carrie Fidler.
     p. ; cm. -- (Methods in molecular medicine ; 68)
   Includes bibliographical references and index.
   ISBN 978-1-61737-102-8   e-ISBN 978-1-59259-135-0
     1. Cancer--Genetic aspects--Research--Methodology. 2. Cancer--Molecular aspects--Research--Methodology. I. Boultwood, Jacqueline. II. Fidler, Carrie. III. Series.
   [DNLM: 1. Neoplasms--genetics. 2. Cell Transformation, Neoplastic--genetics. 3. Gene Expression Regulation, Neoplastic. 4. Genetic Techniques. QZ 200 M7175 2001]
   RC268.4 .M627 2001
   616.99'4042--dc21

2001024306

Preface

Over the past 20 years, technological advances in molecular biology have proven invaluable to the understanding of the pathogenesis of human cancer. The application of molecular technology to the study of cancer has not only led to advances in tumor diagnosis, but has also provided markers for the assessment of prognosis and disease progression. The aim of *Molecular Analysis of Cancer* is to provide a comprehensive collection of the most up-to-date techniques for the detection of molecular changes in human cancer. Leading researchers in the field have contributed chapters detailing practical procedures for a wide range of state-of-the-art techniques.

Molecular Analysis of Cancer includes chapters describing techniques for the identification of chromosomal abnormalities and comprising: fluorescent *in situ* hybridization (FISH), spectral karyotyping (SKY), comparative genomic hybridization (CGH), and microsatellite analysis. FISH has a prominent role in the molecular analysis of cancer and can be used for the detection of numerical and structural chromosomal abnormalities. The recently described SKY, in which all human metaphase chromosomes are visualized in specific colors, allows for the definition of all chromosomal rearrangements and marker chromosomes in a tumor cell. Protocols for the detection of chromosomal rearrangements by PCR and RT-PCR are described, as well as the technique of DNA fingerprinting, a powerful tool for studying somatic genetic alterations in tumorigenesis. A number of approaches to identify mutations are detailed, and include SSCP, DGGE, the nonisotopic RNase cleavage assay, the protein truncation assay, and DNA sequencing. A change in DNA methylation status is commonly observed in cancer, and specific methodology for methylation analysis is also provided by this volume.

The analysis of gene expression represents a key area of research in the study of human cancer and a number of chapters in *Molecular Analysis of Cancer* address this subject. Global RNA expression analysis using microarray technology allows the identification of genes that are differentially expressed in tumor versus normal tissues. This is a powerful approach for identifying genes that are central to disease development or progression and can also identify new prognostic markers.

v

A reduction in telomere length, together with expression of the telomere maintenance enzyme, telomerase, has been described in a wide range of human cancers. To complete the volume, we include chapters describing the measurement of telomere length and telomerase levels, an area of extensive study in the field of cancer research.

We wish to thank the authors of the various chapters of *Molecular Analysis of Cancer* for their excellent contributions. Clearly, they share our hope that this volume will assist other researchers in the analysis and detection of genetic abnormalities occurring in human malignancy, and lead to a better understanding of the molecular pathogenesis of cancer.

Jackie Boultwood
Carrie Fidler

Contents

Preface v

Contributors ix

1 Molecular Analysis of Cancer: *An Overview*
Ken Mills *1*

2 Detection of Chromosome Abnormalities in Leukemia Using
Fluorescence *In Situ* Hybridization
Lyndal Kearney, Sabrina Tosi, and Rina J. Jaju *7*

3 Spectral Karyotyping in Cancer Cytogenetics
**Eva Hilgenfeld, Cristina Montagna, Hesed Padilla-Nash,
Linda Stapleton, Kerstin Heselmeyer-Haddad,
and Thomas Ried** *29*

4 Comparative Genomic Hybridization Analysis
Binaifer R. Balsara, Jianming Pei, and Joseph R. Testa *45*

5 Detection of Chromosomal Deletions by Microsatellite Analysis
Rachel E. Ibbotson and Martin M. Corcoran *59*

6 Detection and Quantification of Leukemia-Specific Rearrangements
Andreas Hochhaus *67*

7 Detection of t(2;5)(p23;q35) Translocation by Long-Range PCR
of Genomic DNA
Yunfang Jiang, L. Jeffrey Medeiros, and Andreas H. Sarris *97*

8 Use of DNA Fingerprinting to Detect Genetic Rearrangements
in Human Cancer
**Vorapan Sirivatanauksorn, Yongyut Sirivatanauksorn,
Arthur B. McKie, and Nicholas R. Lemoine** *107*

9 Mutation Analysis of Large Genomic Regions in Tumor DNA Using
Single-Strand Conformation Polymorphism: *Lessons from
the* ATM *Gene*
Igor Vorechovsky *115*

10 Mutational Analysis of Oncogenes and Tumor Suppressor Genes
in Human Cancer Using Denaturing Gradient Gel Electrophoresis
**Per Guldberg, Kirsten Grønbæk, Jesper Worm, Per thor Straten,
and Jesper Zeuthen** *125*

vii

11 Detection of Mutations in Human Cancer Using Nonisotopic RNase Cleavage Assay
Marianna Goldrick and James Prescott 141

12 Mutational Analysis of the Neurofibromatosis Type 1 Gene in Childhood Myelodysplastic Syndromes Using a Protein Truncation Assay
Lucy Side 157

13 Mutation Analysis of Cancer Using Automated Sequencing
Amanda Strickson and Carrie Fidler 171

14 Detection of Differentially Expressed Genes in Cancer Using Differential Display
Yineng Fu 179

15 Genomewide Gene Expression Analysis Using cDNA Microarrays
Chuang Fong Kong and David Bowtell 195

16 Gene Expression Profiling in Cancer Using cDNA Microarrays
Javed Khan, Lao H. Saal, Michael L. Bittner, Yuan Jiang, Gerald C. Gooden, Arthur A. Glatfelter, and Paul S. Meltzer 205

17 Wilms Tumor Gene *WT1* as a Tumor Marker for Leukemic Blast Cells and Its Role in Leukemogenesis
Haruo Sugiyama 223

18 Detection of Aberrant Methylation of the *p15^{INK4B}* Gene Promoter
Toshiki Uchida 239

19 Clonality Studies in Cancer Based on X Chromosome Inactivation Phenomenon
John T. Phelan II and Josef T. Prchal 251

20 Telomere Length Changes in Human Cancer
Dominique Broccoli and Andrew K. Godwin 271

21 Measurement of Telomerase Activity in Human Hematopoietic Cells and Neoplastic Disorders
Kazuma Ohyashiki and Junko H. Ohyashiki 279

Index 301

Contributors

BINAIFER R. BALSARA • *Human Genetics Program, Division of Population Sciences, Fox Chase Cancer Center, Philadelphia, PA*

MICHAEL L. BITTNER • *Cancer Genetics Branch, National Human Genome Research Institute, National Institutes of Health, Bethesda, MD*

JACQUELINE BOULTWOOD • *Leukaemia Research Fund Molecular Haematology Unit, University of Oxford, NDCLS, John Radcliffe Hospital, Oxford, UK*

DAVID BOWTELL • *Research Division, Peter MacCallum Cancer Institute, Melbourne, Australia*

DOMINIQUE BROCCOLI • *Medical Sciences Division, Department of Medical Oncology, Fox Chase Cancer Center, Philadelphia, PA*

MARTIN M. CORCORAN • *Molecular Biology Laboratory, Royal Bournemouth Hospital, Bournemouth, UK*

CARRIE FIDLER • *Leukaemia Research Fund Molecular Haematology Unit at the University of Oxford, NDCLS, John Radcliffe Hospital, Oxford, UK*

YINENG FU • *Department of Pathology, Beth Israel-Deaconess Medical Center and Harvard Medical School, Boston; and Department of Pathology, Ardais Corporation, Lexington, MA*

ARTHUR A. GLATFELTER • *Cancer Genetics Branch, National Human Genome Research Institute, National Institutes of Health, Bethesda, MD*

ANDREW K. GODWIN • *Medical Sciences Division, Department of Medical Oncology, Fox Chase Cancer Center, Philadelphia, PA*

MARIANNA GOLDRICK • *Ambion RNA Diagnostics, Austin, TX*

GERALD C. GOODEN • *Cancer Genetics Branch, National Human Genome Research Institute, National Institutes of Health, Bethesda, MD*

KIRSTEN GRØNBÆK • *Department of Tumour Cell Biology, Institute of Cancer Biology, Danish Cancer Society, Copenhagen, Denmark*

PER GULDBERG • *Department of Tumour Cell Biology, Institute of Cancer Biology, Danish Cancer Society, Copenhagen, Denmark*

KERSTIN HESELMEYER-HADDAD • *Genetics Department, Center for Cancer Research, National Cancer Institute, National Institutes of Health, Bethesda, MD*

EVA HILGENFELD • *Genetics Department, Center for Cancer Research, National Cancer Institute, National Institutes of Health, Bethesda, MD* x Contributors

ANDREAS HOCHHAUS • *III. Medizinische Universitätsklinik, Klinikum Mannheim der Universität Heidelberg, Mannheim, Germany*

RACHEL E. IBBOTSON • *Molecular Biology Laboratory, Royal Bournemouth Hospital, Bournemouth, UK*

RINA J. JAJU • *Leukaemia Research Fund Molecular Haematology Unit, University of Oxford, NDCLS, John Radcliffe Hospital, Oxford, UK*

YUAN JIANG • *Cancer Genetics Branch, National Human Genome Research Institute, National Institutes of Health, Bethesda, MD*

YUNFANG JIANG • *Laboratory of Lymphoma Biology, Department of Lymphoma and Myeloma, University of Texas MD Anderson Cancer Center, Houston, TX*

LYNDAL KEARNEY • *MRC Molecular Haematology Unit, Weatherall Institute of Molecular Medicine, Oxford, UK*

JAVED KHAN • *Oncogenomics Section, Pediatric Oncology Branch, Center for Cancer Research, National Cancer Institute, National Institutes of Health, Bethesda, MD*

CHUANG FONG KONG • *Research Division, Peter MacCallum Cancer Institute, Melbourne, Australia*

NICHOLAS R. LEMOINE • *Imperial Cancer Research Fund Oncology Unit, Imperial College School of Medicine, Hammersmith Hospital, London, UK*

ARTHUR B. MCKIE • *Imperial Cancer Research Fund Oncology Unit, Imperial College School of Medicine, Hammersmith Hospital, London, UK*

L. JEFFREY MEDEIROS • *Department of Hematopathology, University of Texas MD Anderson Cancer Center, Houston, TX*

PAUL S. MELTZER • *Cancer Genetics Branch, National Human Genome Research Institute, National Institutes of Health, Bethesda, MD*

KEN MILLS • *Department of Haematology, University of Wales College of Medicine, Heath Park, Cardiff, Wales, UK*

CRISTINA MONTAGNA • *Genetics Department, Center for Cancer Research, National Cancer Institute, National Institutes of Health, Bethesda, MD*

KAZUMA OHYASHIKI • *First Department of Internal Medicine, Tokyo Medical University, Tokyo, Japan*

JUNKO H. OHYASHIKI • *First Department of Internal Medicine, Tokyo Medical University, Tokyo, Japan and the Division of Virology, Medical Research Institute, Tokyo Medical and Dental University, Tokyo, Japan*

HESED PADILLA-NASH • *Genetics Department, Center for Cancer Research, National Cancer Institute, National Institutes of Health, Bethesda, MD*

JIANMING PEI • *Human Genetics Program, Division of Population Sciences, Fox Chase Cancer Center, Philadelphia, PA*

JOHN T. PHELAN II • *Rochester General Hospital, Rochester, NY*

Contributors

JOSEF T. PRCHAL • *Department of Medicine Hematology and Oncology, Baylor College of Medicine, Houston, TX*

JAMES PRESCOTT • *UroCor, Inc., Oklahoma City, OK*

THOMAS RIED • *Genetics Department, Center for Cancer Research, National Cancer Institute, National Institutes of Health, Bethesda, MD*

LAO H. SAAL • *Cancer Genetics Branch, National Human Genome Research Institute, National Institutes of Health, Bethesda, MD*

ANDREAS H. SARRIS • *Laboratory of Lymphoma Biology, Department of Lymphoma and Myeloma, University of Texas MD Anderson Cancer Center, Houston, TX*

LUCY SIDE • *Leukaemia Research Fund Molecular Haematology Unit at the University of Oxford, NDCLS, John Radcliffe Hospital, Oxford, UK*

VORAPAN SIRIVATANAUKSORN • *Imperial Cancer Research Fund Oncology Unit, Imperial College School of Medicine, Hammersmith Hospital, London, UK*

YONGYUT SIRIVATANAUKSORN • *Department of Surgery, Anaesthetics and Intensive Care, Imperial College School of Medicine, Hammersmith Hospital, London, UK*

LINDA STAPLETON • *Genetics Department, Center for Cancer Research, National Cancer Institute, National Institutes of Health, Bethesda, MD*

AMANDA STRICKSON • *Leukaemia Research Fund Molecular Haematology Unit at the University of Oxford, NDCLS, John Radcliffe Hospital, Oxford, UK*

PER THOR STRATEN • *Department of Tumour Cell Biology, Institute of Cancer Biology, Danish Cancer Society, Copenhagen, Denmark*

HARUO SUGIYAMA • *Department of Clinical Laboratory Science, Osaka University Medical School, Yamada-Oka, Suita City*

JOSEPH R. TESTA • *Human Genetics Program, Division of Population Sciences, Fox Chase Cancer Center, Philadelphia, PA*

SABRINA TOSI • *MRC Molecular Haematology Unit, Weatherall Institute of Molecular Medicine, Oxford, UK*

TOSHIKI UCHIDA • *First Department of Internal Medicine, Nagoya University School of Medicine, Showa-ku, Nagoya, Japan*

IGOR VORECHOVSKY • *Department of Biosciences at NOVUM, Karolinska Institute, Huddinge, Sweden*

JESPER WORM • *Department of Tumour Cell Biology, Institute of Cancer Biology, Danish Cancer Society, Copenhagen, Denmark*

JESPER ZEUTHEN • *Department of Tumour Cell Biology, Institute of Cancer Biology, Danish Cancer Society, Copenhagen, Denmark*

1

Molecular Analysis of Cancer

An Overview

Ken Mills

1. Introduction

Cancer is a complex disease occurring as a result of a progressive accumulation of genetic aberrations and epigenetic changes that enable escape from normal cellular and environmental controls *(1)*. Neoplastic cells may have numerous acquired genetic abnormalities including aneuploidy, chromosomal rearrangements, amplifications, deletions, gene rearrangements, and loss-of-function or gain-of-function mutations. Recent studies have also highlighted the importance of epigenetic alterations of certain genes that result in the inactivation of their functions in some human cancers. These aberrations lead to the abnormal behavior common to all neoplastic cells: dysregulated growth, lack of contact inhibition, genomic instability, and propensity for metastasis.

The genes affected by mutations in cancer may be divided into two main classes: genes that have gain-of-function (activating) mutations, which are known as oncogenes; and genes for which both alleles have loss-of-function (inactivating) mutations, which are known as tumor suppressor genes. Close to 100 genes have been shown to play a role in the development or progression of human cancers, some of which have been implicated in a broad spectrum of malignancies, whereas others are unique to a specific type. Cancers can arise via the aberration of different combinations of genes, which in turn may be mutated, overexpressed, or deleted. The order in which these events occur has also proved to be important. For example, in breast cancer it has been proposed that at least 10 distinct gene alterations may be involved in disease initiation and progression *(2)*. The study of colon cancer has shown that carcinogenesis

From: *Methods in Molecular Medicine, vol. 68: Molecular Analysis of Cancer*
Edited by: J. Boultwood and C. Fidler © Humana Press Inc., Totowa, NJ

is a multistage process involving the activation of cellular oncogenes, the deletion of multiple chromosomal regions, and the loss of function of tumor suppressor genes *(3)*.

Technologic advances in molecular biology over the past 20–25 yr have led to a dramatic increase in the identification of the molecular processes involved in tumorigenesis. Over this period, the molecular basis of cancer no longer holds the mystery that it once did *(1)*. It is, however, also clear that the knowledge that has been accumulated is insufficient to claim a total understanding of the mechanism of cancer development. This volume has brought together a number of relevant techniques by which genetic abnormalities occurring in cancer can be detected and analyzed. This, in turn, will give rise to other avenues of study, such as: how mutations affect function, how these genes are regulated, and how they interact with each other.

The mutational analysis of oncogenes and tumor suppressor genes can provide evidence for a specific association between these genes and tumor type. These genes can be altered during carcinogenesis by different mechanisms such as point mutations, chromosomal translocations, gene amplification, or deletion. Furthermore, these genes may be analyzed at different levels—DNA, RNA, or expressed proteins.

2. DNA Analysis

Mutational analysis can be performed using a variety of techniques, and the majority of these are highlighted in this volume. The amplification of specific regions of DNA or RNA (Chapters 5–8) by the polymerase chain reaction (PCR) has opened endless possibilities that can be used for the rapid and efficient detection of alterations, even single nucleotide changes. These PCR-based techniques rely on changes in electrophoretic mobility induced by altered single-stranded secondary structure (single-strand conformation polymorphism) (Chapter 9), by altered dissociation rates of the DNA fragments (denaturing gradient gel electrophoresis) (Chapter 10), or by RNase cleavage assays (Chapter 11). PCR can also be used for the rapid and quantitative detection of chromosomal rearrangements, such as commonly observed in leukemia (Chapter 7). PCR is designed to specifically amplify genomic fragments that are not normally contiguous and are, therefore, unique to that type of gene rearrangement. Converting the RNA to DNA with reverse transcriptase (RT) prior to the PCR stage is usually required for this assay. However, in some cases, genomic DNA can be used for the direct amplification of translocation break points (Chapter 7). A variation on the PCR theme involves the use of DNA fingerprints to detect genetic rearrangements in cancer (Chapter 8). The primers are often arbitrary or repeat (e.g., ALU) sequences, which will give, after electrophoresis, a DNA fingerprint that can be used for the detection of genetic abnormalities. Microsatellite repeats occur throughout the

Overview of Molecular Cancer Genetics

genome and can be used as markers for genetic alterations, usually for the loss of heterozygosity, which will indicate that a deletion has occurred that overlaps that specific marker (Chapter 5). For specific genes involved in certain cancers, the mutational analysis can be carried out using a protein truncation assay (Chapter 12). This assay involves the identification of abnormal polypeptides synthesized in vitro from RT-PCR products, and the truncating mutations are usually confirmed by sequence analysis.

3. RNA Expression Analysis

DNA microarray technology, which makes use of high-density two-dimensional oligonucleotide probe arrays containing hundreds or thousands of oligonucleotide probes, represents a powerful new DNA sequence analysis tool to test for a variety of genetic mutations (Chapters 15 and 16). Hybridization to cDNA microarrays allows the simultaneous parallel expression analysis of thousands of genes. High-throughput gene expression profiling increasingly is becoming a valuable method for identifying genes differentially expressed in tumor vs normal tissues. Gene expression microarrays hold great promise for studies of human tumorigenesis, and the large gene expression data sets produced have the potential to provide novel insights into fundamental cancer biology at the molecular level (Chapter 16). Indeed, cDNA microarray technology has already begun to aid in the elucidation of the genetic events underlying the initiation and progression of some human cancers. Differentially expressed genes can also be detected by other techniques such as differential display (Chapter 14), which involves a random primed RT-PCR display or fingerprint of subsets of expressed RNA, or subtractive hybridization, which involves the enrichment of genes preferentially expressed in one tissue compared with a second.

4. Chromosomal Analysis

Fluorescence *in situ* hybridization (FISH) is one of the techniques with an expanding role in the molecular analysis of cancer (Chapter 2). It can be used for the simple detection of numerical and structural chromosomal abnormalities that may occur in cancer cells and is particularly useful as a tool for the diagnosis of nonrandom translocations in leukemia and numerous other cancers. To date, most FISH studies have involved the use of single whole-chromosome or gene probes. This has been taken to new levels by the development of spectral karyotyping, which involves the hybridization of 24 fluorescently labeled chromosome painting probes to metaphase spreads in such a manner that simultaneous visualization of each of the chromosomes in a different color is accomplished (Chapter 3). Using this method, it is possible to define all chromosomal rearrangements and identify all of the marker chromosomes in tumor cells. Comparative genomic hybridization (CGH) is a FISH-based technique that can detect gains and losses of whole chromosomes and subchromosomal regions (Chapter 4). CGH is based on a two-color, competitive FISH of differentially labeled tumor and reference DNA to normal metaphase chromosomes and can scan the whole genome without prior knowledge of specific chromosomal abnormalities.

5. Analysis of Methylation Status

Some molecular methods will analyze specific changes to the DNA structure or genomic modifications. Changes in the DNA methylation status are one of the most common detectable abnormalities in human cancer. Hypermethylation within the promoters of selected genes is especially common and is usually associated with inactivation of the involved gene or genes and may be an early event in the pathogenesis of some cancers, whereas other genes become methylated during disease progression (Chapter 18).

6. Telomere and Telomerase Activity

Telomeres are repetitive DNA sequences at chromosome ends, which are necessary for maintaining chromosomal integrity. A reduction in telomere length has been described in a wide range of human cancers, including both solid tumors and leukemias. The enzyme telomerase synthesizes *de novo* telomeric repeats and incorporates them onto the DNA 3' ends of chromosomes. Telomere shortening in normal cells is a result of DNA replication events, and reduction beyond a critical length is a signal for cellular senescence. However, the maintenance of telomere length, by the activation of the enzyme telomerase, is thought to be essential for immortalization of human cancer cells to compensate for the loss of DNA from the ends of chromosomes. Therefore, the measurement of telomere length (Chapter 20) and telomerase enzyme activity levels (Chapter 21) are important in monitoring disease progression or response to therapy. Recently, the possible manipulation of telomerase has generated some excitement as an anticancer strategy.

7. Clonal Origin of Cancer

The methods I have described allow the investigator to study the myriad of genetic alterations that can occur during the initiation, development, and progression of cancer. However, it is also possible to provide insight into the transition from somatic cell mutation to neoplasia. The clonal origin of cells can be assessed in patients with X chromosome-linked polymorphisms, taking advantage of the random inactivation of the X chromosome (Chapter 19). The inactivation is related to the differentially methylated patterns on the active and inactive X chromosomes.

8. Summary

Human cancers are generally characterized by acquisition of a series of somatic mutations. Molecular techniques, such as those described in this volume, have been used to identify a plethora of chromosomal translocations and mutations associated with carcinogenesis. The analysis and comparison of the array of genetic changes occurring in malignancy will enable a move toward a better understanding of cancer development. This will eventually lead to the development of improved therapies tailored to take into account the cytogenetic and molecular characteristics of specific human cancers.

References

1. Weinberg, R. A. (1996) How cancer arises. *Sci. Am.* **275,** 62–70.
2. Devilee, P., Schuuring, E., van de Vijver, M. J., and Cornelisse, C. J. (1994) Recent developments in the molecular genetic understanding of breast cancer. *Crit. Rev. Oncogen.* **5,** 247–270.
3. Goyette, M. C., Cho, K., Fasching, C. L., Levy, D. B., Kinzler, K. W., Paraskeva, C., et al. (1992) Progression of colorectal cancer is associated with multiple tumor suppressor gene defects but inhibition of tumorigenicity is accomplished by correction of any single defect via chromosome transfer. *Mol. Cell. Biol.* **12,** 1387–1395.

2

Detection of Chromosome Abnormalities in Leukemia Using Fluorescence *In Situ* Hybridization

Lyndal Kearney, Sabrina Tosi, and Rina J. Jaju

1. Introduction

Cytogenetic analysis plays a pivotal role in the diagnosis and management of patients with hematologic malignancies. In research, the identification of specific chromosomal rearrangements associated with defined clinical groups has led to an explosion in the knowledge of basic mechanisms contributing to leukemogenesis. The strength of cytogenetic analysis is as a direct method for screening the whole genome. However, the interpretation of the banding pattern of highly rearranged chromosomes is often unreliable. Since the advent of molecular cytogenetic technologies based around fluorescence *in situ* hybridization (FISH), the accuracy of cytogenetic diagnosis has been considerably enhanced. Specific problems hampering the accurate analysis of leukemic karyotypes such as the low mitotic index, heterogeneity of the sample, and often poor morphology of chromosomes are also largely overcome by FISH. One of the most significant advances is the use of interphase FISH, which permits the use of nondividing cells as DNA targets and enables a large number of cells to be evaluated *(1–4)*. This has advantages for monitoring disease progression, response to treatment, and success of bone marrow transplantation. The simultaneous identification of cell type (by morphology or immunophenotype) and chromosome abnormality (by FISH) is also possible, allowing the identification of cell lineages involved in the neoplastic clone *(5)*.

The application of FISH to metaphase chromosomes provides unequivocal evidence of chromosome rearrangements. Whole-chromosome painting probes, derived from chromosome-specific libraries, or polymerase chain reaction (PCR) amplification of flow-sorted or microdissected chromosomes can be used to identify accurately the components of complex rearrangements and marker chromosomes *(6–10)*. Chromosome-specific centromeric probes,

From: *Methods in Molecular Medicine, vol. 68: Molecular Analysis of Cancer*
Edited by: J. Boultwood and C. Fidler © Humana Press Inc., Totowa, NJ

targeting the tandemly repeated alpha (or beta) satellite sequences present in the heterochromatin of chromosome centromeres, are invaluable for the rapid visualization of numerical chromosome abnormalities. Specific gene probes for the detection of leukemia-associated translocations and inversions *(11–13)* allow accurate detection of these rearrangements, especially in complex or masked versions of the translocation, and are particularly useful for interphase analysis. A significant advance in the resolution of FISH for the visualization of translocations is provided by hybridization to extended DNA fibers, so-called fiber-FISH. This is particularly valuable for the analysis of chromosome rearrangements with highly variable breakpoints, provided there is a well-characterized contig of the region *(14,15)*.

One of the most appealing aspects of FISH is the ability to identify several targets simultaneously using different colors (so-called multicolor FISH) (*see* **Fig. 1A**). The most recent developments in this area are those that enable "color karyotyping," using whole-chromosome painting probes that delineate each of the 22 pairs of autosomes and the sex chromosomes in a different color. The related techniques of multiplex-FISH (M-FISH) and spectral karyotyping (SKY) *(16,17)* provide the prospect of a molecular analysis of karyotype. One of these, SKY, is detailed in Chapter 3. Herein we outline the basic FISH methodologies, as well as some of the more advanced techniques, with particular reference to specific applications in hematologic malignancy. Further specialized *in situ* hybridization methods are given in **ref.** *18*.

Fig. 1. Examples of applications for FISH in leukemia. (**A**) Dual-color FISH using whole chromosome painting probes for chromosomes 7 (green) and 12 (red) to a leukemic metaphase from an acute myeloid leukemia patient. This identified a cryptic translocation between chromosomes 7 and 12. In this metaphase chromosome 12 material is visible on the der(7) (arrow); however, the reciprocal chromosome 7 material is not visible on the der(12). (**B**) Dual-color FISH to map the extent of the 5q deletion in a leukemic metaphase from a patient with 5q- syndrome. A 5p subtelomeric probe (red) was cohybridized to tag both chromosomes 5, to ensure that only metaphases containing the del(5q) were evaluated. Green fluorescent signal corresponding to a probe containing the *CSF1R* gene is present on the normal homolog, but absent from the del(5q) (arrow). (**C,D**) Combined immunophenotyping and FISH (using a YAC probe containing the *CSF1R* gene) to bone marrow cells from a patient with a del(5q) clonal chromosome marker. In each case, the APAAP positive cells show bright red fluorescence. In (C) the CD3 antibody identifies a T cell with two green fluorescent FISH signals corresponding to the YAC. In (D) the glycophorin A antibody identifies an erythroid precursor with only one fluorescent signal. This confirms that the erythroid, but not the T-lymphocyte, lineage is involved in the malignant

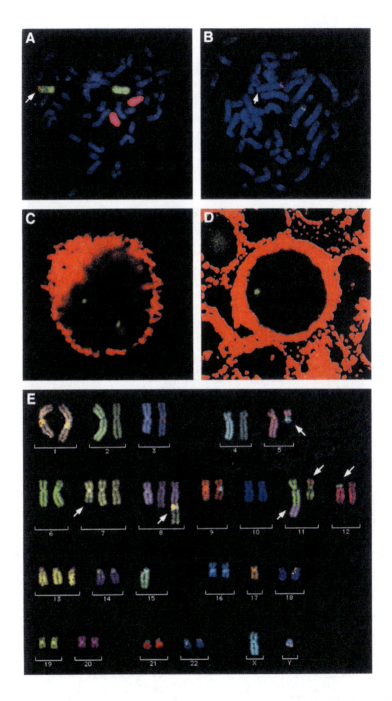

clone in this patient. (**E**) M-FISH karyotype of a metaphase from the leukemia-derived cell line GF-D8. Metaphases were hybridized with a set of combinatorially labeled whole chromosome painting probes, and chromosomes assigned a pseudocolor according to their unique fluorochrome composition using Powergene M-FISH software (Applied Imaging, Newcastle, UK). Structurally abnormal chromosomes thus identified are indicated by arrows.

2. Materials

2.1. Preparation of Bone Marrow Metaphase Chromosomes

1. Bone marrow aspirate collected into sterile bottles containing transport medium (RPMI 1640 plus 50 U/mL of penicillin, 50 μg/mL of streptomycin, and 10 U/mL of preservative-free lithium heparin).
2. Thymidine, crystalline (Sigma, St. Louis, MO): 100 μM stock.
3. 5-Fluorodeoxyuridine (Sigma): 100 μM stock.
4. Uridine (Sigma): 400 μM stock.
5. Colcemid (10 μg/mL) (Gibco).
6. Culture medium: RPMI 1640, 50 U/mL of penicillin, 50 μg/mL of streptomycin, 2 mM L-glutamine, 20% fetal calf serum (FCS) (all from Gibco-BRL).
7. Hypotonic solution: 0.075 M KCl.
8. Fixative: 3:1 AnalaR methanol:glacial acetic acid, at 4°C.
9. Precleaned microscope slides (Superfrost, BDH).

2.2. Pretreatment of Chromosomes and Nuclei

1. Pepsin (100 mg/mL) (Sigma).
2. Phosphate-buffered saline (PBS)/50 mM MgCl$_2$: 50 mL of 1 M MgCl$_2$ + 950 mL of 1X PBS.
3. PBS/50 mM MgCl$_2$/1% formaldehyde (make up fresh each time): 2.7 mL of formaldehyde in 100 mL of PBS/MgCl$_2$.
4. PBS (1X): 8 g of NaCl, 0.2 g of KCl, 1.44 g of Na$_2$HPO$_4$, 0.2 g of KH$_2$PO$_4$ in 800 mL of H$_2$O, pH to 7.4 with HCl. Add H$_2$O to 1 L.
5. RNase A (10 mg/mL) (Sigma) (boiled for 10 min to remove contaminating DNase).
6. Formaldehyde (40% [w/v]).

2.3. Preparation of Probe DNA

2.3.1. Cosmids, P1 Artificial Chromosomes (PACs)

1. 2X TY medium (1 L): 16 g of Bacto tryptone, 10 g of yeast extract, 5 g of NaCl.
2. Glucose/EDTA/Tris (GET): 0.9% glucose, 10 mM EDTA, 25 mM Tris-HCl, pH 7.0.
3. NaOH/sodium dodecyl sulfate (SDS): 0.2 M NaOH, 1% SDS.
4. 3 M KOAc, pH 5.5.
5. RNase A (DNase free) (10 mg/mL) (Sigma).

2.3.2. Yeast Artificial Chromosomes (YACs)

1. YEPD medium (1 L): 10 g of Bacto yeast extract, 20 g of Bactopeptone, 20 g of dextrose, 10 mL of adenine sulfate (0.5% in 0.5 M of HCl).
2. GDIS: 2% Triton X-100, 1% SDS, 100 mM NaCl, 10 mM Tris-HCl, pH 7.4, 1 mM EDTA.
3. Phenol:chloroform:isoamyl alcohol (25:24:1).
4. RNase A (DNase free) (10 mg/mL) (Sigma).
5. Glass beads, 710–1180 μm, acid washed (Sigma).

FISH to Detect Abnormalities in Leukemia

2.4. Nick Translation Labeling

1. Purified probe DNA (1 μg).
2. 10X Nick translation buffer: 0.5 M Tris-HCl, pH 7.5, 50 mM MgCl$_2$, 0.5 mg/mL of nuclease-free bovine serum albumin (BSA).
3. 1 mM Biotin-16-dUTP (bio-16-dUTP), 1 mM digoxigenin-11-dUTP (dig-11-dUTP) (Roche Diagnostics).
4. 100 mM Dithiothreitol (DTT) (Sigma).
5. dNTP mix: 0.5 mM each dATP, dCTP, dGTP, and 0.1 mM dTTP (Roche Diagnostics).
6. DNase 1 (200,000 U) (Roche Diagnostics).
7. DNase 1 dilution buffer: 50% glycerol, 0.15 M NaCl, 20 mM sodium acetate, pH 5.0.
8. DNA polymerase 1 (10 U/μL) (New England Biolabs).
9. MicroSpin G50 columns (Amersham Pharmacia Biotech).
10. *Escherichia coli* tRNA (10 mg/mL) (Roche Diagnostics).
11. Salmon sperm DNA (5 mg/mL, sonicated to 200–500 bp) (Sigma).
12. TE: 10 mM Tris-HCl, pH 7.5, 1 mM EDTA.
13. Gel-loading buffer (5X bromophenol blue): 10% (w/v) Ficoll, 0.1 M Na$_2$ EDTA, 0.5% (w/v) SDS, 0.1% (w/v) bromophenol blue.
14. Electrophoresis buffer (10X TBE): 108 g of Tris base (89 mM), 55 g of boric acid (89 mM), 40 mL of 0.5 M EDTA, pH 8.0 (2 mM) per liter.
15. *Phi*X174 *Hae*III size marker (BRL Life Technologies).

2.5. Competitive In Situ Suppression Hybridization

1. Human Cot-1 DNA (BRL Life Technologies).
2. 3 M Sodium acetate.
3. Denaturing solution: 70% (v/v) formamide, 2X saline sodium citrate (SSC), 0.1 mM EDTA, pH 7.0.
4. Hybridization buffer: 50% (v/v) formamide, 10% (w/v) dextran sulfate, 1% (v/v) Triton X-100, 2X SSC, pH 7.0.
5. Formamide (purified) (Fluka).
6. 50% Dextran sulfate.
7. 20X SSC: 1X SSC = 150 mM sodium chloride, 15 mM sodium citrate, pH 7.0.
8. Blocking solution: 3% (w/v) BSA in 4X SSC, 0.05% (v/v) Triton X-100 (make up fresh).
9. Wash solution: 4X SSC, 0.05% (v/v) Triton X-100.

2.6. Detection of Bound, Labeled Probe

1. Fluorescence microscope (epifluorescence illumination), with suitable fluorescence objectives and filter sets (usually need separate filter sets for fluorescein isothiocyanate [FITC], Texas red/rhodamine and 4,6-diamidino-2-phenylindole [DAPI]/AMCA, as well as a double or triple filter block).
2. Avidin-DCS-FITC (1 mg/mL) (Vector).
3. Biotinylated anti-avidin D (0.5 mg/mL) (Vector).
4. Propidium iodide (Sigma).

5. DAPI (Sigma).
6. Vectashield mountant (Vector).
7. Avidin DCS-Texas red (2.5 mg/mL stock) (Vector).
8. Diluent for antibodies: blocking solution, filtered through a 0.45-μm syringe filter. Stock antibody solutions are stored at –20°C.
9. Monoclonal antidigoxigenin (Sigma).
10. Rabbit antimouse Ig-FITC (Sigma).
11. Monoclonal antirabbit-FITC (Sigma).

2.7. Degenerate Oligonucleotide Primer-PCR Amplification of Flow-Sorted Chromosomes

1. Flow-sorted chromosomes (approximate concentration: 500/μL).
2. 2X PCR buffer: 10 mM MgCl$_2$, 100 mM KCl, 20 mM Tris-HCl, pH 8.4, 0.2 mg/mL of gelatin.
3. dNTP mix: 2 mM each dATP, dCTP, dGTP, dTTP.
4. 6-MW primer: 5' CCGACTCGAGNNNNNNATGTGG 3' (30 μM).
5. *Taq* 1 (2.5 U/μL) polymerase (Roche Diagnostics).
6. 1 mM Biotin-16-dUTP or 1 mM dig-11-dUTP (Roche Diagnostics).

2.8. Alkaline Phosphatase Antialkaline Phosphatase Staining

1. Thin bone marrow smears (store unfixed wrapped in foil at –20°C).
2. Tris-buffered saline (TBS): 1 M Tris, 0.5 M NaCl.
3. Appropriate primary monoclonal antibody.
4. Rabbit antimouse antibody (Z259; Dako, Cambridge, UK) diluted 1:500 in TBS.
5. Monoclonal alkaline phosphatase antialkaline phosphatase (APAAP) complex (1:500 dilution) (Roche Diagnostics).
6. Alkaline phosphatase substrate: Dissolve 2 mg of naphthol AS mix (Sigma) into 10 mL of 0.1 M Tris buffer (pH 8.2). To this add 10 mg of Fast Red TR mix (Sigma) and dissolve. Then add levamisole (0.1 M) (Sigma) to block endogenous alkaline phosphatase. Filter before use.

3. Methods
3.1. Preparation of Target Material

3.1.1 Culture and Harvesting of Mitotic Chromosomes from Leukemic Bone Marrow (see ref. 19)

1. Set up between one and four cultures, depending on the white cell count. Each culture should contain approx 1×10^6 cells/mL. In most cases, the following will suffice:
   a. Direct harvesting after 1 h exposed to colcemid (0.1 μg/mL).
   b. A 24-h incubation with the addition of colcemid for the last hour.
   c. Twenty-four hour synchronized cultures. For these, add fluorodeoxyuridine (0.1 μM) and uridine (4 μM) after 24 h and reincubate the cultures overnight (16–18 h). Finally, add thymidine (10 μM), and reincubate for 5 to 6 h before adding of colcemid for 10 min before harvesting.

FISH to Detect Abnormalities in Leukemia

13

2. Centrifuge at 100*g* for 5 min. Discard the supernatant and resuspend the pellet in hypotonic solution (prewarmed to 37°C). Incubate at 37°C for 20 min.
3. Centrifuge, discard the supernatant, and mix the pellet in the small volume of hypotonic solution remaining. Add freshly made fixative dropwise, with mixing. Add the first milliliter of fixative slowly, and then make up to 10 mL.
4. Leave in fixative for 30 min at 4°C. Centrifuge at 100*g* for 5 min, then wash in three to five changes of fixative before making slides.
5. Wipe Superfrost slides clean with absolute ethanol just before use.
6. Place a drop of cell suspension on each slide and air-dry. Monitor the quality of chromosome spreading under phase contrast. Chromosomes should be well spread without visible cytoplasm and should appear dark gray under phase contrast (not black and refractile or light gray and almost invisible).

The "direct" culture can be replaced by overnight incubation with colcemid (0.5 μg/mL). For cell lines, culture according to their specified growth requirements, then harvest when growing logarithmically, usually 24–48 h after a change of medium. Add colcemid for the final 1 h before harvesting.

3.1.2. Preparation of Interphase Nuclei

Interphase nuclei are present in large numbers on slides from leukemic bone marrow or blood prepared as in **Subheading 3.1.1.** Interphase nuclei can also be prepared from fresh bone marrow after Ficoll separation of mononuclear cells. After washing pellets in culture medium (RPMI, without FCS), fix the cell pellet in several changes of methanol:acetic acid (3:1). Drop onto clean slides. Nuclei from a variety of tissues and culture types can be prepared by cytospin, then fixed in methanol (10–20 min). Bone marrow smears are prepared in the usual way and stored unfixed, wrapped in foil at –20°C until required.

3.2. Pretreatment of Chromosomes and Nuclei

The methanol/acetic acid fixation of metaphase chromosomes removes some basic proteins that might interfere with hybridization. However, there is still a variable amount of other protein and cytoplasmic contaminants on metaphase chromosome preparations that may block hybridization, or cause nonspecific background. We routinely use an RNase treatment and postfixation with formaldehyde. For interphase FISH, it may be necessary to add a proteolytic digestion (e.g., pepsin) treatment to this, to aid access of the probe and detection reagents. However, overdigestion can cause loss of cells from slides, so use only when absolutely necessary.

1. Place 100 μL of RNase A (100 μg/mL) on slides under a 24 × 50 mm coverslip and incubate at 37°C for 30 min to 1 h.
2. Wash three times (3 min each) in 2X SSC (with agitation).

3. Pepsin treatment (optional): 50 μg/mL in 0.01 M HCl. Incubate for 10 min at RT.
4. Wash (two times for 5 min each) in 1X PBS.
5. Wash (once for 5 min) in 1X PBS/50 mM MgCl$_2$.
6. Fix in PBS/50 mM MgCl$_2$/1% formaldehyde (2.7 mL of formaldehyde in 100 mL of 1X PBS/50 mM MgCl$_2$ [fresh solution]) for 10 min.
7. Wash in 1X PBS for 5 min (with agitation).
8. Dehydrate slides through an alcohol series (70%, 95%, absolute) and allow to air-dry. Slides can be stored desiccated at 4°C for up to 1 mo before use (*see* **Note 1**).

3.3. Preparation of Probe DNA

3.3.1. Cosmid, P1, and PAC DNA

Any DNA purification method that produces DNA suitable for sequencing will generally also work for FISH. The following medium-scale alkaline lysis method gives a high yield of cosmid, PAC, or P1 DNA. However, this is relatively impure and may require additional purification steps. As a guide, if the DNA fails to cut with DNase I, purify with phenol/chloroform or CsCl gradient centrifugation.

1. Inoculate 250 mL of 2X YT medium plus antibiotic (final concentration: 30 μg/mL of kanamycin, 50 μg/mL of ampicillin) in a 500-mL sterile plugged flask with a single well-separated colony.
2. Grow at 37°C with shaking (300 rpm) until approaching saturation (approx 18 h)
3. Transfer to a 250-mL bottle. Centrifuge at 4000g for 10 min.
4. Discard the supernatant medium and drain briefly. Add 50 mL of cold glucose/EDTA/Tris (GET). Resuspend by drawing up in a 10-mL pipet.
5. Add 50 mL of NaOH/SDS at room temperature. Mix by very gentle, minimal inversions. Leave for 5 min (room temperature).
6. Add 50 mL of cold 3 M KoAc. Mix by very gentle, minimal inversions. Place on ice for 20 min.
7. Centrifuge at 9000g for 20 min (4°C).
8. Carefully transfer the supernatant to a fresh 250-mL bottle through a mesh.
9. Add 90 mL of isopropanol (0.7X vol) and mix. Leave at room temperature for 5 min.
10. Centrifuge at 5000g for 15 min at room temperature. Discard supernatant.
11. Add 25 mL of 70% ethanol, and rotate the bottle to rinse the inner surface. Transfer pellet to 50-mL Falcon tubes.
12. Centrifuge at 5000g for 5 min (4°C). Discard the supernatant.
13. Allow to stand for 1 min, and then remove final traces of 70% ethanol with a Gilson.
14. Air-dry. Resuspend in approx 200 μL of H$_2$O (or TE).
15. Incubate with RNase A (final concentration: 30 μg/mL) at 37°C for 30 min.

3.3.2. Yeast Artificial Chromosome DNA (20)

The following method yields high quantities of total yeast DNA suitable for FISH (*see* **Note 2**). The average yield from a 10-mL culture is 10–20 μg.

FISH to Detect Abnormalities in Leukemia

1. Culture cells at 30°C for up to 2 d in 10 mL of YEPD medium (grow to saturation).
2. Centrifuge (1500g, 10 min) to pellet the cells, and discard the supernatant. Transfer to an Eppendorf tube, and wash the cells with 500 µL of distilled water.
3. Centrifuge and then resuspend in 200 µL of GDIS. Add 0.35 g of glass beads and 200 µL of phenol. Vortex continuously for 5 min.
4. Add 200 µL of distilled water to the suspension, mix well, and spin for 4 min in a microcentrifuge.
5. Extract once more with phenol, then once with phenol:chloroform:isoamyl alcohol.
6. Precipitate the DNA as usual (0.1X sodium acetate, 2X absolute ethanol) followed by a 70% ethanol rinse.
7. Remove the aqueous layer and treat this with 50 µg/mL of RNase A for 20 min at 37°C.
8. Dry the pellet and resuspend in 20 µL of distilled water.
9. Measure the DNA concentration accurately, preferably in a fluorometer (*see* **Note 3**).

3.4. Nick Translation Labeling of Probes

Nick translation is the most widely used method for labeling probes for *in situ* hybridization, because the fragment size can be controlled by the amount of DNase I in the reaction mixture. As nick translation is highly efficient for labeling double-stranded circular DNA molecules, there is no need to isolate the insert from the vector sequences. The size of labeled probe fragments is a critical factor in *in situ* hybridization protocols, with an average size of 300 bp being optimal (range 100–500 bp). Larger probe fragments will result in bright background fluorescence all over the slide, obscuring any specific signal. If the labeled probe fragments are too small (<50 bp), the site of hybridization may not be visible owing to the resulting weak fluorescent signal. To ensure the correct size of labeled fragments, it is necessary to run a small aliquot of labeled probe on a 2% agarose gel. Other labeling methods (e.g., random primer labeling, PCR) can be used to produce labeled probes for FISH. However, in all cases the size of the labeled fragments must be checked, and recut with DNase I, if necessary. Probes for localization by FISH are usually labeled with either biotin or digoxigenin, available conjugated to dUTPs by a spacer arm of variable length (e.g., bio-16-dUTP, dig-11-dUTP). Various fluorochromes including FITC, and the cyanine dyes Cy3, and Cy5 are now available directly conjugated to dUTP (Amersham Pharmacia Biotech), enabling direct labeling of DNA.

1. Add the following (in order) to a 1.5-mL Eppendorf tube on ice:
   a. 1 µg of probe DNA.
   b. 1.2 µL of 1 m*M* bio-16-dUTP, dig-11-dUTP, or fluorochrome-dUTP.
   c. 5 µL of dNTP mix.
   d. 5 µL of 10X nick translation buffer.
   e. 5 µL of 100 m*M* DTT.
   f. Sterile-distilled water to make up to a final volume of 50 µL.

16   *Kearney et al.*

    g. 3–5 µL of 100 U/mL DNase I (need to establish amount for each new batch).

    h. 1 µL of 10 U/µL DNA Polymerase I.

2. Mix well.

3. Incubate at 15°C for 90 min.

4. Stop reaction by placing tubes on ice.

5. Check the size of the labeled products by running an aliquot on a 2% agarose gel (in TBE and containing 5 µL of 5 mg/mL ethidium bromide/100 mL) as follows:

    a. 5 µL of labeled probe (approx 100 ng).

    b. 4 µL of gel-loading buffer (5X bromophenol blue).

    c. 11 µL of sterile distilled water.

6. Run at 50 V for 1–1.5 h with *Phi*X174 *Hae*III (20 µL = 250 ng) as a size marker.

7. View on a transilluminator and photograph. The optimal size range for *in situ* hybridization is 50–500 bp (*see* **Note 4**). A smear of products from 100 to 300 (corresponding to the six smallest bands of *Phi*X174) is suitable. If the size range is larger than this, add a further 5 µL of DNase I, place at 15°C for an additional 30–60 min, and run another aliquot on a gel to test the size.

8. Purify to remove unincorporated nucleotides by passing the labeled probe through a MicroSpin G50 column (designed for biotinylated probes) according to the manufacturer's instructions.

9. Measure the volume of eluate and then ethanol precipitate the purified, labeled probe by adding the following:

    a. 50 µg of *E. coli* tRNA.

    b. 50 µg of salmon sperm DNA.

    c. 0.1 vol of 3 *M* sodium acetate, pH 5.6.

    d. 2–2.25 vol of ice-cold ethanol.

    Mix well and place at –70°C for 1–2 h or –20°C overnight.

10. Centrifuge in a microcentrifuge for 15–25 min at 4°C. Pour off the supernatant and dry the pellet (either air-dry or dry in a vacuum desiccator). Resuspend the pellet in 20 µL TE pH 8.0 to give a final concentration of 50 ng/µL. Allow the DNA to dissolve at room temperature for 1 to 2 h or at 4°C overnight with occasional mixing. Purified, labeled probes are stable for several years when stored at –20°C.

3.5. Competitive In Situ Suppression Hybridization (see Note 5)

    Clones containing large DNA fragments (i.e., phage, cosmid, YAC, P1) and whole-chromosome paints require an additional step before hybridization to remove ubiquitous repetitive sequences (*see* **Table 1**) This is achieved by a short incubation prior to hybridization, with unlabeled human competitor DNA, in the form of either total human DNA (placental DNA, sheared and sonicated to 50–300 bp) or human Cot-1 DNA (Gibco-BRL). When all of the probe sequences contribute to the hybridization signal (e.g., repetitive DNA probes, unique cDNA probes), there is no need to add competitor DNA. Suggested amounts of probe and competitor DNA are given in **Table 1**. Hybridization is carried out in a moist chamber. This can be achieved by using a plastic micro-

FISH to Detect Abnormalities in Leukemia

Table 1
Suggested Amount of Probe and Competitor (10 μL Hybridization Volume)

Type of probe	Amount	Cot-1 DNA (μg)
Single fragment cloned in plasmid[a]	200 ng	
Single fragment cloned in phage	200 ng	2.5
Single fragment cloned in cosmid	50–100 ng	2.5
YAC, total yeast DNA	400 ng–1 μg	5–7.5
PAC, P1	200–400 ng	3–5
Alphoid DNA repeat (centromere)[a]	10 ng	
Whole-chromosome paint, libraries[b]	100–400 ng	5–7.5
Whole-chromosome paint, PCR amplified flow-sorted chromosomes	100 ng	6.25

[a]Whole probe contributes to signal: no competitor required.
[b]DNA from flow-sorted chromosome libraries cloned in plasmids.

scope slide box containing moist tissue paper (wring out excess water), placed in an incubator or floated in a water bath. Alternatively, we use metal trays (Lamb's immunoslide staining trays, Raymond Lamb, UK) for both hybridization and detection steps.

1. Dry down the appropriate concentration of probe and competitor either in a vacuum desiccator (Speedivac) or by ethanol precipitation; e.g., for cosmids:
   a. 100 ng of labeled probe.
   b. 2.5 μg (2.5 μL) of Cot-1 DNA.
   c. 0.1 vol of 3 M sodium acetate.
   d. 2 vol of ice-cold ethanol.
   Allow to precipitate for 1 to 2 h at –70°C.
2. Centrifuge and dry down the pellet as for labeled probes. Resuspend the pellet in 11 μL of hybridization buffer (warmed to room temperature).
3. Denature the probe mixture at 95°C in a hotblock for 10 min. Plunge the tubes on ice for a few minutes, and then centrifuge briefly in a microcentrifuge.
4. Place the probe mixture at 37°C for 15 min to 2 h.
5. Just prior to hybridization, denature the chromosomal DNA as follows:
   a. Incubate the slides in denaturing solution (in a water bath in a fume hood) at 70°C for 5 min.
   b. Wash the slides in cold 2X SSC, followed by two changes of 2X SSC.
   c. Dehydrate through a cold alcohol series (70%, 90%, absolute).
6. Air-dry the slides and place on a hot plate at approx 42°C.
7. Centrifuge the probe mixture quickly to get the liquid to the bottom of the tube. Place this mixture on the previously treated slide containing chromosomes and cover with a 22 × 32 mm coverslip (do not let drop dry). Seal the coverslip with rubber solution, and place the slides in a moist chamber at 37°C for overnight to 4 d.

8. Remove the rubber solution. The coverslips can then be removed either by soaking in 2X SSC or by gently tipping them off into the glass disposal bin (never pull them off).
9. Carry out the following washes (*see* **Note 6**):
   a. Three washes (3 min each) in 2X SSC at room temperature (with agitation).
   b. Two washes (20 min each) in 0.1X SSC at 65°C.
   c. One 5-min wash in 0.1X SSC at room temperature (with agitation).
10. Wash the slides in wash solution for 3 min.
11. Incubate the slides in blocking solution for 10–20 min (room temperature).
12. Wash in wash solution for 3 min before carrying out the appropriate detection steps.

3.6. Detection of Bound, Labeled Probe

For directly fluorochrome labeled probes, no immunologic detection steps are required. For repetitive centromeric probes and whole-chromosome paints, usually only one layer of detection reagent is required (i.e., fluorochrome-conjugated avidin or antibody). For single-copy probes, we use the following protocols, using three detection layers. The signal can be amplified further by adding several layers of detection reagents. However, increasing the number of layers to more than three will result in high background and reduced signal:noise ratio.

3.6.1. Biotin-Labeled Probes

1. Dilute 2.5 µL of stock avidin DCS-FITC in 1 mL of blocking solution (final concentration: 5 µg/mL). Add 100 µL of this under a 24 × 50 mm coverslip. Incubate in a moist chamber at 37°C for 30 min.
2. Flick off the coverslips and wash the slides three times (for 3 min each) in wash solution (*see* **Subheading 2.5.**).
3. Dilute 10 µL of stock biotin anti-avidin D in 1 mL of blocking solution (final concentration: 5 µg/mL). Add 100 µL of this under a 24 × 50 mm coverslip. Incubate in a moist chamber at 37°C for 30 min.
4. Flick off the coverslips and wash the slides three times (for 3 min each) in wash solution.
5. Add 100 µL of avidin-FITC (same as the first layer). Incubate for 30 min as before.
6. Carry out the following final washes:
   a. Wash once for 3 min in wash solution.
   b. Wash twice (5 min each) in PBS.
   c. Dehydrate the slides through an ethanol series. Air-dry.
7. Mount the slides in 40 µL of Vectashield containing 1.5 µg/mL of DAPI and 0.75 µg/mL of propidium iodide under a 24 × 50 mm coverslip. Seal the edges of the coverslip with rubber solution or nail varnish. The signal keeps well for several weeks when slides are stored at 4°C.

FISH to Detect Abnormalities in Leukemia

3.6.2. Digoxigenin-Labeled Probes

1. Prepare all antibody dilutions in blocking solution, filtered before use. Make up the following antibody dilutions in 1 mL of blocking solution:
   a. First layer: 1.5 µL of mouse monoclonal antidigoxigenin.
   b. Second layer: 1 µL of rabbit antimouse-FITC.
   c. Third layer: 10 µL of monoclonal antirabbit-FITC.
2. Incubate in each antibody layer (100 µL under a 24 × 50 mm coverslip) for 30 min at 37°C in a moist chamber.
3. After each antibody layer, wash three times (3 min each) in wash solution.
4. Carry out the final washes as for biotin detection
5. Mount in Vectashield containing 1.5 µg/mL of DAPI and 0.75 µg/mL of propidium iodide.

3.6.3. Dual-Color Detection of Biotin- and Digoxigenin-Labeled Probes

1. Prepare all antibody dilutions in blocking solution, filtered before use. Make up the following antibody dilutions in 1 mL of blocking solution:
   a. First layer: 1 µL of avidin-Texas red + 1.5 µL of mouse monoclonal antidigoxigenin.
   b. Second layer: 10 µL of biotin antiavidin + 1 µL of rabbit antimouse-FITC.
   c. Third layer: 1 µL of avidin-Texas red + 10 µL of monoclonal antirabbit-FITC.
2. Incubate in each antibody layer for 30 min at 37°C in a moist chamber.
3. After each antibody layer, wash three times (3 min each) in wash solution.
4. Carry out the final washes as for biotin detection.
5. Mount in Vectashield containing only 1.5 µg/mL of DAPI.

3.7. Microscopy

For the majority of FISH signals, the only equipment required is an epifluorescence microscope equipped with the appropriate filter sets (*see* **Table 2** for commonly used fluorochromes and their spectral characteristics). Both metaphase and interphase FISH analysis can be performed directly at the microscope, with photographic recording of representative images. However, photomicroscopy of multicolor FISH images may be difficult, owing to the long exposure times and loss of registration of images when changing filters. Digital imaging fluorescence systems such as confocal laser scanning microscopes and charge-coupled device (CCD) cameras provide significant advantages in terms of both image storage and the ability for image processing. Confocal laser scanning microscopes provide complete and accurate registration of fluorescent signals on chromosomes by the simultaneous scanning of each fluorochrome through separate filter blocks. These systems are also highly suitable for three-dimensional FISH applications. However, confocal systems are limited for multicolor imaging because most standard lasers only allow excitation of up to three fluorochromes.

Table 2
Fluorescent Dyes Commonly Used for FISH

Fluorochrome	Color	Absorbance (nm)	Emission (nm)
DAPI	Blue	350	456
SpectrumAqua[a]	Blue	433	480
FITC	Yellow/green	490	520
SpectrumGreen[a]	Green	497	524
Rhodamine	Red	550	575
Cy3[b]	Red	554	568
SpectrumOrange[a]	Orange	559	588
Cy3.5[b]	Red	581	588
SpectrumRed[a]	Red	587	612
Texas red	Deep red	595	615
Cy5[b]	Far red	652	672
Cy5.5[b]	Near infrared	682	703
Cy7[b]	Near infrared	755	778

[a]Vysis.
[b]Amersham.

High-performance, highly cooled (–30°C) CCD cameras are extremely sensitive to photons over a wide range of wavelengths and are now the instrument of choice for FISH, particularly for multicolor applications. Problems with image registration owing to the movement of microscope filter blocks can be overcome by the use of a filter wheel containing the excitation filters and situated between the lamp and the microscope. For most FISH applications ambient temperature (+15°C), video-rated CCD cameras are probably sufficient, and for whole-chromosome painting, relatively inexpensive video cameras will suffice. When purchasing a FISH imaging system, it is important to consider requirements for hardware (i.e., compatibility and storage) and software (i.e., sophisticated packages for multicolor FISH and comparative genomic hybridization in addition to standard image capture and enhancement facilities).

3.8. Interpretation of Results

3.8.1. Metaphase FISH

For mapping purposes and also for the assessment of yeast artificial chromosome (YAC) chimerism, FISH is carried out to normal male metaphase spreads. To determine the number of metaphases that need to be evaluated for these applications, it is important to consider the hybridization efficiency, which decreases proportionately with probe size. For whole-chromosome painting probes and centromeric alphoid repeats, only a few metaphases need to be evaluated. Single-copy probes cloned in cosmids, YACs, bacterial artificial chromosomes (BACs), P1, and PACs also hybridize very efficiently (>80% of cells with signal on all four chromatids), so that usually only a few cells (5–10) need to be scored. Small single-copy sequences (<3 kb) hybridize less efficiently (30% of cells with signal on all four chromatids), and, thus, many more metaphases need to be evaluated.

In addition to these considerations, it should be borne in mind that all leukemic cell preparations (with the possible exception of cell lines) are heterogeneous mixtures, with variable numbers of normal and clonal cells. Therefore, for assessing the presence of numerical or structural rearrangements in leukemic bone marrow, it is important to screen as many metaphases as possible. The percentage of abnormal cells from G-banding can be used as a guide. For the presence of deletions, the normal chromosome homolog serves as an internal control. For mapping the extent of chromosome deletions, it is necessary to include a probe to tag the appropriate chromosome, so that only metaphases with the abnormal chromosome are scored (*see* **Fig. 1B**).

3.8.2. Interphase FISH

Probes used for interphase analysis should be chosen to hybridize with high efficiency (>90%). Also note that in dual- or triple-color FISH experiments, three probes with 90% efficiency will hybridize simultaneously to only 73% of nuclei. Centromeric probes are most suitable for detecting numerical abnormalities in interphase, because these exhibit compact, unambiguous signals. Choosing suitable probes is particularly important for the assessment of deletions. In this case, cohybridization with a control probe in a second color will increase the sensitivity. The control probe should be of similar complexity, localized to a region not likely to be affected by a chromosome rearragement in the particular type of leukemia being studied. However, because of the established occurrence of false monosomy (owing to inefficient hybridization or the overlap of signals viewed in two dimensions), diagnostic cutoff levels need to be established for each probe. DNA probes are now available commercially for the majority of specific translocations in leukemia. Differential labeling and dual-color detection of these allow the direct visualization of the fusion gene. However, it is important to establish "in-house" cutoff levels for false positivity for such probes. This can be quite high for some translocations, owing to the variability of breakpoints.

3.9. Advanced Methods and Applications

3.9.1. Whole-Chromosome Painting Probes by Degenerate Oligonucleotide Primer-PCR Amplification of Flow-Sorted Chromosomes (8)

One of the most significant advances in probe generation has been the ability to selectively amplify genomic regions by PCR. Whole-chromosome paints can be produced by interspersed repetitive sequence element-PCR (e.g., Alu-PCR) by selectively amplifying the human DNA content of somatic cell hybrids *(21)*. However, because of the distribution of these sequences across the genome, the resultant chromosome paints produce an R-banded pattern, which may not be optimal for the detection of some rearrangements. The technique of degenerate oligonucleotide primer (DOP)-PCR can be used to obtain more evenly distributed whole-chromosome or region-specific chromosome paints *(8,9)*. This technique is also the basis for the production of 24 color paint sets for SKY (*see* Chapter 3) and M-FISH.

3.9.1.1. FIRST-ROUND DOP-PCR AMPLIFICATION

All reagents except chromosomal DNA and *Taq* 1 polymerase can be sterilized by exposure to short-wave ultraviolet irradiation (5 min on a transilluminator). All solutions, microcentrifuge tubes, and tips should be autoclaved and kept for only PCR. Use aerosol-resistant tips and add all reagents in a laminar flow hood to minimize contamination. Prepare positive (2.5 pg of genomic DNA) and negative (all of the reagents except chromosomes) controls in the same way.

1. Combine in a sterile 0.5-mL microcentrifuge tube: x μL (= 500 flow-sorted chromosomes), 50 μL of 2X PCR buffer, 10 μL of dNTP mix, 6.6 μL of 30 mM 6-MW primer, 0.5 μL of (1.25 U) *Taq* 1 polymerase, and distilled water to a final volume 100 μL.
2. Overlay with 100 μL of mineral oil and run the following program in a DNA thermal cycler: Denature for 10 min at 93°C. 5 cycles of: 1 min at 94°C, 1.5 min at 30°C, 3 min at 30–72°C transition, and 3 min at 72°C; 35 cycles of 1 min at 94°C, 1 min at 62°C, and 3 min at 72°C, with an additional 1 s/cycle and final extension time of 10 min.
3. Run a 10-μL aliquot of the amplified products on a 1.2% agarose gel with *Phi*X174 to check the success of the amplification. There should be no amplification in the negative control.

3.9.1.2. SECOND-ROUND DOP-PCR AND PROBE LABELING

1. Add the following to a new sterile 0.5-mL microcentrifuge tube: 5 μL of amplified products from first round, 25 μL of 2X PCR buffer, 5 μL of nucleotide mix, 3.3 μL of 6-MW primer, 2.5 μL *Taq* 1 polymerase, and 12 μL of 1 mM biotin-16-dUTP.
2. Mix well, overlay with 50 μL of mineral oil, and run the following PCR program: Denature for 10 min at 93°C. 25 cycles of 1 min at 94°C, 1 min at 62°C, and 3 min at 72°C, with a final extension time of 10 min.
3. Remove the mineral oil. Run 10 μL of labeled products on a 1.2% agarose gel to check the size range. If the labeled fragments are too large, recut with 5 μL of DNase I for 30–60 min.
4. Purify the labeled DNA through a MicroSpin G50 (or Sephadex G50) column. Measure the DNA concentration of the purified, labeled DNA in a fluorimeter

FISH to Detect Abnormalities in Leukemia

(usually 20–50 ng/mL). Ethanol precipitate the labeled DNA with tRNA and single-stranded DNA as usual, and dry and resuspend in distilled water or TE to a suitable concentration; this is now ready for use as a chromosome paint. Use 100 ng of probe + 6 μg of Cot-1 DNA per slide.

3.9.2. Combined Immunophenotyping and FISH

The following technique relies on the ability of the reaction product of the APAAP immunophenotyping method to remain throughout subsequent harsh FISH procedures *(22)*. Staining with Fast red produces autofluorescence visible through all filter sets and can be viewed at the same time as the FISH signal. We have used this to identify the cell lineages carrying the del(5q) clonal chromosome abnormality in myelodysplastic syndrome patients *(see* **Fig. 1C,D).** After immunostaining, FISH is carried out essentially as described in **Subheadings 3.5.** and **3.6.,** using a pepsin pretreatment to aid probe penetration.

1. Allow bone marrow smears to reach room temperature and then unwrap.
2. Fix in either acetone:methanol (1:1) for 90 s or acetone alone for 10 min. Then transfer immediately to TBS for 5 min at room temperature.
3. Add the appropriate primary mouse monoclonal antibody and incubate the slides in a moist chamber at room temperature for 30 min. Also incubate a negative control slide (no antibody added) in PBS for 30 min.
4. Add the second layer, rabbit antimouse antibody, and incubate for 30 min in a humid chamber.
5. Add the third antibody, mouse monoclonal APAAP complex, and incubate for 30 min in a moist chamber at room temperature.
6. Wash for 5 min in TBS between each antibody layer.
7. To enhance staining, repeat the antimouse antibody and APAAP steps (**steps 4** and **5**) with reduced incubation times of 10 min.
8. Finally, add alkaline phosphatase substrate to the slides and incubate for 10–20 min.
9. Wash the slides in TBS, then distilled water, and allow to air-dry.

3.9.3. Multicolor FISH

The simplest approach to multicolor FISH uses two probes labeled with different haptens or fluorochromes, and the third probe labeled separately with both, mixed in a 1:1 ratio. An extension of this approach can be used to detect up to seven different targets using three fluorochromes *(23)*. Increasing the number of fluorochromes to five allows the identification of all 24 pairs of human chromosomes *(16,17)*. Both M-FISH and SKY use a set of whole-chromosome paints combinatorially labeled with five fluorochromes, but differ in their method for the discrimination of the fluorochrome combinations. The SKY approach is detailed in Chapter 3. The second detection method, M-FISH, uses a filter-based detection system, capturing the separate fluorochrome images for each of five fluorochromes using specifically selected narrow bandpass filter sets. We have used M-FISH and a set of combinatorially labeled whole-chromosome paints to analyze the complex karyotype in the myeloid leukemia-derived cell line GF-D8 *(24)* (*see* **Fig. 1E**).

4. Notes

1. Proper storage of slides is important to maintain good-quality chromosomal DNA. Slides can be used for hybridization the day after they are made, or kept for up to 1 mo at room temperature. For long-term storage, keep slides in a sealed container with desiccant at −20°C.
2. Alu-PCR amplification of total yeast DNA can be used to increase the yield of YAC DNA *(25)*. However, Alu-poor YACs may not amplify, and the sensitivity for determining YAC chimerism is not known. Isolation of the YAC from the yeast background by pulsed-field gel electrophoresis can be used, but this has a low yield and may be difficult if the YAC is not visible by ethidium bromide staining.
3. It is important to have an accurate measurement of DNA concentration for nick translation labeling. Spectrophotometric measurements are often inaccurate, owing to RNA and other contaminants. We measure probe DNA concentration using a fluorometer (e.g., Hoeffer DynaQuant 200; Amersham Pharmacia Biotech), which measures the fluorescence of a DNA-binding dye, compared to a known standard.
4. These are frequently encountered problems:
   a. *No hybridization signal.* This may be owing to insufficient probe DNA in the hybridization mix. The DNA concentration of any new probe should be measured accurately. This may also be owing to inadequate denaturation of probe and/or chromosomes.
   b. *Probe fragment size too small.* Always check the labeled fragment size on a 2% (1.2% for PCR products) gel with *PhiX174 HaeIII* size marker. The optimum fragment size is 100–500 bp.
   c. *High background.* High background with strong specific signal may be owing to low stringency of hybridization or posthybridization washes or incomplete competition. The stringency of hybridization can be increased by either increasing the hybridization temperature, increasing the formamide concentration of the hybridization mix and/or posthybridization washes to 60%, or decreasing the SSC concentration to 0.1% in the posthybridization washes. Alternatively, increase the Cot-1 DNA concentration: This is already present in large excess so that any increase should be substantial (up to 10-fold).
   d. *Brightly fluorescent signal all over the slide.* This occurs when the labeled probe fragments are too large: If labeled probe is >500 bp, it should be recut with DNase I. High background of this type also may be caused by insufficient blocking with BSA.
   e. *Cells lost from slide.* Handle slides with care at all stages especially during removal of cover slips (never pull them off). Agitation during posthybridization washes should be carried out on a rocking platform set at minimum speed.

FISH to Detect Abnormalities in Leukemia

f. *Poor chromosome morphology/banding*. If chromosomes look "blown," they may have been overdenatured: Always check the temperature of the denaturing solution inside the coplin jar. Overdenatured chromosomes give a C-banding pattern with DAPI staining.

5. These are important hybridization parameters:

a. *Temperature*. The temperature at which two DNA strands separate (T_m) is in the range of 85–95°C. The optimal DNA-DNA reassociation temperature (T_r) is approx 25°C below the T_m of the native duplex. However, fixed chromosome preparations on microscope slides will not tolerate temperatures >65°C for long periods. The presence of formamide in the hybridization buffer lowers the T_r, allowing hybridization to take place at 37–42°C, and preserving chromosome morphology.

b. *Time of hybridization*. This depends on the size and copy number of the target sequence, as well as the complexity of the probe. Repetitive sequence probes such as alphoid centromeric probes require only 1 h for hybridization. Unique sequence probes cloned in plasmid, cosmid, or phage vector require hybridization overnight (16–18 h). Larger insert probes (large YACs) may benefit from longer times to (1–2 d), and very complex probes such as multicolor painting sets and whole genomes in comparative genomic hybridization require 2 to 3 d.

c. *Denaturation of chromosomal DNA*. The optimal time for denaturation needs to be determined for each batch of slides. Overdenaturation results in loss of chromosome morphology and very poor DAPI banding after hybridization. Underdenaturation results in little or no signal. The pH of the denaturation solution is also important: This should be checked when the solution is up to temperature and adjusted if necessary. It is preferable to prepare the denaturing solution and use it as soon as it has reached the desired temperature to prevent pH fluctuations. Alternatively, use EDTA (final concentration of 0.1 m*M*) to stabilize the denaturing solution against pH changes.

d. *Stringency of hybridization conditions*. Renaturation depends on specific base pairing between two complementary DNA strands and can be controlled by the stringency of the hybridization conditions. Increasing the hybridization temperature or decreasing the salt concentration increases the stringency, which has a direct effect on the accuracy of base pairing.

6. The low salt washes used in **Subheading 3.5.** are comparable to the following formamide washes: 50% formamide in 2X SSC (three times for 5 min each), followed by 2X SSC (three times for 5 min each) at 45°C.

Acknowledgments

We wish to thank Margaret Jones and David Mason, LRF Immunodiagnostic Unit, John Radcliffe Hospital, Oxford, for providing us with antibodies for the immunophenotyping and FISH studies. This work was supported by the Leukaemia Research Fund, UK, and Medical Research Council.

References

1. Bentz, M., Schroder, M., Herz, M., Stilgenbauer, S., Lichter, P., and Dohner, H. (1993) Detection of trisomy 8 on blood smears using fluorescence *in situ* hybridization. *Leukemia* **7,** 752–757.
2. Poddighe, P. J., Van Der Lely, N., Vooijs, P., De Witte, T., and Ramaekers, F. C. S. (1993) Interphase cytogenetics on agar cultures: a novel approach to determine chromosomal aberrations in hematopoietic progenitor cells. *Exp. Hematol.* **21,** 859–863.
3. Mühlmann, J., Thaler, J., Hilbe, W., Bechter, O., Erdel, M., Utermann, G., and Duba, H.-C. (1998) Fluorescence in situ hybridization (FISH) on peripheral blood smears for monitoring Philadelphia chromosome-positive chronic myeloid leukemia (CML) during interferon treatment: a new strategy for remission assessment. *Genes Chromosomes Cancer* **21,** 90–100.
4. Kearney, L. (1999) The impact of the new FISH technologies on the cytogenetics of haematological malignancies. *Brit. J. Haemat.* **104,** 648–658.
5. Knuutila, S. (1997) Lineage specificity in haematological neoplasms. *Brit. J. Haemat.* **96,** 2–11.
6. Collins, C., Kuo, W. L., Segraves, R., Fuscoe, J., Pinkel, D., and Gray, J. W. (1991) Construction and characterization of plasmid libraries enriched in sequences from single human chromosomes. *Genomics* **11,** 997–1006.
7. Vooijs, M., Yu, L.-C., Tkachuk, D., Pinkel, D., Johnson, D., and Gray, J. W. (1993) Libraries for each human chromosome, constructed from sorter-enriched chromosomes by using linker-adaptor PCR. *Am. J. Hum. Genet.* **52,** 586–597.
8. Telenius, H., Pelmear, A. H., Tunnacliffe, A., Carter, N. P., Behmel, A., Ferguson-Smith, M. A., et al. (1992) Cytogenetic analysis by chromosome painting using degenerate oligonucleotide-primed-polymerase chain reaction amplified flow-sorted chromosomes. *Genes Chromosomes Cancer* **4,** 257–263.
9. Guan, X. Y., Meltzer, P. S., and Trent, J. M. (1994) Rapid generation of whole chromosome painting probes (WCPs) by chromosome microdissection. *Genomics* **22,** 101–107.
10. Ried, T., Schröck, E., Ning, Y., and Wienberg, J. (1998) Chromosome painting: a useful art. *Hum. Mol. Genet.* **7,** 1619–1626.
11. Tkachuk, D. C., Westbrook, C. A., Andreeff, M., Donlon, T. A., Cleary, M. L., Suryanarayan, K., et al. (1990) Detection of bcr-abl fusion in chronic myelogeneous leukemia by in situ hybridization. *Science* **250,** 559–562.
12. Sacchi, N., Magnani, I., Kearney, L., Wijsman, J., Hagemeijer, A., and Darfler, M. (1995) Interphase cytogenetics of the t(8;21)(q22;q22) associated with acute myelogenous leukemia by two color fluorescence in situ hybridisation. *Cancer Genet. Cytogenet.* **79,** 97–103.
13. Dauwerse, J. G., Kievits, T., Beverstock, G. C., van der Keur, D., Smit, E., Wessels, H. W., et al. (1990) Rapid detection of chromosome 16 inversion in acute nonlymphocytic leukemia, subtype M4: regional localization of the breakpoint in 16p. *Cytogenet. Cell Genet.* **53,** 126–128.

FISH to Detect Abnormalities in Leukemia 27

14. Vaandrager, J.-W., Schuuring, E., Zwikstra, E., de Boer, C. J., Kleiverda, K. K., van Krieken, J. H. J. M., et al. (1996) Direct visualization of dispersed 11q13 chromosomal translocations in mantle cell lymphoma by multicolor DNA fiber fluorescence in situ hybridization. *Blood* **88,** 1177–1182.
15. Raap, A. K. (1998) Advances in fluorescence in situ hybridization. *Mut. Res.* **400,** 287–298.
16. Speicher, M. R., Ballard, S. G., and Ward, D. C. (1996) Karyotyping human chromosomes by combinatorial multi-fluor FISH. *Nat. Genet.* **12,** 368–375.
17. Schröck, E., du Manoir, S., Veldman, T., Schoell, B., Wienberg, J., Ferguson-Smith, M. A., et al. (1996) Multicolor spectral karyotyping of human chromosomes. *Science* **273,** 494–497.
18. Choo, K. H. A. (1994) *Methods in Molecular Biology: In Situ Hybridization Protocols.* Humana, Totowa, NJ.
19. Czepulkowski, B. H., Bhatt, B., and Rooney, D. E. (1992) Basic techniques for the preparation and analysis of chromosomes from bone marrow and leukaemic blood, in *Human Cytogenetics* (Rooney, D. E. and Czepulkowski, B. H., eds.), Oxford University Press, Oxford, pp. 1–25.
20. Heng, H. H. Q., Tsui, L.-C. (1994) FISH detection on DAPI-banded chromosomes, in In Situ *Hybridization Protocols* (Choo, K. H. A., ed.), Humana, Totowa, NJ, pp. 35–50.
21. Lichter, P., Ledbetter, S. A., Ledbetter, D. H., and Ward, D. C. (1990) Fluorescence *in situ* hybridization with *Alu* and L1 polymerase chain reaction probes for rapid characterization of human chromosomes in hybrid cell lines. *Proc. Natl. Acad. Sci. USA* **87,** 6634–6638.
22. Jaju, R. J., Jones, M., Boultwood, J., Mason, D. Y., Wainscoat, J. S., and Kearney, L. (2000) Combined immunophenotyping and FISH identifies the involvement of B cells in 5q- syndrome. *Genes Chromosomes Cancer* **29,** 276–280.
23. Ried, T., Baldini, A., Rand, T. C., and Ward, D. C. (1992) Simultaneous visualization of seven different DNA probes by *in situ* hybridization using combinatorial fluorescence and digital imaging microscopy. *Proc. Natl. Acad. Sci. USA* **89,** 1388–1392.
24. Tosi, S., Giudici, G., Rambaldi, A., Scherer, S. W., Bray-Ward, P., Dirscherl, L., et al. (1999) Characterisation of the human myeloid leukaemia-derived cell line GF-D8 by multiplex fluorescence *in situ* hybridisation, subtelomeric probes and comparative genomic hybridisation. *Genes Chromosomes Cancer* **24,** 213–221.
25. Lengauer, C., Speicher, M. R., and Cremer, T. (1994) FISH of *Alu*-PCR-amplified YAC clones and applications in tumor cytogenetics, in In Situ *Hybridization Protocols* (Choo, K. H. A., ed.), Humana, Totowa, NJ, pp. 85–94.

3

Spectral Karyotyping in Cancer Cytogenetics

Eva Hilgenfeld, Cristina Montagna, Hesed Padilla-Nash, Linda Stapleton, Kerstin Heselmeyer-Haddad, and Thomas Ried

1. Introduction

Cancer is a genetic disease. Gene mutations are not only responsible for rare hereditary forms of human cancer, but for the sporadic forms of human malignancies as well. Many of these specific genetic defects in cancer cells can be visualized as chromosomal aberrations. Conventional cytogenetic analysis of metaphase chromosomes from human malignancies is a first screening step to identify chromosomal aberrations. Since the introduction of chromosome banding techniques in 1970 by Caspersson et al. *(1)*, significant knowledge of chromosomal aberrations especially in hematologic malignancies as well as sarcomas has been gained. In these malignancies, specific balanced translocations were identified and have led to the cloning of the genes involved at many breakpoints. These aberrations have proven to be of significant etiologic, diagnostic, prognostic, as well as therapeutic relevance, especially in leukemias. While cytogenetic analyses have been exceedingly valuable for the description of chromosomal abnormalities in hematologic malignancies and in sarcomas, epithelial cancers were more difficult to study. This is owing, in part, not only to the accessibility of malignant cells and subsequently metaphases for cytogenetic analysis in leukemias, but also to the nature of reciprocal translocations, which provided more immediate entry points for positional cloning efforts.

Although cytogenetic methodologies for the analysis of solid tumor specimens have improved, the difficulty in obtaining good-quality metaphase chromosomes remains *(2)*. The interpretation of cytogenetic abnormalities in epithelial cancers is further confounded by the often vast number and complex nature of chromosomal aberrations in these tumors. Still, recurrent aberrations

From: *Methods in Molecular Medicine, vol. 68: Molecular Analysis of Cancer*
Edited by: J. Boultwood and C. Fidler © Humana Press Inc., Totowa, NJ

and recurrent chromosomal imbalances have been identified, but their clinical relevance is less firmly established *(2–4)*.

Some of the limitations of chromosome banding techniques were overcome by the introduction of molecular cytogenetic techniques such as fluorescence *in situ* hybridization (FISH) with chromosome-painting probes and comparative genomic hybridization (CGH) *(5–7)*. For example, in hematologic malignancies, the t(12;21)(p13;q22) was detected by chromosome painting, because the telomeric regions involved in this translocation are indistinguishable by banding techniques *(8)*. The 12;21 translocation was ascertained to be the most common chromosomal aberration in pediatric B-ALL and has been associated with a favorable prognosis *(9)*. In solid tumors, the application of CGH has led to the identification of recurring patterns of genomic imbalances, both for different tumors and for distinct tumor stages *(10,11)*.

Herein we focus on recently introduced molecular cytogenetic screening techniques that allow one to visualize all human metaphase chromosomes in specific colors.

1.1. Methodology of SKY

Two alternative techniques were developed for color karyotyping: combinatorial multifluor FISH (M-FISH) and spectral karyotyping (SKY) *(12,13)*. Whereas M-FISH employs a conventional imaging approach requiring multiple exposures through a series of single bandpass filters *(12)*, SKY utilizes a novel approach by combining Fourier spectroscopy with epifluorescence microscopy and charge-coupled device (CCD)-imaging, thereby measuring the entire spectrum at all points in a single exposure *(13,14)*.

For SKY, 24 differentially labeled chromosome libraries are produced by amplifying flow-sorted chromosomes utilizing a degenerate oligonucleotide primed polymerase chain reaction (DOP-PCR) *(15)*. Subsequently, the probes are labeled through the incorporation of either haptenized (biotin and digoxigenin) or directly labeled nucleotides, again via PCR. The use of five fluorochromes, either alone or in combination, allows one to discern up to 31 targets simultaneously. The generated chromosome-specific probes are pooled, precipitated with an excess of Cot-1 DNA to suppress repetitive sequences (suppression hybridization), and hybridized onto metaphase chromosomes. The use of an epifluorescence microscope equipped with a single, custom-designed triple bandpass filter allows for the simultaneous excitation of all fluorochromes as well as measurement of the entire emission spectrum of one metaphase in a single exposure. The emitted light from each point of the metaphase is passed through the collection optics and subsequently the Sagnac interferometer, where an optical path difference is created. The resulting interferogram is measured for every pixel of the CCD camera and, using Fourier transformation, is converted to spectral information. The spectral image can be displayed first in RGB colors (obtained by assigning red, green, and blue to specific sections of the emission spectrum) to evaluate the quality of the hybridization (i.e., homogeneity). Every pixel with the same spectral information is subsequently assigned a pseudo-color allowing the spectral classification of all chromosomes *(14)*. **Figure 1A–C** shows a metaphase of the human bladder carcinoma cell line HT1197 displayed in the RGB colors with the accompanying 4,6-diamidino-2-phenylindole (DAPI)-image, and the SKY classification colors.

1.2. Advantages and Limitations

SKY, which is a screening tool, combines the respective advantages of chromosome banding techniques with the advantages of FISH. SKY is especially useful for the detection of interchromosomal structural aberrations that lead to color changes of the aberrant chromosome, such as translocations and insertions. It therefore facilitates the identification of cryptic translocations as well as the clarification of complex aberrations. In addition, SKY assists in the identification of material not recognizable by banding techniques such as marker and ring chromosomes. Other aberrations important in tumor cytogenetics such as double minute chromosomes as well as homogeneously staining regions, which are aberrations that harbor amplified DNA sequences, can be better resolved and contribute to the identification of critical oncogenes. Since its introduction, the value of SKY for use in cancer cytogenetics has been amply demonstrated (for a review, *see* **ref. *16***).

Limitations of the technique pertain to intrachromosomal changes, such as para- or pericentric inversions as well as small deletions or duplications that do not lead to a color change or change in size of the respective aberrant chromosome, which then can be identified more readily in conjunction with the inverted DAPI image or other banding techniques. However, very small marker chromosomes or double minute chromosomes cannot in all instances be classified unambiguously, perhaps owing to the fact that their euchromatin content is low. Therefore, for a comprehensive analysis of tumor metaphases, a combination of molecular cytogenetic methods and banding techniques is advocated.

1.3. Applications of SKY

The usefulness of SKY for cancer cytogenetics, of hematologic malignancies as well as solid tumors, has been shown (for a review, *see* **ref. *16***). Although the difficulty in obtaining good metaphase chromosomes from primary solid tumors remains, SKY analysis of the often complex karyotypes contributes to a more comprehensive cytogenetic analysis and might assist in the identification of stage-specific aberrations *(17–19)*.

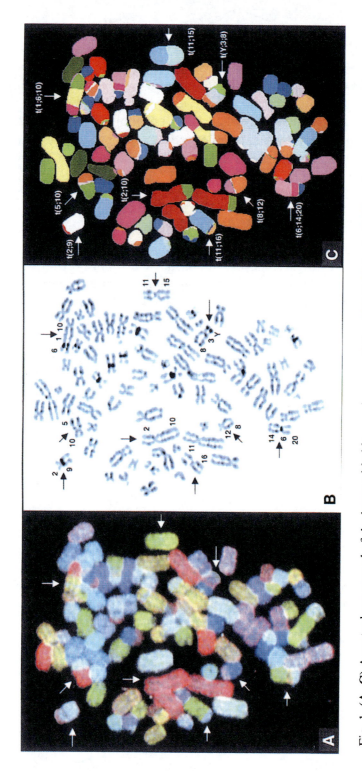

Fig. 1. (A–C) A metaphase spread of the human bladder carcinoma cell line HT 1197 in the RGB-colors (A), the corresponding inverted DAPI image (B), and the SKY classification colors (C). Some, but not all aberrations present within this complex karyotype are marked by arrows.

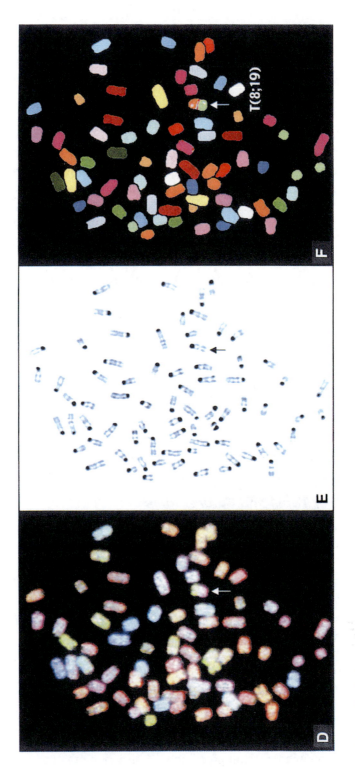

Fig. 1. (**D–F**) Depicts a metaphase prepared from a cell line derived from a mouse mammary tumor. (D) Shows the metaphase in RGB colors, (E) in the corresponding inverted DAPI image, and (F) in the SKY classification colors. The T(8;19) is identified in all three images.

In contrast to the common assumption that cytogenetic changes in cell lines are frequently the result of culture artifacts, the molecular cytogenetic analysis of tumor cell lines showed that the karyotype is surprisingly stable after years of culturing *(20–22)*. Furthermore, results of the SKY analysis of pancreatic cell lines correlated well with those of the CGH analysis of primary tumors *(21)*. In contrast to CGH, SKY can detect the specific type of aberrations that result in chromosomal gains, the amplification of putative oncogenes (e.g., duplications, double minute chromosomes, homogeneously staining regions, jumping translocations), as well as loss of chromosomal material that may harbor tumor suppressor genes [e.g., deletions, isochromosomes such as i(17)(q10)]. Therefore, SKY analysis might not only contribute to the comprehensive analysis of complex aberrations, but also to our understanding of the mechanisms leading to these changes *(23)*.

Mouse models of human disease become more and more important for our understanding of malignancies. As they often can be studied at earlier stages of carcinogenesis, they hold the promise for identification of tumor-initiating events as well as the dissection of genetic events responsible for tumor progression. Nevertheless, the analysis of mouse chromosomes is challenging because mouse chromosomes are all acrocentric and of similar size. The adaptation of SKY to the mouse karyotype by Liyanage et al. *(24,27)* has proven to be a very valuable tool in the analysis of several mouse models *(24–28)*. Comprehensive SKY analyses have shown that chromosomal aberrations in the aforementioned mouse tumors are similar to the changes in the respective human tumors, thereby validating these models. **Figure 1D–F** displays a mouse metaphase in the RGB, inverted DAPI, and SKY classification colors.

1.4. Further Tools and Future Goals

To collect the increasing amount of emerging SKY data and to expedite the identification of new recurrent tumor or tumor stage-specific aberrations, a database has been developed (www.ncbi.nlm.nih.gov/sky/skyweb.cgi).

This database is linked to the Cancer Chromosome Aberration Project (CCAP) (www.ncbi.nlm.nih.gov/CCAP), which integrates the physical and sequence maps with the cytogenetic map of the human genome *(29)*. This project provides STS-tagged and sequenced BAC clones for the entire human genome, whose cytogenetic location has been determined by high-resolution FISH mapping with a resolution of 1 to 2 Mb. CCAP facilitates the high-resolution mapping of chromosomal breakpoints and the subsequent cloning of the genes located at the breakpoints, and potentially will provide new diagnostic tools for interphase cytogenetics *(29)*.

Furthermore, the combination of a comprehensive cytogenetic analysis with gene and protein expression profiling will provide in the near future a wealth

SKY in Cancer Cytogenetics

of information on the consequences of chromosomal aberrations in cancer, and it is hoped that this will identify entry points for the identification of new therapeutic targets and strategies.

2. Materials

2.1. Preparation of SKY Kits

1. PCR cycler.
2. Gel electrophoresis setup.
3. Speedvac.
4. Temperature-controlled microcentrifuge.
5. Primer: Telenius 6 MW(5'-CCGACTCGAGNNNNNNATGTGG-3') (100 μM).
6. Nucleotides for DNA amplification: 100 mM dNTPs, 2 mM stock solution (Boehringer Mannheim, Indianapolis, IN).
7. Nucleotides for labeling:
   a. Spectrum Orange dUTP (Vysis, Downers Grove, IL); dilute 1:5 to 0.2 mM.
   b. Texas Red dUTP (Molecular Probes, Eugene, OR); dilute 1:5 to 0.2 mM.
   c. 0.1 mM Rhodamine 110-dUTP (Perkin-Elmer, Foster City, CA).
   d. 1 mM Biotin-16-dUTP (Boehringer Mannheim).
   e. 1 mM Digoxigenin-11-dUTP (Boehringer Mannheim).
   f. For the labeling PCR, prepare a stock solution of dNTPs with a final concentration of dATP, dCTP, and dGTP of 2 mM, but only 1.5 mM of dTTP.
8. Polymerase: native *Taq* (5 U/μL) (MBI Fermentas).
9. Buffer: 10X PCR Buffer (MBI Fermentas).
10. Human Cot-1 DNA (1 mg/mL) (Life Technologies, BRL, Grand Island, NY).
11. Salmon sperm DNA (9.7 mg/mL) (Sigma, St. Louis, MO).
12. 3 M Na-acetate.
13. Deionized formamide (pH 7.0).
14. Master mix: 20% dextran sulfate in 2X saline sodium citrate (SSC), pH 7.0; autoclave and store aliquots at −20°C.

2.2. Pretreatment, Denaturation, and Hybridization of Slides for SKY

1. Thermomixer or water bath.
2. Hot plate.
3. Shaker.
4. Hybridization chamber at 37°C.
5. 2X SSC.
6. RNase A (stock solution: 20 mg/mL) (Boehringer Mannheim).
7. Pepsin (stock solution: 100 mg/mL) (Sigma).
8. 0.01 N HCl.
9. 1X Phosphate-buffered saline (PBS).
10. 1X PBS/MgCl$_2$ (50 mM).
11. 1% Formaldehyde in 1X PBS/MgCl$_2$ (50 mM).
12. Ethanol (70, 90, 100%).
13. 70% Formamide/2X SSC (pH 7.0).

2.3. Detection

1. 50% Formamide/2X SSC (adjust to pH 7.0).
2. 1X SSC.
3. 4X SSC/Tween-20 (0.1%).
4. Blocking Solution: 3% bovine serum albumine (BSA) (Boehringer Mannheim) in 4X SSC/Tween-20; store at 4°C.
5. 1% BSA (Boehringer Mannheim) in 4X SSC/Tween-20.
6. DAPI: 80 ng/mL in 2X SCC (stock solution: 2 mg of DAPI/10 mL of sterile water).
7. Antifade: Dissolve 100 mg of 1,4-phenylenediamine in 2 mL of 1X PBS. Adjust pH with carbonate-biocarbanate buffer (pH 9.0) to 8.0, add 1X PBS to 10 mL, mix with 90 mL of 86% glycerol, aliquot and store at −20°C, and protect from light during use.
8. Mouse antidigoxin (Sigma).
9. Fluorolink-Cy5-avidin (Jackson Immuno Research, West Grove, PA).
10. Fluorolink-Cy5.5-sheep-antimouse-IgG (Amersham Pharmacia Biotech, Buckinghamshire, UK).

2.4. Image Acquisition and Analysis

1. Epifluorescence microscope equipped with a DAPI filter and SKY filter V 3.0 (Chroma Technology, Brattleboro, VT).
2. 150-W Xenon lamp (Opti-Quip, Highland Mills, NY).
3. SpectraCube™SD200, Spectral Imaging Acquisition Software, and SkyView™ software (Applied Spectral Imaging, Migdal Ha'Emek, Israel).

3. Methods

The protocols in this chapter are for SKY analysis of human chromosomes. Nevertheless, the procedure is quite similar for the mouse genome. Further information and protocols can be obtained from the following website: www.riedlab.nci.nih.gov.

3.1. Preparation of SKY Kits

3.1.1. Primary DOP-PCR

Flow-sorted chromosomes are amplified by PCR using a DOP as described by Telenius et al. *(15)*. The DNA amplification with DOPs is sequence unspecific. Therefore, employment of sterile techniques is extremely important in order to avoid contamination with genomic DNA.

Each chromosome-specific primary PCR product is labeled with a single fluorescent dye in a second DOP-PCR step for quality control purposes. Individual hybridization of all painting probes onto normal control slides should result only in specific hybridization signals for the respective pair of homologous chromosomes with low overall background. Otherwise, the primary PCR product cannot be used for the secondary and labeling DOP-PCR.

SKY in Cancer Cytogenetics

3.1.2. Secondary DOP-PCR

The primary PCR products are further amplified in a second DOP-PCR. Great precautions should be taken to avoid contamination also during this step.

1. Mix the following components for the PCR reaction: 2 µL of DNA (150–200 ng), 10 µL of PCR buffer (10X), 8 µL of MgCl$_2$ (25 mM), 10 µL of dNTP (2 mM), 65 µL of dH$_2$O, 4 µL of primer (100 mM), 1 µL of *Taq* polymerase (5 U/µL) for a total volume of 100 µL.
2. Run the following DOP-PCR program:
   a. Step 1: 94°C for 1 min.
   b. Step 2: 56°C for 1 min.
   c. Step 3: 72°C for 3 min with addition of 1 s/cycle.
   d. Step 4: Repeat **steps 1–3**, 29 times.
   e. Step 5: 72°C for 10 min.
   f. Step 6: 4°C for ∞.
3. Of the PCR product, run 2 µL on a 1% agarose gel as a quality control (intense smear between 500 bp and 2 kb).
4. Freeze DNA at –20°C.

3.1.3. DOP-PCR for Labeling

Five different fluorochromes (either directly labeled or haptenized nucleotides) are used to accomplish the differential labeling of 24 painting probes. **Table 1** was devised in order to achieve good color differences among chromosomes.

1. The setup in **Table 1** leads to 57 reactions. Label 57 autoclaved PCR tubes accordingly.
2. Mix the following components for the PCR reaction: 4 µL of DNA (400–600 ng), 10 µL of PCR buffer (10X), 8 µL of MgCl$_2$ (25 mM), 5 µL of dNTP (2 mM), dTTP (1.5 mM), 65 µL (for direct)/67 µL (for indirect) of dH$_2$O, 2 µL of primer (100 mM), 1 µL of *Taq* polymerase (5 U/mL); x-dUTP: 5 µL of Rhodamine 110 (0.1 mM), 5 µL of Spectrum Orange (0.1 mM), 5 µL of Texas Red (0.2 mM), 3 µL of biotin (1 mM), 3 µL of digoxigenin (1 mM) for a total volume of 100 µL.
3. Run the following PCR program:
   a. Step 1: 94°C for 1 min.
   b. Step 2: 56°C for 1 min.
   c. Step 3: 72°C for 3 min with addition of 1 s/cycle.
   d. Step 4: Repeat **steps 1–3**, 29 times.
   e. Step 5: 72°C for 10 min.
   f. Step 6: 4°C for ∞.
4. Run 2 µL of each DNA on a 1% agarose gel as a quality control (intense smear between 500 bp and 2 kb).
5. One SKY Kit should be precipitated according to the protocol in **Subheading 3.1.4.** and hybridized onto normal chromosomes to assess the quality. If the SKY

Table 1
Labeling Scheme

Chromosome	Rhodamine 110	Spectrum Orange	Texas Red	Cy 5 (biotin)	Cy 5.5 (digoxigenin)
1		X			X
2					X
3	X			X	X
4			X	X	
5	X	X	X		X
6			X		X
7	X			X	
8	X				
9	X	X			X
10				X	X
11		X			
12	X		X	X	X
13	X	X			
14			X		
15		X	X	X	
16	X		X	X	
17				X	
18	X	X	X		
19		X		X	
20	X	X		X	
21	X				X
22		X	X	X	X
X	X		X		
Y	X	X		X	X

Kit is of good quality, the automated classification of a normal metaphase using the SkyView software should be correct. The following points should be evaluated for quality assessment:

a. The overall painting homogeneity as well as the suppression of heterochromatin.

b. The signal-to-noise ratio: Using the software for image acquisition, the highest and lowest values for the fluorescence intensity within the image are displayed. A difference of at least 100 counts between the intensity along chromosomes and background must be achieved.

c. The color separation between chromosomes displayed in red, green or blue in the RGB image.

d. The spectra of the single dyes: The spectra of this test hybridization should be compared with and should match the reference spectra stored in the combinatorial table (ctb)-file.

SKY in Cancer Cytogenetics

6. If the quality of the test hybridization was good, all SKY Kits can be precipitated and stored at –20°C until further use.

3.1.4. Precipitation of SKY Kits

1. Combine 4 µL of each chromosome-painting probe (400–600 ng), 20 µL of human Cot-1 DNA and 1 µL of salmon sperm DNA in an Eppendorf tube for every SKY Kit.
2. Add 1/10 vol of 3 M Na-acetate and 2.5 to 3.0 times the total volume of cold 100% ethanol.
3. Vortex and precipitate at –20°C overnight or at –80°C for 30 min.
4. Centrifuge the precipitated DNA at 4°C and 11,700g for 30 min.
5. Remove the supernatant and dry the DNA pellet in a Speedvac for 5–10 min.
6. Add 6 µL of deionized formamide (pH 7.0), and shake in a thermomixer at 37°C until the pellet is completely dissolved (at least 1 h).
7. Add 6 µL of Master Mix, vortex, and spin briefly.
8. Store SKY Kits at –20°C until used for hybridization.

3.2. Preparation of Metaphase Chromosomes

Metaphase chromosome preparation for SKY follows standard cytogenetic protocols *(30)*. Best hybridization results are generally obtained with slides aged for 1 wk either at room temperature or in a drying oven at 37°C, if they are exposed to humidity at room temperature. Prepared slides can be stored for several years in an airtight container with desiccant at –20 or –80°C after dehydration through an ethanol series.

3.3. Pretreatment, Denaturation, and Hybridization of Slides for SKY

3.3.1. Pretreatment of Slides

1. Equilibrate slides in 2X SSC (room temperature).
2. Dilute the RNase stock 1:200 in 2X SSC, apply 120 µL per slide, and cover with a 24 × 60 mm coverslip.
3. Incubate at 37°C for 60 min.
4. Prepare 100 mL of 0.01 N HCl, adjust to pH 2.0, and prewarm at 37°C.
5. Remove the coverslips and wash three times for 5 min each in 2X SSC on a shaker at room temperature.
6. Pepsin treatment: Add 5–30 µL of pepsin to a Coplin jar, and then add 100 mL of prewarmed HCl, and incubate the slides at 37°C for 2 min (*see* **Note 1**).
7. Wash twice for 5 min each in 1X PBS at room temperature, shaking.
8. Wash once for 5 min in 1X PBS/MgCl$_2$.
9. Incubate the slides for 10 min at room temperature in 1% formaldehyde in 1X PBS/MgCl$_2$ for postfixation.
10. Wash again one time for 5 min in 1X PBS at room temperature, shaking.
11. Dehydrate the slides in 70, 90, and 100% ethanol for 3 min each.
12. Let the slides air-dry (*see* **Note 1**).

3.3.2. Denaturation of SKY Kit

1. Prewarm SKY Kits at 37°C for 30 min.
2. Denature SKY Kits at 80°C for 5 min in a thermomixer or water bath,
3. Before applying to the slide, allow the SKY Kit to preanneal at 37°C for 1 to 2 h.

3.3.3. Slide Denaturation

1. Apply 120 μL of 70% formamide/2X SSC to a 24 × 60 mm coverslip and touch slide to coverslip.
2. Denature the slides at 75°C on a slide warmer for 1 min, 30 s. Denaturation of slides can also be performed by preheating 70% formamide/2X SSC in a Coplin jar in a water bath to 72°C. This is especially applicable for G-banded slides, for which denaturation times are shorter (10–30 s).
3. Shake off the coverslips and immediately place the slides in freshly prepared 70% ethanol (precooled to 0°C) for 3 min, followed by 3 min in 90% and 100% ethanol each.
4. Let the slides air-dry.

3.3.4. Hybridization

1. After preannealing, add the SKY Kit to the preselected hybridization area on the denatured slides and cover with an 18-mm^2 coverslip.
2. Seal the coverslips with rubber cement and incubate in a hybridization chamber at 37°C for 48 h. Drying out of the SKY Kit during the hybridization time should be avoided.

3.4. Detection

1. Prepare solutions (formamide/SSC, 1X SSC, 4X SSC/Tween-20) and prewarm at 45°C for 30 min before starting the detection.
2. After the hybridization time, carefully remove the rubber cement and dip the slides in formamide/SSC until the coverslips slide off (*see* **Note 2**).
3. Wash the slides three times for 5 min each in formamide/SSC, shaking.
4. Wash the slides three times for 5 min each in 1X SSC, shaking.
5. Dip the slides in 4X SSC/Tween-20.
6. Incubate the slides with blocking solution (120 μL/slide, covered with a 24 × 60 mm coverslip) in a hybridization chamber at 37°C for 30 min.
7. Spin all the fluorescent dyes for 3 min at 13,000 rpm.
8. Dip the slides in 4X SSC/Tween-20.
9. Add 120 μL of antibody solution containing mouse antidigoxin (1:200 dilution in 1% BSA) per 24 × 60 mm coverslip, touch the slide to the coverslip, and incubate in a hybridization chamber for 1 h at 37°C.
10. Wash the slides three times for 5 min each in 4X SSC/Tween-20, shaking.
11. Add 120 μL of antibody solution containing avidin-Cy5 and Cy5.5 antimouse (1:200 dilution in 1% BSA each) per coverslip (24 × 60 mm), touch the slide to the coverslip, and incubate in a hybridization chamber for 1 h at 37°C.

SKY in Cancer Cytogenetics

12. Wash the slides three times for 5 min each in 4X SSC/Tween-20, shaking.
13. Stain with DAPI for 5 min in a light-protected Coplin jar.
14. Wash for 5 min in 2X SSC, shaking.
15. Dehydrate the slides in an ethanol series (70, 90, 100%) for 3 min each.
16. Let the slides air-dry in the dark.
17. When the slides are completely dry, apply 30 µL of antifade, cover with 24 × 60 mm coverslips, and store in the dark at 4°C until image acquisition.

3.5. Image Acquisition and Analysis

For each metaphase, a spectral image and the corresponding DAPI image is acquired using an epifluorescence microscope connected to the SpectraCube (Applied Spectral Imaging; a combination of a Sagnac-Interferometer and a CCD-camera). For the spectral image, a custom-designed SKY filter (Chroma) is employed; the DAPI image is acquired using the TR1-filter (Chroma). The subsequently inverted DAPI-image gives a chromosomal banding pattern comparable with the one obtained by G-banding (**Fig. 1B,E**). During image acquisition, heat protection filters should normally be placed into the light pass but can be removed if the intensity of the fluorescent dyes with emission in the far red range (Cy5 and Cy5.5) is weak.

For image analysis, the spectral image is first displayed in RGB (red-green-blue) colors. This allows for the evaluation of hybridization quality (**Fig. 1A,C**). Using the SkyView software, both the spectral and the DAPI image are then analyzed simultaneously. Through correlation of the spectral information with the labeling scheme and the reference spectra of the five fluorescent dyes (stored in a ctb–file) a specific pseudocolor is assigned to each image point. Thus, all material belonging to the same chromosome will be displayed in the same pseudocolor, and chromosomal aberrations will be easily visible (**Fig. 1C, F**).

4. Notes

1. Pretreatment with pepsin to remove residual cytoplasm is a crucial step because overtreatment with pepsin leads to reduced signal intensity and impaired chromosome morphology and therefore compromises SKY results. Pepsin concentration and time must therefore be adjusted according to the amount of cytoplasm; that is, use low concentrations of pepsin (5–10 µL; 2 min) if there is little cytoplasm, and 20–30 µL, 5 min, for cells with high amounts of cytoplasm. Cytoplasm is visible as opaque material around the metaphase chromosomes. If no cytoplasm is present, pepsin treatment may not be necessary at all.
2. During the detection avoid exposure to light as much as possible and avoid air-drying of the slides between the different steps. Slides should be handled carefully in order to avoid scratching the surfaces.

Acknowledgments

We gratefully acknowledge Prof. M. A. Ferguson-Smith and Dr. J. Wienberg for providing high-quality flow-sorted chromosomes. E. H. received a postdoctoral fellowship from the Deutsche Krebshilfe.

References

1. Caspersson, T., Zech, L., and Johansson, C. (1970) Differential banding of alkylating fluorochromes in human chromosomes. *Exp. Cell Res.* **60**, 315–319.
2. Thompson, F. H. (1997) Cytogenetic methods and findings in human solid tumors, in *The AGT Cytogenetics Laboratory Manual*, 3rd ed., (Barch, M. J., Knutsen, T., and Spurbeck, J., eds.), Lippincott-Raven, Philadelphia, PA, pp. 375–30.
3. Heim, S. and Mitelman, F. (eds.) (1995) *Cancer Cytogenetics,* 2nd ed., Wiley-Liss, New York.
4. Mertens, F., Johansson, B., Höglund, M., and Mitelman, F. (1997) Chromosomal imbalance maps of malignant solid tumors: a cytogenetic survey of 3185 neoplasms. *Cancer Res.* **57**, 2765–2780.
5. Cremer, T., Lichter, P., Borden, J., Ward, D. C., and Manuelidis, L. (1988) Detection of chromosome aberrations in metaphase and interphase tumor cells by in situ hybridization using chromosome-specific library probes. *Hum. Genet.* **80**, 235–246.
6. Pinkel, D., Landegent, J., Collins, C., Fuscoe, J., Segraves, R., Lucas, J., and Gray, J. W. (1988) Fluorescence in situ hybridization with human chromosome specific libraries: detection of trisomy 21 and translocation of chromosome 4. *Proc. Natl. Acad. Sci. USA* **85**, 9138–9142.
7. Kallioniemi, A., Kallioniemi, O.-P., Sudar, D., Rutovitz, D., Gray, J. W., Waldman, F., and Pinkel, D. (1992) Comparative genomic hybridization for molecular cytogenetic analysis of solid tumors. *Science* **258**, 818–821.
8. Romana, S. P., Le Coniat, M., and Berger, R. (1994) t(12;21): A new recurrent translocation in acute lymphoblastic leukemia. *Genes Chromosomes Cancer* **9**, 186–191.
9. Shurtleff, S. A., Buijs, A., Behm, F. G., Rubnitz, J. E., Raimondi, S. C., Hancock, M. L., et al. (1995) TEL/AML1 fusion resulting from a cryptic t(12;21) is the most common genetic lesion in pediatric ALL and defines a subgroup of patients with an excellent prognosis. *Leukemia* **9**, 1985–1989.
10. Forozan, F., Karhu, R., Kononen, J., Kallioniemi, A., and Kallioniemi, O. P. (1997) Genome screening by comparative genomic hybridization. *Trends Genet.* **13**, 405–409.
11. Ried, T., Heselmeyer-Haddad, K., Blegen, H., Schröck, E., and Auer, G. (1999) Genomic changes defining the genesis, progression, and malignancy potential in solid human tumors: a phenotype/genotype correlation. *Genes Chromosomes Cancer* **25**, 195–204.
12. Speicher, M., Ballard, S. G., and Ward, D. C. (1996) Karyotyping human chromosomes by combinatorial multi-fluor FISH. *Nat. Genet.* **12**, 368–375.
13. Schröck, E., du Manoir, S., Veldman, T., Schoell, B., Wienberg, J., Ferguson-Smith, M. A., et al. (1996) Multicolor Spectral Karyotyping of human chromosomes. *Science* **273**, 494–497.

SKY in Cancer Cytogenetics

14. Garini, Y., Macville, M., du Manoir, S., Buckwald, R.A., Lavi, M., Katzir, N., et al. (1996) Spectral karyotyping. *Bioimaging* **4**, 65–72.

15. Telenius, H., Pelear, A. H., Tunnacliffe, A., Carter, N. P., Behmel, A., Ferguson-Smith, M. A., et al. (1992) Cytogenetic analysis by chromosome painting using DOP-PCR amplified flow-sorted chromosomes. *Genes Chromosomes Cancer* **4**, 257–263.

16. Knutsen, T. and Ried, T. (2000) SKY: a comprehensive diagnostic and research tool: a review of the first 300 published cases. *J. Assoc. Genet. Technol.* **26**, 3–15.

17. Adeyinka, A., Kytola, S., Mertens, F., Pandis, N., and Larsson, C. (2000) Spectral karyotyping and chromosome banding studies of primary breast carcinomas and their lymph node metastases. *Int. J. Mol. Med.* **5**, 235–240.

18. Wong, N., Lai, P., Pang, E., Wai-Tong Leung, T., Wan-Yee Lau, J., and Johnson, P. J. (2000) A comprehensive karyotypic study on human hepatocellular carcinoma by spectral karyotyping. *Hepatology* **32**, 1060–1068.

19. Phillips, J. L., Ghadimi, B. M., Wangsa, D., Padilla-Nash, H., Worrell, R., Hewitt, S., Linehan, W. M., et al. (2001) Cytogenetic characterization of early and late renal cell carcinomas in von Hippel-Lindau (VHL) disease. *Genes Chromosomes Cancer* **31**, 1–9.

20. Macville, M., Schröck, E., Padilla-Nash, H., Keck, C., Ghadimi, B. M., Zimonjic, D., et al. (1999) Comprehensive and definitive molecular cytogenetic characterization of HeLa cells by spectral karyotyping. *Cancer Res.* **59**, 141–150.

21. Ghadimi, B. M., Schröck, E., Walker, R. L., Wangsa, D., Jauho, A., Meltzer, P. S., and Ried, T. (1999) Specific chromosomal aberrations and amplification of the *AIB1* Nuclear Receptor Coactivator Gene in pancreatic carcinomas. *Am. J. Pathol.* **154**, 525–536.

22. Ghadimi, B. M., Sackett, D. L., Difilippantonio, M. J., Schröck, E., Neumann, T., Jauho, A., et al. (2000) Centrosome amplification and instability occurs exclusively in aneuploid, but not in diploid colorectal cancer cell lines, and correlates with numerical chromosomal aberrations. *Genes Chromosomes Cancer* **27**, 183–190.

23. Padilla-Nash, H. M., Heselmeyer-Haddad, K., Wangsa, D., Zhang, H., Ghadimi, B. M., Macville, M., et al. (2001) Jumping translocations (JT) are common in solid tumor cell lines and result in recurrent fusions of whole chromosome arms. *Genes Chromosomes Cancer* **30**, 349–363.

24. Liyanage, M., Coleman, A., du Manoir, S., Veldman, T., McCormack, S., Dickson, R. B., et al. (1996) Multicolour spectral karyotyping of mouse chromosomes. *Nat. Genet.* **14**, 312–315.

25. Coleman, A. E., Schrock, E., Weaver, Z., du Manoir, S., Yang, F., Ferguson-Smith, M. A., et al. (1997) Previously hidden chromosome aberrations in T(12;15)-positive BALB/c plasmacytomas uncovered by multicolor spectral karyotyping. *Cancer Res.* **57**, 4585–4592.

26. Weaver, Z. A., McCormack, S. J., Liyanage, M., du Manoir, S., Coleman, A., Schröck, E., et al. (1999) A recurring pattern of chromosomal aberrations in mammary gland tumors of MMTV-*cmyc* transgenic mice. *Genes Chromosomes Cancer* **25**, 251–260.

27. Liyanage, M., Weaver, Z., Barlow, C., Coleman, A., Pankratz, D. G., Anderson, S., et al. (2000) Abnormal rearrangement within the a/d T-cell receptor locus in lymphomas from Atm-deficient mice. *Blood* **96,** 1940–1946.
28. Difilippantonio, M. J., Zhu, J., Chen, H. T., Meffre, E., Nussenzweig, M. C., Max, E. E., et al. (2000) DNA repair protein Ku80 suppresses chromosomal aberrations and malignant transformation. *Nature* **404,** 510–514.
29. Kirsch, I. R., Green, E. D., Yonescu, R., Strausberg, R., Carter, N., Bentley, D., et al. (2000) A systematic, high-resolution linkage of the cytogenetic and physical maps of the human genome. *Nat. Genet.* **24,** 339–340.
30. Barch, M. J., Knutsen, T., and Spurbeck, J. L. (eds.) (1997) *The AGT Cytogenetics Laboratory Manual*, 3rd ed., Lippincott-Raven, Philadelphia, PA.

4

Comparative Genomic Hybridization Analysis

Binaifer R. Balsara, Jianming Pei, and Joseph R. Testa

1. Introduction

Molecular genetic investigations of human tumors have increased our understanding of the mechanistic relationship between chromosome abnormalities and cancer. In leukemias and lymphomas, for which extensive karyotypic analysis has been possible, specific translocations and inversions have been identified that result in the deregulation of protooncogenes or the creation of aberrant fusion genes *(1,2)*. Similarly, certain sarcomas (e.g., Ewing and synovial sarcomas) are characterized by specific translocations *(3,4)*. In many cases, these translocations represent the only chromosome alteration present in the tumor cells, consistent with the notion that such changes play a critical role in the pathogenesis of these neoplasms.

Unlike the aforementioned malignancies, in the common epithelial tumors of adults, such as lung and breast carcinomas, conventional karyotyping has proven difficult. Many of these solid tumors have a low mitotic index, limiting the number of metaphase spreads suitable for detailed chromosome banding analysis. Moreover, the karyotypes of epithelial tumors are often complicated, with many additional chromosomes and complex markers, hindering efforts to identify chromosome segments that are consistently lost or gained. Although other techniques permit the detection of allelic loss, mutations, or DNA amplification, such methods are highly focused in that they target one specific gene or chromosome region at a time, leaving the majority of the genome unexamined. These limitations can be circumvented through the use of a molecular cytogenetic approach referred to as comparative genomic hybridization (CGH) analysis *(5)*. This invaluable technique permits the assessment of genomic imbalances (gains, losses, and DNA amplifications) within the entire tumor genome in a single experiment.

From: *Methods in Molecular Medicine, vol. 68: Molecular Analysis of Cancer*
Edited by: J. Boultwood and C. Fidler © Humana Press Inc., Totowa, NJ

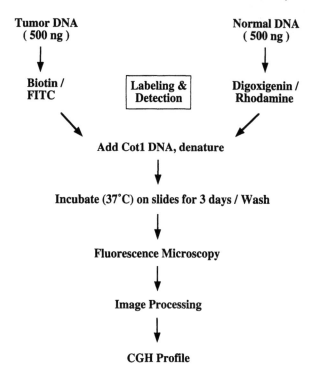

Fig. 1. Schematic representation depicting steps involved in CGH analysis. Equimolar amounts of tumor and normal reference DNAs are labeled differentially, denatured, and cohybridized to normal human metaphase spreads. Cot-1 DNA is added to block ubiquitous repetitive sequences. Hybridization is allowed to take place for several days, followed by washing to remove unbound probe. Chromosomes are counterstained with DAPI and observed with a fluorescence microscope equipped with a cooled charge-coupled device (CCD) camera operated by a computer workstation. Images of 4',6'-diamidino-2-phenylindole (DAPI) staining, fluorescein isothiocyanate, and rhodamine signals are acquired, digitized, and merged using interactive software. This software also performs ratio computations and profile averaging to detect genomic imbalances.

The CGH procedure involves competitive *in situ* hybridization of differentially labeled tumor DNA and normal reference DNA to normal human metaphase spreads (**Fig. 1**). More important, this technique does not require mitotic tumor cells, so that archival as well as fresh specimens can be examined. Moreover, only a small amount (≤500 ng) of genomic DNA is needed for a genomewide analysis. Furthermore, CGH accounts for all chromosomal segments in the tumor cell genome, including those present in marker chromosomes whose origin cannot be determined by conventional karyotyping. Application of the CGH procedure has permitted the identification of recurrent

CGH Analysis

imbalances in a wide variety of human cancers, especially the common epithelial tumors. In the last decade, CGH analyses of more than 2200 solid tumor specimens, involving 27 different tumor types, have been reported (*6*).

2. Materials

2.1. Preparation of Normal Metaphase CGH Target Slides

1. Peripheral blood (5–10 mL) from a normal male donor collected in preservative-free heparin-sodium salt. Note that 10 U of heparin is sufficient as an anticoagulant for each milliliter of blood.
2. Tissue culture flasks (25 cm^2).
3. Complete medium: RPMI 1640 medium supplemented with 15% fetal bovine serum, antibiotics (100 U/mL of penicillin sodium salt and 50 mg/mL of streptomycin), and L-glutamine (2 mM).
4. Phytohemagglutinin (PHA-M) (cat. no. 10576-015; Gibco).
5. Colcemid (cat. no. 15210-040; Gibco).
6. Centrifuge tubes (10 mL).
7. Hypotonic KCl (0.075 M).
8. Fixative (methanol:acetic acid, 3:1).
9. Glass slides (Fisher Premium Superfrost microscope slides; cat. no. 12-544-7). Preclean the slides by soaking in detergent, scrubbing gently, and rinsing thoroughly in distilled water. Chill the slides in 70% ethanol before use.

2.2. Labeling of Test and Reference Genomic DNA

1. Test DNA: High molecular weight genomic DNA from fresh, frozen, or paraffin-embedded tumor tissue. Be sure that the specimen has a high percentage of tumor cells (*see* **Note 1**). Tumor cell line DNA may also be used.
2. Reference DNA: High molecular weight genomic DNA from peripheral blood lymphocytes of a normal individual.

2.2.1. Indirect Labeling by Random Priming

1. BioPrime DNA Labeling System (cat. no. 18094-011; Gibco) with the following components:
   a. 2.5X Random Primers Solution: 125 mM Tris-HCl (pH 6.8), 12.5 mM MgCl$_2$, 25 mM 2-mercaptoethanol, 750 µg/mL of oligodeoxyribonucleotide primers (random octamers).
   b. 10X dNTP mixture: 1 mM biotin-14-dCTP, 1 mM dCTP, 2 mM dATP, 2 mM dGTP, 2 mM dTTP in 10 mM Tris-HCl (pH 7.5), 1 mM Na$_2$EDTA.
   c. Klenow fragment (large fragment of DNA polymerase I): 40 U/µL of Klenow fragment in 50 mM potassium phosphate (pH 7.0), 100 mM KCl, 1 mM dithiothreitol, 50% glycerol.
   d. Stop Buffer: 0.2 M Na$_2$EDTA (pH 8.0).
2. 10X Digoxigenin DNA Labeling Mix (cat. no. 1277 065; Boehringer Mannheim).
3. Distilled water.

2.2.2. Direct Labeling by Random Priming

Use the same kit as in the indirect labeling protocol, with the following additions:

1. Fluoro Green (fluorescein-11-dUTP) (cat. no. RPN 2121; Amersham Pharmacia).
2. Fluoro Red (rhodamine-4-UTP) (cat. no. RPN 2122; Amersham Pharmacia).
3. 10X dNTP mixture: 1.2 mM dCTP, 1.2 mM dATP, 1.2 mM dGTP, 0.6 mM dTTP in 58 mL of distilled water.

2.3. Hybridization Reagents, Probe Precipitation, and Pretreatment of Target Slides

1. Human Cot-1 DNA (cat. no. 15279-011; Gibco).
2. 3 M Sodium acetate.
3. Absolute alcohol.
4. Hybrisol VII (50% formamide/2X saline sodium citrate [SSC]) (cat. no. S1390-10; Ventana).
5. RNase A (100 mg/mL) (cat. no. 109169; Boehringer-Mannheim). Boil for 20 min after dissolving 100 mg in 1 mL of distilled water; immediately cool on ice.
6. 70% Formamide (cat. no. 47670; Fluka)/2X SSC.
7. Coverslips (18 mm × 18 mm).
8. Glass coverslip sealant (cat. no. S1370-12; Oncor).

2.4. Posthybridization Washing and Probe Detection

1. Capped Corning centrifuge tubes (50 mL).
2. Coplin jars.
3. 50% Formamide (cat. no. 47670; Fluka), 2X SSC.
4. 20X SSC: 3.0 M NaCl, 0.3 M Na citrate, pH 7.0. Dilute 1:10 for 2X SSC.
5. 1X PBD: 4X SSC, pH 7.0/0.05% Tween-20.
6. Rhodamine antidigoxigenin (cat. no. 1207750; Boehringer-Mannheim)/fluorescein-labeled avidin (cat. no. S1370-9; Oncor); 5 µg/mL.
7. Antiavidin antibody (cat. no. S1370-10; Oncor).
8. Plastic coverslips (cat. no. S1370-13; Oncor).
9. DAPI (cat. no. D9542; Sigma). Stock solution is 1 mg/mL in distilled water.
10. Mounting medium (cat. no. H1000; Vector).

2.5. Image Analysis

1. Zeiss Axioplan microscope equipped with a ×63 plan neofluor objective (1.25 na), 100-W mercury arc lamp, Chroma Technology "P1" multiband pass beam splitter and emission filter, and single band excitation filters for each fluorochrome, mounted in a computer-controlled filter wheel.
2. Cooled CCD camera (Photometrics SenSys Grade 2) with 12-bit resolution (4096 gray scales).
3. QUIPS software (Quantitative Image Processing System) for acquisition and analysis of multicolor fluorescence images (Vysis).

3. Methods

3.1. Preparation of Metaphase Slides

3.1.1. Peripheral Blood Cultures, Harvesting, and Fixation of Cells

1. Set up 5–10 whole blood cultures from a young donor (*see* **Note 2**) by adding 1 mL of whole blood to 9 mL of complete medium in a 25-cm^2 flask. Add 150 µL of PHA-M to each culture and incubate at 37°C. Note that we routinely culture cells in 5% CO_2.
2. After 69 h, add 30 µL of colcemid. Incubate for another 2 to 3 h.
3. Transfer the cell culture to a 10-mL tube and centrifuge at 1500 rpm (300g on a regular table-top swing bucket centrifuge) for 10 min.
4. Remove the supernatant and suspend the pellet in 1 to 2 mL of hypotonic KCl (37°C). Slowly add another 10 mL of KCl, cap the tube, and gently invert several times. Incubate for 20–25 min in a water bath at 37°C.
5. Add 1 mL of fresh fixative and centrifuge at 1500 rpm for 10 min. Remove the supernatant and resuspend the pelleted cells in 1 to 2 mL of fixative. Add an additional 10 mL of fixative. Pipet gently to disperse all the clumps.
6. Centrifuge at 1500 rpm for 10 min, remove the supernatant, and add 10 mL of fresh fixative. Allow the cells to remain in the fixative overnight at –20°C.

3.1.2. Preparation of Lymphocyte Metaphase Spreads

Normal metaphase spreads serve as targets for the hybridization. More important, good hybridization and optimal CGH analysis depend, to a large extent, on the quality of the target metaphase preparations.

1. Centrifuge the fixed cells at 1500 rpm for 10 min and remove the supernatant.
2. Resuspend the pellet in a small volume (~0.5 mL) of fresh fixative. Note that the cell suspension should not be too dilute; a slightly milky suspension generally gives good results.
3. Swipe a precleaned, chilled glass slide with tissue paper to remove excess 70% ethanol. Using a fine-bore glass pipet, place three to four drops of the cell suspension on the slide.
4. Allow the fixative to dry by placing the slide at room temperature or on a rack over a beaker of boiling water (30–60 s), depending on the humidity (*see* **Note 3**).

Criteria for acceptable slides for CGH experiments are as follows: slides with moderate cell density and high mitotic index, adequate chromosome length (i.e., neither too contracted nor too elongated), minimal overlapping of chromosomes, and absence of visible cytoplasm around the chromosomes (too much cytoplasm prevents optimal denaturation and hinders hybridization of the genomic DNA probes to the target chromosomes) *(7)* (*see* **Note 3**). The quality of the chromosome preparations should be assessed under a phase-contrast microscope. If the conditions are acceptable, prepare a batch of slides and store them at room temperature in a desiccator. Slides can be used as needed for up to 2 mo. Metaphase preparations can be kept longer, if stored at −20°C. The remaining suspension of fixed cells can also be kept at −20°C. Centrifuge and add fresh fixative before preparing new slides.

3.2. Labeling of Test and Reference Genomic DNAs by Random Priming

Test DNA is usually labeled with biotin-14-dCTP, and reference DNA is labeled with digoxigenin-dUTP. Each reaction typically consists of 600 ng of genomic DNA in a total volume of 100 μL.

1. Dilute the DNA sample to a total volume of 20 μL with distilled water, denature by heating for 5 min in a boiling water bath, and immediately cool on ice.
2. Perform the following additions on ice:
   a. Indirect labeling: 10 μL of 10X dNTP mixture, 40 μL of 2.5X Random Primers Solution, and distilled water to a total volume of 96 μL; for reference DNA, substitute the 10X dNTP mixture with digoxigenin 10X labeling mix.
   b. Direct labeling: 10 μL of 10X dNTP mixture, 40 μL of 2.5X Random Primers Solution, 6 μL of Fluoro Green, and distilled water to a total volume of 96 μL; for reference DNA, substitute the Fluoro Green with Fluoro Red.
3. Mix briefly and add 4 μL of Klenow fragment. Mix thoroughly but gently. Centrifuge for 15–30 s.
4. Incubate overnight at room temperature for test DNA and for 1 h at 37°C for reference DNA (*see* **Note 4**).
5. Add 10 μL of Stop Buffer. Check the fragment size by running 100 ng of the probe on an agarose gel (*see* **Note 4**).
6. Store labeled probes at −20°C until needed.

3.3. Hybridization of Labeled Genomic DNA Probes to Target Slides

3.3.1. Probe Precipitation and Denaturation

Note that genomic DNA contains repeat sequences that require preannealing with excess DNA of the same species to prevent nonspecific hybridization. Human Cot-1 DNA is normally used for this purpose (*see* **Note 5**).

1. Mix 500 ng each of labeled test DNA and reference DNA with 22 μL of human Cot-1 DNA (1 mg/mL) and coprecipitate using 0.1 vol of sodium acetate and 2 to 3 vol of chilled 100% ethanol.
2. Vortex and store at −20°C overnight or at −80°C for 30 min.
3. Centrifuge at 14,000 rpm (18,400g on a table-top centrifuge for Eppendorf tubes) at 4°C for 20 min. Pour off the supernatant.
4. Wash the pellet with 500 mL of 70% ethanol. Centrifuge at 14,000 rpm at 4°C for 10 min.
5. Air-dry the pellet (~10 min).
6. Resuspend the pellet in 10 μL of Hybrisol VII, mix thoroughly, and centrifuge briefly.
7. Denature the probe at 75°C for 5 min and preanneal at 37°C for 1 h.

CGH Analysis 51

3.3.2. Pretreatment of Target Slides

1. Incubate the slides in RNase (40 μL in 40 mL of 2X SSC) for 1 h in a water bath at 37°C.
2. Rinse the slides four times in 40 mL of 2X SSC at room temperature (2 min per wash).
3. Dehydrate in ethanol series (70, 80, and 95%; 2 min each).
4. Allow the slides to air-dry.
5. Denature the slides by incubating for 5 min in 70% formamide at 73°C.
6. Immediately dehydrate in cold series of ethanol (70, 80, 95, and 100%; 2 min each).
7. Air-dry and place the slides at 37°C.

3.3.3. Hybridization

1. Mix the probe and centrifuge briefly. Apply to a denatured, prewarmed slide. Cover with a glass coverslip, being careful not to create air bubbles. Each slide can be used for two hybridizations. Etching a line across the middle of the slide can designate the two separate hybridization areas.
2. Incubate at 37°C for at least 72 h in a humidified chamber.

3.4. Posthybridization Washing and Probe Detection

3.4.1. Indirect Labeling

1. Prewarm 35 mL of 50% formamide/2X SSC in each of two 50-mL Corning centrifuge tubes in a water bath set at 43°C.
2. Carefully remove the sealant and coverslip to avoid scratching the metaphase spreads. If the coverslip cannot be removed easily, moisten the slide surface with 50% formamide/2X SSC.
3. Dip the slides in the tubes and wash twice for 10 min each. Two slides may be placed back-to-back and washed in the same tube. Further washing is carried out in Coplin jars.
4. Wash twice in 2X SSC at 37°C, 4 min in each wash.
5. Wash the slides in 1X PBD at room temperature for 5 min. At this stage, the slides may be stored in 1X PBD at 4°C for several days.
6. Remove the slides from 1X PBD; do not allow the slides to dry. Apply 60 μL of rhodamine antidigoxigenin/fluorescein-labeled avidin onto the slides. Cover with a plastic coverslip and incubate in the dark at 37°C for 20 min.
7. Remove the coverslip and wash three times in 1X PBD at room temperature, 2 min each.
8. Apply 60 μL of antiavidin antibody. Cover with a plastic coverslip and incubate in the dark at 37°C for 20 min.
9. Remove the coverslip and wash three times in 1X PBD at room temperature, 2 min each.
10. Repeat **steps 6** and **7**.
11. Apply 60 μL of DAPI (1 μL of stock/mL of phosphate-buffered saline). Cover with a plastic coverslip and incubate in the dark at room temperature for 5 min.

52   Balsara, Pei, and Testa

12. Remove the coverslip, apply mounting medium, and cover with a glass coverslip.
13. Gently blot the mounted slide with a paper towel to remove extra mounting medium. At this stage, the slide may be stored at 4°C in the dark until examined.

3.4.2. Direct Labeling

1. Wash the slides twice in 2X SSC, 5 min each, in a water bath set at 45°C.
2. Wash in 0.1X SSC twice, 5 min each, in a water bath at 45°C.
3. Wash the slides in 1X PBD at room temperature for 5 min.
4. Rinse in distilled water for 2 min.
5. Follow **steps 11–13** of **Subheading 3.4.1.**

3.5. Image Analysis

3.5.1. Fluorescence Microscopy and Acquisition of Multicolor Digital Images

Metaphases are located by visual scanning, and then a sequence of counterstained, test, and reference images is acquired under software control, by selecting appropriate excitation filters. Exposures are determined automatically and range from 0.5 to 5 s. Each multicolored image is directly filed to an electronic disk for subsequent analysis. The DAPI-counterstained image is displayed in blue, the test DNA image in green, and the reference DNA in red. Thus, in the composite image, those regions of the test genome that have a higher copy number than normal appear greener, whereas those that are at a lower copy number than normal appear to be redder than the yellowish orange hue typical of chromosomal regions exhibiting a balanced state. The DAPI-counterstained image is included to permit visual identification of each chromosome.

3.5.2. Chromosome Segmentation

Chromosomes are segmented automatically. Chromosome clusters not segmented by the software are resolved interactively using a computer mouse to draw separate lines. Chromosomes with overlaps are not analyzed. Typically, more than 75% of the chromosomes are suitable for analysis, so that 8–10 profiles for each individual chromosome type can be obtained from five to seven metaphase cells. The CGH analysis program is interactive. Chromosomes are identified based on DAPI banding after chromosome segmentation. Chromosomes are selected for profiling depending on the quality of the hybridization. Poor hybridization results in an unacceptable level of noise. Judgment can be made by a variety of display options, which include enlarged images of the counterstained, test, and reference versions.

3.5.3. Normalization of Hybridization Intensities

In CGH analysis, the absolute fluorescence intensity of any of the fluorophores is governed by illumination brightness, filter bandwidth, dye absorbance and

CGH Analysis 53

quantum efficiency, camera sensitivity and exposure time, bleaching, hybridization efficiency, DNA labeling efficiency, and metaphase quality *(8)*. Normalization is necessary to compare information among different copies of the same chromosome type in different metaphases and in different experiments. The image analysis system includes a background correction, which is essential in order to obtain ratio values that are directly proportional to copy number.

3.5.4. Ratio Computation and Profile Averaging

Digital image analysis techniques are essential for accurate CGH assessment. Calculation of ratio profiles for each chromosome coupled with statistical analysis of the profiles allows the investigator to detect and map DNA sequence copy number changes throughout the genome. Profiles from at least five metaphases are included to improve the signal-to-noise ratio.

The reference and test intensity profiles for each chromosome are obtained by integrating the pixel values along slices orthogonal to the chromosomal axis *(8)*. The average ratio profile (**Figs. 2** and **3**) is constructed by averaging the individual ratio profiles. This method provides a straightforward way to estimate a confidence interval for the mean ratio at any part of the genome, and it is therefore chosen because such confidence intervals are important for the interpretation of the mean profiles *(8)*. A copy number increase of 50% (i.e., one additional copy in a basically diploid DNA sample) should be visible if the amplified region is at least 2 Mbp in size *(8)*. The smallest deleted segment detected by CGH is on the order of 10 Mbp *(9)*.

3.6. Applications of CGH Analysis

In cancer genetics, CGH analysis permits the detection of consistent chromosomal imbalances in a given type of cancer. These recurrent gains/amplifications and losses represent entry points for the characterization and isolation of pathogenetically relevant genes such as protooncogenes and tumor suppressor genes, respectively. Other applications of CGH analysis include identification of genomic imbalances of prognostic relevance; subclassification of tumors involving a particular organ; localization of chromosomal sites associated with drug resistance (e.g., owing to amplification of a target drug resistance gene); identification of chromosomal imbalances associated with tumor progression (e.g., amplicons involving new or known putative oncogenes) (**Fig. 2B**); and identification of the location of cancer susceptibility genes, to facilitate subsequent genetic linkage analysis *(10)*.

4. Notes

1. DNA should be isolated from tumor tissue with a high percentage of malignant cells. Contaminating normal cells significantly inhibit detection of copy number

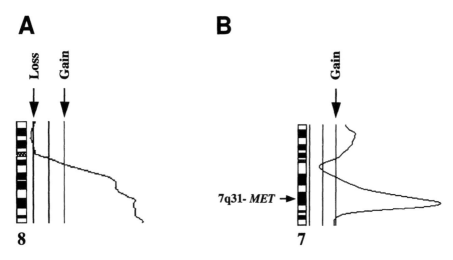

Fig. 2. Examples of average fluorescence ratio profiles of chromosomes 8 and 7 from two different lung carcinoma cell lines. (**A**) Profile depicting loss of the short arm (p) and gain of the long arm (q) of chromosome 8. This abnormality was observed in a lung cancer cell line with two copies of an isochromosome of the long arm of chromosome 8, i(8q), as well as a single copy of a normal chromosome 8. Averaged values are plotted as profiles alongside individual chromosome ideograms. The three vertical lines next to the individual chromosome ideograms indicate different threshold values between tumor DNA and normal reference DNA. The line on the left corresponds to a threshold value of 0.75, which would exist if 50% of the cells from a near diploid tumor had monosomy of a given chromosome or chromosome segment. The center line indicates a balanced state. The line on the right represents a threshold value of 1.25, which would occur if 50% of the cell population exhibited trisomy for a particular chromosome region. (**B**) Ratio profile from a lung tumor cell line showing amplification of part of 7q. The amplification peak resides at 7q31, the location of the *MET* protooncogene, which was found in subsequent molecular studies to be amplified and overexpressed in this cell line.

Fig. 3. *(opposite page)* CGH fluorescence ratio profile of a non–small cell lung carcinoma specimen displaying overrepresentation (gains) of part or all of chromosome arms 1q, 3q, 5p, 6p, 18p, 18q, Xp, Xq, and Yq and underrepresentation (losses) of part or all of 1p, 3p, 4p, 5q, 8p, 10q, 13q, 14q, 16q, and 17p. Gains of 1q, 3q, and 5p and losses of 3p, 8p, and 17p are common in non–small cell lung cancer *(12)*, suggesting the involvement of known or suspected oncogenes and tumor suppressor genes, respectively, at these locations. Note that ratio profile deviations at or near the constitutive heterochromatin are not interpreted. The profile shown represents the average fluorescence ratios calculated for each chromosome from a total of 10 metaphase spreads.

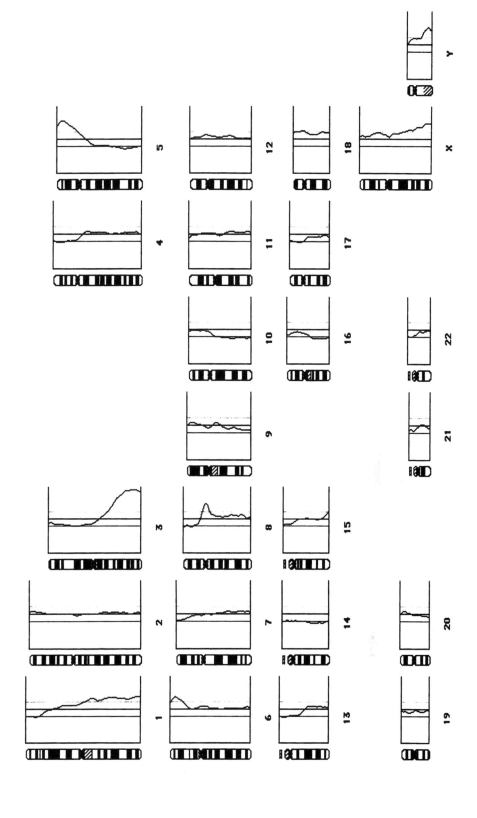

imbalances. Whenever possible, tumor specimens should be microdissected to enrich for the malignant cell population.

2. A high yield of metaphase spreads depends on stimulation of T-lymphocytes with the mitogen PHA-M. We have noticed that lymphocytes from younger age (20–25 yr) donors have a better response to PHA-M stimulation than those from older individuals.

3. Room temperature and relative humidity during metaphase slide preparation are critical considerations in order to obtain cytoplasm-free metaphase preparations. To remove debris, we add a postfixation step in which new slide preparations (before the fixative has evaporated) are gently squirted with 2 to 3 mL of fresh methanol:acetic acid (3:1). Also, note that when conditions are very dry, the quality of the chromosome preparations can be improved considerably by allowing the slides to dry for 30–45 s on a rack placed above a container of boiling water. If the chromosomes tend to overlap, steam may improve the spreading. On the other hand, by allowing preparations to dry at room temperature, overspreading can be minimized.

4. The optimum fragment size of the labeled DNA is 500–1000 bp. DNA samples with an abundance of larger-sized fragments can be treated with DNase to achieve this size range.

5. Ratio changes at the centromeric regions are not interpreted, especially those involving the constitutive heterochromatin of chromosomes 1, 9, 16, and Y, because blockage of repetitive DNA sequences in these regions by the unlabeled Cot-1 DNA is variable *(11)*.

Acknowledgments

This work was supported in part by National Cancer Institute (NCI) Grant U19CA40737 and by NCI Lung Cancer SPORE Grant P50 CA58184.

References

1. Roulston, D. and Le Beau, M. M. (1997) Cytogenetic analysis of hematologic malignant diseases, in *The AGT Cytogenetics Laboratory Manual* (Barch, M. J., Knutsen, T., and Spurbeck, J., eds.), Lippincott-Raven, Philadelphia, PA, pp. 325–372.

2. Rowley, J. D. (1998) The critical role of chromosome translocations in human leukemias. *Annu. Rev. Genet.* **32,** 495–519.

3. Mitelman, F., Martens, F., and Johansson, B. (1997) A breakpoint map of recurrent chromosomal rearrangements in human neoplasia. *Nat. Genet.* **15,** 417–474.

4. Bridge, J. A. and Sandberg, A. A. (2000) Cytogenetic and molecular genetic techniques as adjunctive approaches in the diagnosis of bone and soft tissue tumors. *Skel. Radiol.* **29,** 249–258.

5. Kallioniemi, A., Kallioniemi, O. P., Sudar, D., Rutovitz, D., Gray, J. W., Waldman, F., et al. (1992) Comparative genomic hybridization for molecular cytogenetic analysis of solid tumors. *Science* **258,** 818–-821.

6. Rooney, P. H., Murray, G. I., Stevenson, D. A., Haites, N. E., Cassidy, J., and McLeod, H. L. (1999) Comparative genomic hybridization and chromosomal instability in solid tumours. *Brit. J. Cancer* **80,** 862–873.

CGH Analysis

7. Karhu, R., Kahkonen, M., Kuukasjarvi, T., Pennanen, S., Tirkkonen, M., and Kallioniemi, O. (1997) Quality control of CGH: impact of metaphase chromosomes and the dynamic range of hybridization. *Cytometry* **28,** 198–205.
8. Piper, J., Rutovitz, D., Sudar, D., Kallioniemi, A., Kallioniemi, O. P., Waldman, F. M., et al. (1995) Computer image analysis of comparative genomic hybridization. *Cytometry* **19,** 10–26.
9. du Manoir, S., Schrock, E., Bentz, M., Speicher, M. R., Joos, S., Ried, T., et al. (1995) Quantitative analysis of comparative genomic hybridization. *Cytometry* **19,** 27–41.
10. Hemminki, A., Tomlinson, I., Markie, D., Jarvinen, H., Sistonen, P., Bjorkqvist, A. M., et al. (1997) Localization of a susceptibility locus for Peutz-Jeghers syndrome to 19p using comparative genomic hybridization and targeted linkage analysis. *Nat. Genet.* **15,** 87–90.
11. Kallioniemi, O. P., Kallioniemi, A., Piper, J., Isola, J., Waldman, F. M., Gray, J. W., and Pinkel, D. (1994) Optimizing comparative genomic hybridization for analysis of DNA sequence copy number changes in solid tumors. *Genes Chromosomes Cancer* **10,** 231–243.
12. Balsara, B. R., Sonoda, G., du Manoir, S., Siegfried, J. M., Gabrielson, E., and Testa, J. R. (1997) Comparative genomic hybridization analysis detects frequent, often high-level, overrepresentation of DNA sequences at 3q, 5p, 7p, and 8q in human non-small cell lung carcinomas. *Cancer Res.* **57,** 2116–2120.

5

Detection of Chromosomal Deletions by Microsatellite Analysis

Rachel E. Ibbotson and Martin M. Corcoran

1. Introduction

Microsatellites are tandem repeats of simple sequence, 2–6 bp, that occur abundantly and at random throughout most eukaryotic genomes. They are typically short, often <100 bp long, and are embedded within a unique sequence. Thus, they are ideal for in vitro amplification by the polymerase chain reaction (PCR). The high degree of polymorphism, owing to variation in the number of repeat units, and the stability displayed by microsatellites make them perfect markers for use in constructing high-resolution genetic maps to identify susceptibility loci involved in common genetic diseases (1). In addition to their applications in genome mapping and positional cloning, these markers have been applied in fields as diverse as tumor biology, forensic identification, population genetic analysis, and the construction of human evolutionary trees. This chapter is confined to the analysis of chromosomal deletions.

The significance of chromosomal abnormalities such as deletions, translocations, and inversions is well documented, and these somatically acquired genetic changes often are manifest phenotypically as neoplasia. Translocations and inversions are either idiopathic (i.e., they are only found in the tumor from one patient) or are specific, consistently found in all tumors of the same type. By analyzing the exact point of chromosomal breakage, numerous oncogenic genes have been identified (e.g., the *c-myc* oncogene located on chromosome 8 at band q24) (2). However, investigating consistent regions of deletion has generally led to the identification of tumor suppressor genes; of note are the retinoblastoma gene (*RB-1*) on chromosome 13 (3) and the *p16ARF* locus on chromosome 9 (4).

When no candidate gene is available, genetic alterations can be localized to one particular region of a chromosome by the analysis of specific polymorphic

From: *Methods in Molecular Medicine, vol. 68: Molecular Analysis of Cancer*
Edited by: J. Boultwood and C. Fidler © Humana Press Inc., Totowa, NJ

markers for loss or amplification; that is, the region is tested for loss of heterozygosity (LOH). Southern blotting followed by hybridization with a labeled restriction fragment length polymorphism probe is a standard method for determining LOH; however, by employing microsatellites many benefits are gained. The high degree of heterozygosity displayed by many microsatellite markers is especially advantageous because the majority of samples will be heterozygous (otherwise said to be informative) at the locus of interest. In addition, very small amounts of tissue are required for microsatellite analysis (typically 100 ng compared to 10 µg for a Southern blot), and many samples can be processed simultaneously with relative ease. For LOH studies, it is imperative that there be access to matched normal and tumor tissue so that direct comparison between the two can be made. In our own studies of lymphoproliferative malignancies, we have analyzed peripheral blood B-lymphocytes as the tumor population, using granulocytes or T-lymphocytes as matched controls. Sample pairs are scored as follows: heterozygous, not deleted (two different alleles present in both normal and tumor tissue); heterozygous, deleted (two alleles present in normal tissue but only one present in tumor tissue); homozygous, not informative (two alleles of the same size present in both normal and tumor tissue).

2. Materials

2.1. Isolation of (CA)n Polymorphisms Within Series of Cosmids

1. Cosmid DNA, extracted and purified by standard methods.
2. (CA)n probe (Pharmacia).
3. Hybond N+ nucleic acid transfer membrane (Amersham).
4. 20X Saline sodium citrate (SSC): 3 M NaCl, 0.3 M sodium citrate. Dilute accordingly.
5. 50X Denhardt's: 5 g of ficoll, 5 g of bovine serum albumin, 5 g of polyvinylpyrrolidone. Add distilled water to 500 mL.
6. Hybridization solution: 5X SSC, 1% sodium dodecyl sulfate (SDS), 5X Denhardt's, 5% dextran sulfate.
7. [^{32}P]dCTP (10 µCi/µL).
8. Random primed DNA labeling kit (Boehringer Mannheim).
9. Stringent wash solution: 0.5X SSC, 0.1% SDS.
10. Autoradiography film (Kodak Biomax MS, Anachem).
11. Restriction enzymes and appropriate buffers (Boehringer Mannheim).
12. β-Agarase (New England Biolabs).
13. pBluescript (Stratagene).
14. T7-sequencing kit (Pharmacia).

2.2. Microsatellie Amplification, Resolution, and Detection

1. Purified genomic DNA from tumor and normal tissue.
2. dNTP mix (Pharmacia).

Microsatellite Analysis

3. 10X PCR buffer (Applied Biotechnologies).
4. *Taq* DNA Thermopolymerase (Applied Biotechnologies).
5. Microsatellite primers (Oswel).
6. [^{32}P]dCTP (10 µCi/µ:) (ICN).
7. Mineral oil (Sigma).
8. Microcentrifuge tubes (0.5 mL) (Perkin-Elmer, Foster City, CA).
9. PCR machine (Perkin-Elmer).
10. 10X TBE: 0.9 *M* Tris-borate, 20 m*M* EDTA.
11. Sequencing apparatus (Bio-Rad, Hercules, CA).
12. Sequencing gel dryer (Bio-Rad).
13. Hydrotech Vacuum pump (Bio-Rad).

3. Methods
3.1. Microsatellite Selection

Once the genomic region of interest has been identified, appropriate microsatellites for investigation must be selected, either from previously identified microsatellites listed in the databases or from novel microsatellites. Both methods are described.

3.1.1. Isolation of (CA)n Polymorphisms Within Series of Cosmids

1. Dot-blot the purified cosmid DNA onto hybridization membrane. Fix the DNA by exposing to ultraviolet light on a transilluminator and prehybridized at 65°C in hybridization buffer.
2. Label the (CA)n probe, according to the kit protocol, with [^{32}P]dCTP and hybridize overnight at 65°C (*see* **Note 1**).
3. After stringent washing, autoradiograph the blot overnight at –70°C. The autoradiograph will identify which cosmids contain CA repetitive sequences by the strong hybridization of the probe to the cosmid DNA reflected in a dark spot on the film corresponding to the exact position of that same cosmid.
4. Digest DNA from positive cosmids with restriction enzymes (*see* **Note 2**) and resolve the fragments on an agarose gel.
5. Southern blot and probe the gel, as before, with the (CA)n probe to identify which small fragments contain CA repetitive sequences.
6. Run a repeat gel, using low melting point agarose, to resolve the positive fragment. Then excise the fragment from the gel and subject to digestion with β-agarase to release the DNA.
7. Subclone the fragment into pBluescript that has been previously digested with the same enzyme to produce compatible ends for ligation (*see* **Note 3**).
8. Once cloned, sequence the fragment (*see* **Note 4**). Primers are designed from the novel DNA sequence flanking the repetitive sequence, and these can then be used for PCR (*see* **Note 5**).
9. Analyze DNA from 10 individuals for the new microsatellite marker to assess the variation of the allele size and informativity of the new marker.

3.1.2. Clone Sequencing

Sequencing of midscale genomic clones (cosmids, P1 artificial chromosomes, and bacterial artificial chromosomes) within the region of interest will often reveal stretches of simple repetitive DNA. These dinucleotide, trinucleotide, or tetranucleotide repeats, when found, can often be utilized through the design of flanking PCR primers as microsatellite markers *(5)*.

3.1.3. Databases

It is possible to use computer sequence homology searches on raw sequence data compiled through large- or small-scale sequencing efforts in order to search for the presence of known or novel microsatellites. Programs such as the BLAST program can search these sequences against the many sequences present within the Genome Data Base (GDB) in order to find such results. Chromosome-specific websites with listings of known microsatellite loci are also available. These sites generally have links to the GDB accession page for microsatellite markers that may list the location, the type of repeat, the number of alleles, the frequency of heterozygosity, as well as to the primer sequences.

3.2. Microsatellite Analysis

Microsatellite polymorphism is quantified by PCR and polyacrylamide gel electrophoresis, enabling small amounts of poor-quality DNA to be typed to single nucleotide resolution.

3.2.1. Microsatellite Amplification, Resolution, and Detection

1. Extract genomic DNA by standard methods from constitutional and tumor samples.
2. Perform PCR amplification using 100 ng of template DNA; 50 μM each of dCTP, dATP, dTTP, and dGTP; and 2 μCi of [^{32}P]dCTP, using 1 U of *Taq* polymerase in a total volume of 25 μL overlayed with 30 μL of mineral oil *(see* **Note 6**). PCR conditions are generally 25 cycles of denaturation at 94°C for 30 s; annealing at 58°C (the exact annealing temperature depends on the sequence of the primer and should be determined for each primer pair used) for 30 s; and extension at 72°C for 30 s, with a final extension of 10 min at 72°C *(see* **Note 7**).
3. Mix the PCR products 1:1 with formamide loading buffer (denaturing buffer for sequencing gels), and denature at 96°C for 10 min and kept on ice before loading on a 6% polyacrylamide gel run in 1X TBE buffer.
4. Run the gels for between 2 and 5 h at 2000 V depending on the size of the PCR product *(see* **Note 8**).
5. After electrophoresis, dry the gels directly *(see* **Note 9**).
6. Expose the dried gels to autoradiograph film overnight at –70°C.
7. Determine LOH by visual or densitometric inspection of the autoradiograph by comparing the bands resulting from the PCR of the tumor and normal DNA *(see*

Microsatellite Analysis

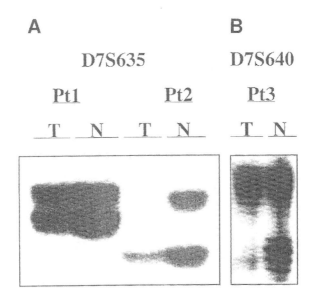

Fig. 1. Examples of microsatellite analysis. DNA extracted from purified tumor and control cells from patients with splenic lymphoma with villous lymphocytes were analyzed for LOH at microsatellite loci on chromosome 7. **(A)** Patient 1 (Pt1) is informative for the microsatellite D7S635 and does not show deletion because both alleles are present in the tumor sample (T) and the control sample (N). Patient 2 (Pt2) is also informative for this microsatellite but shows evidence of heterozygous loss because the upper allele is deleted in the tumor sample in comparison with the control sample. **(B)** Patient 3 (Pt3) is informative for the microsatellite D7S640 and shows heterozygous loss, but in this case the lower allele is deleted.

Note 10). LOH is scored positive if the intensity of one of the polymorphic bands is reduced by >75% (*see* **Fig. 1**). Homozygous loss may not always be determined accurately by this method because the DNA from residual normal cells in the tumor DNA fraction may interfere with the interpretation of the results. It is paramount that the two matched DNA samples be as pure as possible to diminish the chance of incorrect results.

3.3. Recent Advances

Traditionally LOH studies have used radioactive detection methods. However, recent advances made in fluorescent chemistry have seen the widespread introduction of fluorescent microsatellite assays. In addition, the technologic development of automated systems has facilitated the introduction of machines such as those marketed by Perkin-Elmer Applied Biosystems that, when coupled with fluorescent dye-labeled primers, can automatically detect and record electrophoresis data from up to 96 lanes per gel. For linkage analysis

64 Ibbotson and Corcoran

and other high-throughput applications, up to 20 microsatellites can be multiplexed and run in the same lane, and since up to three gels can be processed in 1 d, this could yield 5760 genotypes.

4. Notes

1. Simple repeat probes other than the (CA)n probe are available.
2. A number of different restriction enzymes should be used in order to find a fragment of a suitable size for subcloning and sequencing, ideally <500 bp. Restriction enzymes that have 4-bp recognition sites may be of use. Often an *Sau*3AI digest of a cosmid or PAC clone followed by ligation into *Bam*HI prepared plasmid is ideal for the production of a library of suitably sized fragments for microsatellite identification and sequencing.
3. Stratagene supplies a detailed protocol sheet including ligation conditions, transformations, plating out, and selection of positive clones.
4. Pharmacia supplies a detailed protocol sheet including DNA preparation, sequencing reactions, running the gels, and autoradiography.
5. General rules for primer design are that primers should be approx 50% GC rich, not self-complementary and not complementary, to each other. Primer length should be between 17 and 24 bp, and the size of the target produced for microsatellites should not be >300 bp.
6. An alternative method is to end label one of the PCR primers with $[\gamma\ ^{32}P]ATP$ and T_4-polynucleotide kinase.
7. The annealing temperature should be optimized for each individual microsatellite to be investigated by preliminary nonradioactive PCR and resolution on agarose gels.
8. Typically, a PCR product of 250 bp should be run at 2000 V and 45 W for up to 4 h.
9. There is no need to fix the gel in methanol and acetic acid. This is only required if ^{35}S labeled radionucleotides are used.
10. It is recommended that all experiments be duplicated from the PCR stage through to the final resolution on the gel to verify the LOH results.

Acknowledgments

This work was supported by the Leukaemia Research Fund. We thank Mary Tiller for excellent technical assistance.

References

1. Koreth, J., O'Leary, J. J., and McGee J. (1996) Microsatellites and PCR genomic analysis. *J. Pathol.* **178,** 239–248.
2. Dalla-Favera, R., Bregni, M., Erikson, J., Patterson, D., Gallo, R. C., and Croce, C. M. (1982) Human c-myc oncogene is located in the region of chromosome 8 that is translocated in Burkitt lymphoma cells. *Proc. Natl. Acad. Sci.* USA **79,** 7824–7827.
3. Lee, W.-H., Bookstein, R., Hong, F., Young, L.-J., Shew, J.-Y., and Lee, E. Y. (1987) Human retinoblastoma susceptibility gene: cloning, identification and sequencing. *Science* **235,** 1394–1399.

Microsatellite Analysis

4. Quelle, D. E., Zindy, F., Ashmun, R. A., and Sherr, C. J. (1995) Alternative reading frames of the INK4a tumour suppressor gene encode two unrelated proteins capable of inducing cell cycle arrest. *Cell* **83,** 993–1000.
5. Corcoran, M. M., Rasool, O., Liu, Y., Iyengar, A., Grander, D., Ibbotson, R. E., et al. (1998) Detailed molecular delineation of 13q14.3 loss in B-cell chronic lymphocytic leukaemia. *Blood* **91,** 1382–1390.

6

Detection and Quantification of Leukemia-Specific Rearrangements

Andreas Hochhaus

1. Introduction

A number of leukemia-specific chromosomal translocations have been identified that have been cloned and are appropriate markers for molecular studies (**Table 1**) *(1–4)*. In addition, leukemia nonspecific clonality markers, such as the junctional region of the rearranged immunoglobulin (Ig) and T-cell receptor (TCR) genes can be used for minimal residual disease studies. It is commonly accepted that the Ig heavy chain (IgH) gene junctional regions as well as the junctional regions of rearranged TCR-γ and TCR-δ can be used as targets for polymerase chain reaction (PCR) analysis *(1,2)*. The detection and quantification of leukemia specific rearrangements will be explained on the example chronic myelogenous leukemia (CML), since this disease was the first human tumor associated with a specific chromosomal rearrangement and a specific fusion gene. The spectrum of molecular methods to detect fusion genes and their products has been established on CML during the last 15 years.

1.1. Chronic Myelogenous Leukemia

In many ways, CML serves as a paradigm for the utility of molecular methods to diagnose malignancy or to monitor patient response to therapy *(5)*. CML is a clonal myeloproliferative disorder of the primitive hematopoietic stem cell an annual incidence of approx 1–2 per 100,000. The disease was described by Virchow *(6)* in 1845, introducing the term *Weißes Blut* (Leukämie). CML constitutes a clinical model for molecular detection and therapy surveillance since this entity was the first leukemia known to be associated with a specific chromosomal rearrangement, the Philadelphia (Ph) translocation t(9;22)(q34;q11) *(7,8)* (**Fig. 1**), and the presence of two chimeric genes, *BCR-ABL (9,10)* on

From: *Methods in Molecular Medicine, vol. 68: Molecular Analysis of Cancer*
Edited by: J. Boultwood and C. Fidler © Humana Press Inc., Totowa, NJ

Hochhaus

Table 1
Chromosomal Translocations Observed in Leukemias (Selection) (1–4)

Translocation	Genes	Disease[a]
t(1;19)(q23;p13)	*PBX1, E2A*	B-ALL
t(8;14)(q24;q32)	*MYC*, IgH	B-ALL
t(2;8)(p12;q24)	Igκ, *MYC*	B-ALL
t(8;22)(q24;q11)	*MYK*, Igλ	B-ALL
t(4;11)(q21;q23)	*AF4, MLL*	B-ALL
t(12;21)(p13;q22)	*TEL, AML1*	B-ALL
t(7;19)(q35;p13)	*LYL1, TCR-β*	T-ALL
t(1;14)(p32;q11)	*TAL1, TCR-δ*	T-ALL
t(7;9)(q34;q32)	*TCR-β, TAL2*	T-ALL
t(11;14)(p13;q11)	*RHOM-2, TCR-δ*	T-ALL
t(10;14)(q24;q11)	*HOX11, TCR-δ*	T-ALL
t(15;17)(q22;q21)	*PML, RARα*	AML M3
t(6;9)(p23;q34)	*CAN, DEK*	AML M2, M4
t(8;21)(q22;q22)	*ETO, AML1*	AML M2
inv(16)(p13;q22)	*CBFβ, MYH11*	AML M4Eo
t(9;22)(q34;q11)	*c-ABL, BCR*	CML, ALL
t(8;13)(p11;q12)	*ZNF198; FGFR1*	8p11 MPD
t(9;12)(q34;p13)	*ABL, TEL*	Ph-negative CML, MDS
t(5;12)(q33;p13)	*PDGFR-β, TEL*	CMML

[a]B-ALL, B-lineage acute lymphoblastic leukemia; T-ALL, T-lineage acute lymphoblastic leukemia; AML, acute myelogenous leukemia; CML, chronic myelogenous leukemia; MDS, myelodysplastic syndrome; CMML, chromic myelomonocytic leukemia.

chromosome 22, and *ABL-BCR* on chromosome 9. *BCR-ABL* is transcribed to a specific BCR-ABL mRNA and encodes in most patients a 210-kDa chimeric protein with increased tyrosine kinase activity. The central role of BCR-ABL in several pathways that lead to uncontrolled proliferation has been shown in vitro and in vivo by transfection and transplantation experiments in mice *(11,12)*. *ABL-BCR* is expressed in about 60% of patients with CML but lacks any biologic function *(13)*.

1.2. Detection and Quantification of BCR-ABL-Positive Cells

1.2.1. Cytogenetic Analysis of Bone Marrow Metaphases

The degree of tumor load reduction is an important prognostic factor for patients with CML on therapy. Conventional cytogenetics is considered the "gold standard" for evaluating this response. This method, however, is limited by the requirement of mitotic cells *(14)*. Insufficient metaphases are obtained

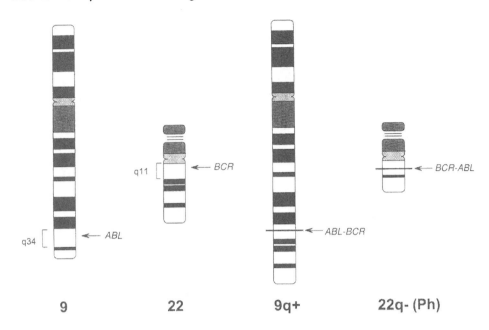

Fig. 1. Philadelphia (Ph) translocation. Reciprocal translocation of genomic material from the long arms of chromosomes 9 and 22. The resulting fusion genes are *ABL-BCR* on chromosome 9q+ and *BCR-ABL* on chromosome 22q–.

in many cases on interferon-α (IFN-α) therapy. Furthermore, cytogenetic analysis is not applicable to patients with Ph-negative, BCR-ABL-positive disease.

Commonly, response is determined according to the Houston classification *(15)*:

1. Complete response (0% Ph-positive metaphases).
2. Partial response (1–34% Ph-positive metaphases).
3. Minor response (35–94% Ph-positive metaphases).
4. Nonresponse ($\geq$95% Ph-positive metaphases).

The Ph chromosome is present in about 90% of patients with a clinical picture consistent with CML. Three to five percent of patients show a normal chromosome 22 with molecular evidence of the *BCR-ABL* translocation. At presentation, cytogenetic analysis usually reveals the Ph chromosome in 100% of cells analyzed with standard 20- to 30-cell analysis.

Major drawbacks of cytogenetics are the requirement of bone marrow cells in mitosis, and the analysis of relatively small numbers of metaphases, resulting in significant sampling errors *(16)*. The advantage of cytogenetics is the early detection of a cytogenetic evolution as a sign for acceleration of the disease *(17,18)*.

The frequency of cytogenetic analysis can be reduced considerably if patients are monitored by other methods, such as quantitative Southern blot, fluorescence *in situ* hybridization (FISH), quantitative Western blot, or quantitative reverse transcription (RT)-PCR. Molecular methods can be performed on peripheral blood specimens and are therefore less invasive than conventional cytogenetic analysis of bone marrow metaphases. Furthermore, these techniques are applicable to Ph-negative, BCR-ABL-positive cases. Results obtained by Southern blotting, Western blotting, and FISH are readily quantifiable, but the sensitivity is not generally superior to that of cytogenetics.

1.2.2. Fluorescence In Situ Hybridization

FISH analysis is typically performed by cohybridization of a BCR and an ABL probe to denatured metaphase chromosomes or interphase nuclei. Probes are large genomic clones, such as cosmids or yeast artificial chromosomes, and are labeled with different fluorochromes.

Dual-color FISH using probes for *BCR* and *ABL* genes allows the specific detection of *BCR-ABL* gene fusion in interphase or metaphase nuclei. Most cells exhibit four distinct signals, two of each color corresponding to the two normal *BCR* and *ABL* alleles. CML cells are recognized by the juxta- or superposition of one of the *BCR* and *ABL* signals *(19)*. FISH analysis does not depend on the presence of the Ph chromosome and will detect rare *BCR* and *ABL* variant fusions *(19–22)*. The lineage of positive and negative cells can be determined in combination with conventional May-Grünwald staining or immunocytochemistry *(23,24)*.

A limitation of the interphase FISH method is the background of a variant proportion of false positive cells, depending on the probe/detection system used *(25,26)*. In practice, the limit of detection of CML cells is typically 1–5% and depends, in part, on which probes are used, the size of the nucleus, the precise position of the breakpoint within the *ABL* gene, and the criteria used to define colocalization *(27)*. The advantage of FISH over conventional cytogenetics is the analysis of a larger number of nuclei, resulting in smaller sampling errors *(28)*. Therefore, FISH is applicable for quantification of residual disease in partial, minor, and nonresponders to IFN-α *(29–31)* as well as for determination of the BCR-ABL positivity of individual cell colonies *(32)* or the proportion of BCR-ABL-positive cells in small samples, such as highly enriched cell fractions *(33)*.

The sensitivity of interphase FISH can be considerably increased by introducing a third probe that permits identification of both the Ph chromosome and the derivative 9 chromosome in Ph-positive cells, thus lowering the rate of false-positive cells *(34)*, or by choosing breakpoint spanning probes that result in two fusion signals *(35,36)*.

Leukemia-Specific Rearrangements

The development of a high-resolution quantitative procedure termed *hypermetaphase FISH* (HMF) should make it possible to distinguish different levels of Ph chromosome positivity at presentation. In HMF, FISH is coupled with procedures for increasing the number of bone marrow cells that can be analyzed *(37–39)*. When readings can be obtained on 500 cells, one can reliably estimate parameters that characterize minimal residual disease (MRD). However, HMF evaluates only cycling cells and cannot count Ph-positive cells that do not enter division.

1.2.3. Southern Blot Analysis

Southern blotting exploits the fact that the breakpoint within the *BCR* gene generally falls in a very limited area, the 5.8-kb major breakpoint cluster region (M-bcr) *(9)* (**Fig. 2**). Genomic DNA extracted from leukocytes from a patient is digested by a set of appropriate restriction enzymes (*Bgl*II, *Xba*I, *Hin*dIII, *Eco*RI, *Bam*HI) (*see* **Table 2**), fractionated on an agarose gel, transferred to a nylon membrane, and hybridized to two labeled DNA probes derived from the 3' and 5' portion of M-bcr (**Fig. 3**). After autoradiography, a band corresponding to the unrearranged BCR allele is visible; for patients with CML, one or two additional bands may also be present. Using this technique, a *BCR* rearrangement is detectable in about 98% of Ph-positive patients and in a significant proportion of Ph-negative cases *(40)*. For routine use, *Bgl*II and *Xba*I are sufficient and are informative in almost all cases.

Because there are rare restriction site polymorphisms in the M-bcr, the finding of a rearrangement with at least two restriction enzymes is generally considered necessary to exclude a false positive result in any new patient *(41,42)*. False negative results may arise because the rearranged band is too large, too small, or coincidentally exactly the same size as the normal allele, as a result of partial deletion of *BCR* sequences on the translocated allele *(43)* or of rare variants that have breakpoints outside the M-bcr *(21,44,45)*. False positive or false negative results are, however, rare *(40)*.

Once a rearrangement is identified, it is almost always stable throughout the course of the disease. Therefore, Southern blot analysis allows quantification of the proportion of cells with *BCR* rearrangement compared to all cells investigated. The proportion of CML cells is determined by twice the intensity of the rearranged band divided by the sum of the intensities of the rearranged plus germline bands (BCR ratio); each CML cell contributes signals from one normal and one rearranged chromosome 22, whereas the normal cells contribute identical signals from two normal chromosomes *(40,46)* (**Fig. 4**). Subsequent samples from the patient after treatment are analyzed with the same restriction enzyme–probe combination to determine whether there has been a change in the proportion of malignant cells. The level of disease detected in contempora-

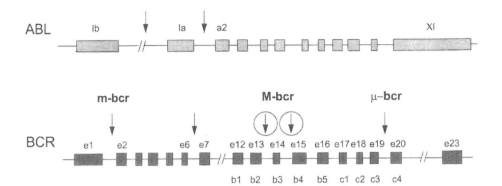

Fig. 2. Map of the exon-intron structure of *ABL* and *BCR*. Arrows indicate genomic break point cluster regions in the first intron of *ABL* and in introns 1, 13, 14, and 19 of *BCR*. The breakpoint cluster region in *BCR* intron 1 is designated minor-bcr (m-bcr), in introns 13 and 14, Major-bcr (M-bcr); and in intron 19, micro-bcr (μ-bcr). Rarely, breakpoints in *BCR* intron 6 have been described.

**Table 2
Fragment Size of *BCR* Germline Allele According
to Restriction Enzymes and Probes Used**

Restriction enzyme	2 kb-*Bgl*II/*Hin*dIII-5'-M-bcr-probe	1.2-kb-*Hin*dIII/*Bgl*II-3'-M-bcr-probe
*Bgl*II	5.0 kbp	
*Eco*RI	18.1 kbp	
*Xba*I	8.9 kbp	
*Bam*HI	12.2 kbp	3.4 kbp
*Hin*dIII	10.1 kbp	4.5 kbp

neous peripheral blood and bone marrow samples is essentially identical *(46,47)*, and, therefore, peripheral blood is normally used for analysis. Quantitative Southern blot allows the detection and quantification of down to 1% leukemic cells *(40,47)*. To evaluate the response to treatment, knowledge of the initial restriction pattern and intensity of the rearranged band is mandatory. Complete cytogenetic responses are associated with the disappearance of rearranged *BCR* bands in most cases *(40,48,49)*.

The BCR ratio is usually lower than the proportion of Ph-positive metaphases. The reason for this is that in Southern blotting analyses there are a large number of dividing and resting cells, including BCR-ABL-negative lymphocytes, and cytogenetics analysis provides information on a small number of dividing myeloid cells *(40,46)*. The main advantage of Southern blotting over

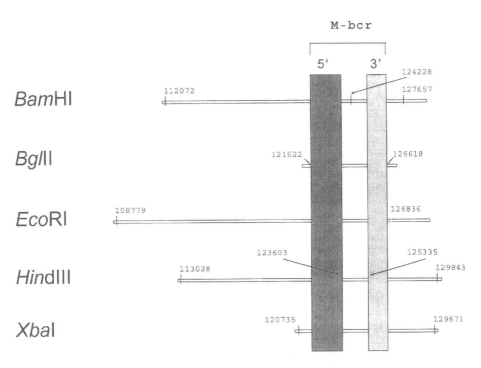

Fig. 3. Restriction enzymes, restriction fragments of the *BCR* germline allele, and 5' and 3' M-bcr probes designed to hybridize these fragments for Southern blot analysis.

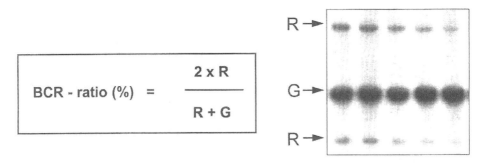

Fig. 4. Southern blot analysis after *Bgl*II digest of genomic DNA labeled with 5' and 3' M-bcr probes and autoradiographed. Arrows indicate the germline band (G) and rearranged bands (R).

cytogenetics is the independence from dividing cells, which permits the use of peripheral blood instead of bone marrow.

The comparison of 235 blood and bone marrow samples analyzed by Southern blot and conventional cytogenetics showed a rank correlation between both methods of $r = 0.82$ ($p < 0.001$). The BCR ratio was significantly different among cytogenetically defined minor, partial, and complete response groups ($p < 0.001$). Empirically derived cutoff points in the BCR ratio were introduced in order to define molecular response groups: A BCR ratio of 0% was defined as a complete response; and ratios of 1–24, 25–50, and >50% were defined as partial, minor, and no molecular response, respectively. Using these cutoff points, a major cytogenetic response could be predicted or excluded in >90% of cases *(40)*.

1.2.4. Western Blot Analysis

Western blotting can be used to detect BCR-ABL proteins directly in cell extracts qualitatively and quantitatively in both bone marrow and in peripheral blood. Leukocytes are lysed in the presence of potent protease inhibitors, fractionated on a polyacrylamide gel, transferred to a nylon membrane, and probed with an anti-ABL antibody. After washing, bound antibody is detected using a labeled secondary antibody. Blots are autoradiographed and a band corresponding to the normal p145 ABL is visualized; BCR-ABL, if present, is larger and therefore migrates more slowly. The limit of sensitivity is about 0.5–1%. The Western blot assay can distinguish the three major types of BCR-ABL proteins, p190, p210, and p230, and is able to detect rare types of BCR-ABL proteins, such as p200 *(21)*. Using a quantitative Western blot assay, a linear correlation between BCR-ABL/ABL protein ratios and contemporaneous conventional cytogenetics has been described in 392 sample pairs ($r = 0.97; p < 0.001$) *(50,51)*.

1.2.5. Reverse Transcriptase PCR

In 1989, first encouraging results concerning the detection of MRD by PCR in CML patients after allogeneic bone marrow transplantation were reported *(52)*. However, conflicting data from a comparative multicenter study revealed serious problems of the method with a high rate of false positive results and provoked an open discussion *(53,54)*. Over the past 10 yr, PCR has been optimized and developed. Specificity has been increased considerably by the partial standardization of methodology and the introduction of rigorous precautions to avoid contamination *(55)*. Sensitivity has been improved by using nested primer pairs and performing two consecutive PCR steps. In view of the limited value of qualitative PCR for monitoring CML patients after therapy, quantitative BCR-ABL PCR assays were developed to monitor patients after bone marrow transplantation *(56,57)* or treatment with IFN-α, and STI571 *(58,59)* and are now in routine clinical use.

1.2.5.1. Screening for BCR-ABL mRNA Transcripts at Diagnosis

For diagnostic samples, the use of multiplex PCR has been suggested to detect simultaneously several kinds of BCR-ABL and BCR transcripts as

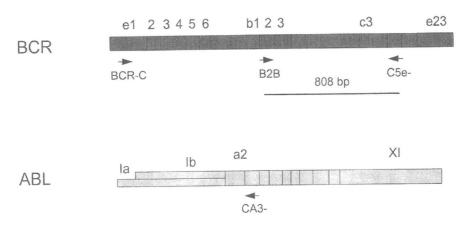

Fig. 5. Primer mapping for multiplex RT-PCR for BCR-ABL and BCR transcripts as internal control. These primer combinations allow the simultaneous amplification of all known types of BCR-ABL and BCR transcripts in one reaction *(60)*.

internal controls in one reaction *(60)* by using three BCR and one ABL primers (**Fig. 5**). This method allows the reliable detection of typical BCR-ABL transcripts, such as b2a2 or b3a2, and atypical types, such as, transcripts lacking *ABL* exon a2 (b2a3 and b3a3), or transcripts resulting from *BCR* breakpoints outside M-bcr, such as e1a2 or e6a2 *(21,22,61)* (**Figs. 6–8**).

1.2.5.2. DETECTION OF MRD: NESTED RT-PCR

The term "minimal residual disease" (MRD) refers to the presence of detectable malignant cells in patients who are in conventional remission. The aim of MRD analysis is to distinguish patients who have differing levels of residual leukemic cells and who may therefore benefit from either reduced or intensified treatment regimens.

Since patients with leukemia at presentation or relapse usually have a total burden of $>10^{12}$ malignant cells *(62)*, and since cytogenetics, Western blot, and conventional FISH have a maximum sensitivity of 1%, a patient with negative results may harbor as much or few as zero or as many as 10^{10} residual leukemic cells. At this point, the patient is judged to be in clinical and hematologic remission, although the term remission refers only to an arbitrary point toward one end of leukemic cell numbers *(63)*.

RT-PCR for BCR-ABL mRNA is by far the most sensitive assay in this context and can detect a single leukemia cell in a background of 10^5–10^6 normal cells. Therefore, PCR is up to four orders of magnitude more sensitive than conventional methods. However, patients who have no MRD detectable by this technique may still harbor up to 1,000,000 malignant cells that could

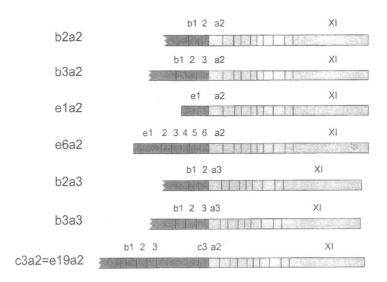

Fig. 6. Types of *BCR-ABL* fusion transcripts. Ninety-eight percent of patients show the typical b2a2 or b3a2 *BCR-ABL* fusion transcripts. Two percent of cases show rare transcripts resulting from genomic breakpoints outside M-bcr (e1a2, e6a2, e19a2) or *BCR-ABL* transcripts lacking *ABL* exon a2 (b2a3 or b3a3).

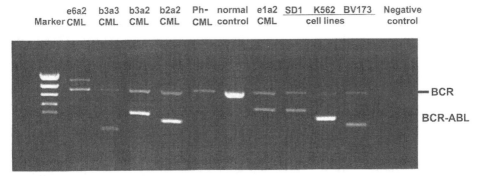

Fig. 7. Multiplex RT-PCR for *BCR-ABL* transcripts and *BCR* transcripts as internal control.

contribute to subsequent relapse. The sensitivity with which MRD can be detected will be limited by the amount of peripheral blood or bone marrow that can be analyzed.

By using nested RT-PCR with two pairs of ("nested") primers corresponding to appropriate *BCR* and *ABL* exons in two rounds of amplification, residual

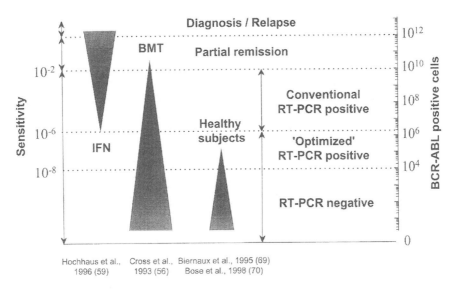

Fig. 8. Schematic illustration of therapeutic response of CML patients on molecular level. Almost all IFN-treated patients remain RT-PCR positive, whereas the majority of patients after allogeneic BMT become RT-PCR negative. Healthy donors may be RT-PCR positive for *BCR-ABL* transcripts using an optimized, very sensitive PCR strategy.

CML cells after treatment can be specifically detected with a sensitivity of up to 1 in 10^6 cells. This qualitative method has been used for the detection of MRD after bone marrow transplantation (BMT). A summary of 700 results from 15 centers *(64)* shows the following:

1. The majority of patients is PCR positive in the first 6 mo after BMT.
2. The graft vs leukemia effect leads to PCR negativity in two-thirds of patients. Persistent PCR negativity after 1 yr is a marker for good prognosis.
3. PCR-positive patients more than 6 mo after BMT have a great risk of relapse; however, qualitative PCR cannot predict relapse in the individual patient *(56,65,66)*.
4. In the majority of cases after BMT, RT-PCR, and DNA-PCR (using patient-specific primers), results are concordant; that is, that patients in remission do not generally harbor a substantial pool of CML cells that do not express BCR-ABL mRNA *(67)*.

Nested PCR is essentially useless in patients after IFN-α therapy, because almost all patients are repeatedly positive *(68)*.

By using an optimized RT-PCR method, BCR-ABL mRNA can be detected at a very low level of 1–10 transcripts/10^8 cells in normal individuals in an age-dependent frequency *(69,70)*. One interpretation of this finding could be that *BCR-ABL*, and probably several other fusion genes, is being formed continuously in mitotic cells in the normal bone marrow, but only the combination of the correct *BCR-ABL* fusion in the correct primitive hematopoietic progenitor has a selective advantage and becomes functional as an expanding clone *(71)* (**Fig. 8**).

1.2.5.3. QUANTITATIVE PCR

In view of the very limited value of qualitative PCR, several groups have developed quantitative PCR assays to estimate the amount of MRD in positive specimens. Most groups have initially used competitive PCR strategies that can effectively control for variations in amplification efficiency and reaction kinetics *(56,58,72–74)*.

In general, nested PCR is performed using serial dilutions of a BCR-ABL competitor construct added to the same volume of patients' cDNA. The equivalence point at which the competitor and sample band would be of equal intensity is determined by densitometry *(56,59)*. To standardize results for both quality and quantity of blood, RNA, and cDNA, quantification of transcripts of normal housekeeping genes, such as *ABL* or glucose-6-phosphate dehydrogenase *(G6PD)*, has been employed. The standardized results are expressed as the ratios of BCR-ABL/ABL or BCR-ABL/G6PD in a percentage. The quantification of the transcript level of control genes is of special importance if different RNA qualities are expected, i.e., particularly when samples are mailed in multicenter trials (**Fig. 9**).

In patients after BMT, rising or persistently high levels of BCR-ABL mRNA can be detected prior to cytogenetic or hematologic relapse. Of 69 patients with low or falling *BCR-ABL* transcripts, 3% relapsed compared with 79% in 29 patients with high or rising BCR-ABL transcript levels *(65,75)*. By contrast, patients who remain in remission have low, stable, or falling BCR-ABL levels *(56,57,75–77)*.

Quantitative PCR is the method of choice to determine the best time point for therapeutic interventions in case of relapse after BMT. Quantitative PCR data have been used to determine the optimum time point to initiate donor lymphocyte transfusions *(78)* and to monitor its response *(79)*. The great majority of patients who respond to donor lymphocyte infusions achieve durable molecular remission (RT-PCR negativity) with a median follow-up of >2 yr *(79)*.

Quantitative RT-PCR for *BCR-ABL* has been shown to be a reliable method for monitoring residual leukemia load in mobilized peripheral blood stem cells, particularly in Ph-negative collections. Quantitative RT-PCR allows selection of the best available collections for reinfusion into patients after myeloablative therapy (autografting) *(80)*.

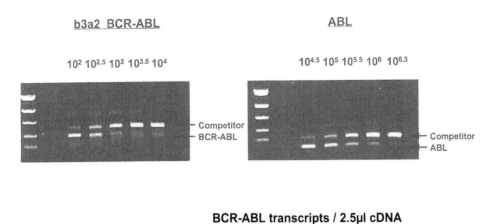

Fig. 9. Quantitative competitive RT-PCR for *BCR-ABL* transcripts. Nested PCR is performed using serial dilutions of a *BCR-ABL* competitor construct added to the same volume of patients' cDNA. The equivalence point at which patients and sample band would be of equal intensity is determined by densitometry. Total ABL transcripts are quantified to standardize the assay for different qualities of patients' blood, RNA, or cDNA *(59)*.

For 96 Ph-positive patients after IFN-α therapy, all were positive for *BCR-ABL* transcripts. The MRD in complete responders spanned a range over four orders of magnitude. The median ratios of complete, partial, minor, and nonresponders differed significantly ($p < 0.0001$). The results of nonresponders on IFN-α therapy and patients at diagnosis were not different *(59,68)*.

Cytogenetic response to IFN-α (complete, partial, minor/none) was compared to molecular response by introducing cutoff points for the BCR-ABL/ABL ratio. Using optimum cutoff points of 2 and 14% (i.e., comparing a ratio up to 2% to complete cytogenetic responders, between 2 and 14% to partial responders, and >14% to minor and nonresponders), the concordance between the two methods was 82%, the χ^2 test was highly significant ($p < 0.001$) *(59)*.

All 54 patients investigated who had achieved complete response (CR) to IFN-α treatment had molecular evidence of MRD during complete remission, although 3 patients were intermittently negative by RT-PCR. In general, *BCR-ABL* transcript numbers were inversely related to the duration of CR. The median ratio of BCR-ABL to ABL at the time of maximal response for each patient was 0.045% (range 0–3.6%). During the period of observation, 14 patients relapsed, 11 cytogenetically to chronic phase disease, and 3 directly to blastic phase. The median ratio of BCR-ABL/ABL at maximal response was significantly higher in patients who relapsed than in those who remained in CR (0.49

vs 0.021%; $p < 0.0001$) *(81)*. The findings show that the level of MRD falls with time in patients who maintain their cytogenetic response to IFN, but molecular evidence of disease is rarely if ever eliminated. The RT-PCR analysis of colony-forming unit granulocyte macrophage colonies grown from bone marrow of eight complete cytogenetic responders demonstrated that residual disease resides in myeloid colony-forming cells, which may have the potential to repopulate the bone marrow and contribute to relapse *(82)*. Therefore, it is unlikely that CML can be cured by IFN-α therapy. The actual level of MRD correlates with the probability of relapse. For patients who reach complete cytogenetic remission should be continued at least until relatively low levels of residual leukemia are achieved *(81)*.

In other series, the frequency of PCR negativity in complete cytogenetic responders is higher in a long-term follow-up using an RT-PCR strategy with a lower sensitivity *(83)*. However, since the actual level of residual *BCR-ABL* transcripts is related to the probability of relapse, molecular monitoring may identify a subset of patients for whom treatment may be safely withdrawn *(81)* (**Fig. 10**).

Rising levels of BCR-ABL mRNA in sequential samples from patients who are not in cytogenetic remission may precede disease progression *(84)*.

The low-level expression of e1a2 BCR-ABL mRNA in patients with M-bcr-positive CML is a common finding *(85)*. Whether increasing levels of e1a2 mRNA transcripts correlate to disease progression is still controversial *(86)*.

Recently, novel real-time PCR procedures have been developed that promise to simplify existing protocols. Several procedures for quantification of BCR-ABL mRNA using the TaqMan™ system have been developed *(87,88)*. The assay is based on the use of the 5' nuclease activity of *Taq* polymerase to cleave a nonextendable hybridization probe during the extension phase of PCR. The approach uses dual-labeled fluorogenic probes. One fluorescent dye serves as a reporter and its emission spectrum is quenched by the second fluorescent dye. The nuclease degradation of the probe releases the quenching, resulting in an increase in fluorescent emission. The fluorescence is monitored by a sequence detector in real time. C_T (threshold cycle) values are calculated by determining the point at which the fluorescence exceeds a threshold limit. C_T corresponds to the amount of target transcripts in the sample *(89)*.

An alternative real-time RT-PCR approach for detection and quantification of *BCR-ABL* fusion transcripts has been established using the new LightCycler™ technology *(90,91)*, which combines rapid thermocycling with on-line fluorescence detection of PCR product formation as it occurs. Fluorescence monitoring of PCR amplification is based on the concept of fluorescence resonance energy transfer between two adjacent hybridization probes carrying donor and acceptor fluorophores. Excitation of a donor fluorophore (fluores-

Leukemia-Specific Rearrangements

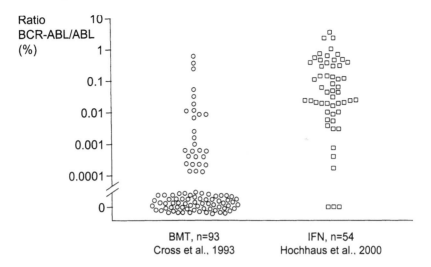

Fig. 10. Quantitative PCR analysis for the ratio to BCR-ABL/ABL in complete cytogenetic responders after allogeneic BMT and IFN therapy. Two-thirds of patients after allogeneic BMT are after 6 mo RT-PCR negative *(56)*, whereas almost all patients after IFN therapy are persistently RT-PCR positive. Only 3 of 54 patients showed transient PCR negativity *(81)*.

cein) with an emission spectrum that overlaps the excitation spectrum of an acceptor fluorophore (e.g., LC Red640; Roche Diagnostics, Mannheim, Germany) results in nonradioactive energy transfer to the acceptor (**Fig. 11**). Once conditions are established, the amount of fluorescence resulting from the two probes is proportional to the amount of PCR product. Owing to amplification in glass capillaries with a low volume/surface ratio, PCR reaction times have been reduced to <30 min.

A pair of probes was designed that is complementary to *ABL* exon 3, thus enabling detection of all known *BCR-ABL* variants and also normal ABL as an internal control (**Fig. 12**). Conditions were established to amplify less than 10 target molecules/reaction, and to detect one CML cell in 10^5 cells from healthy donors and one K562 cell in 10^7 HL60 cells. To determine the utility of the assay, *BCR-ABL* and *ABL* transcripts in a series of 254 samples from 120 patients with CML after therapy were quantified (**Fig. 13**). The level of MRD was expressed as the ratio of BCR-ABL/ABL. This ratio was compared to results obtained by three established methods from contemporaneous specimens. A highly significant correlation was seen among the BCR-ABL/ABL ratios determined by the LightCycler and (1) the BCR-ABL/ABL ratios obtained by nested competitive RT-PCR ($n = 201$; $r = 0.90$; $p < 0.0001$) (**Fig. 14**); (2) the proportion of Philadelphia chromosome positive metaphases determined

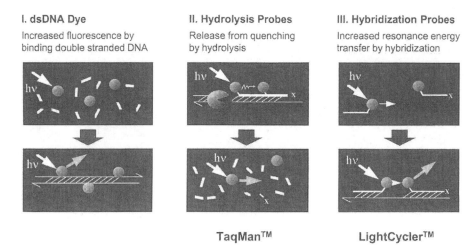

Fig. 11. Real-time fluorescence detection of PCR products during the amplification phase (real-time PCR). Fluorescence labeling can be performed by unspecific binding of an appropriate dye to double-stranded DNA (e.g., SYBR Green), by hybridization of TaqMan probes carrying quencher and reporter dyes that are cleaved during elongation, or by hybridization to a pair of probes labeled with a donor and a reporter dye with increased fluorescence in juxtaposition (LightCycler method).

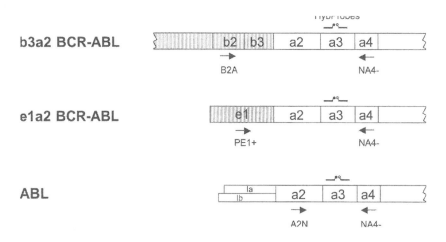

Fig. 12. Schematic map of the amplification and detection of BCR-ABL and ABL transcripts. Specific primer pairs were used to amplify various types of BCR-ABL and ABL transcripts. The detection format was uniform using a pair of adjacent fluorescent labeled hybridization probes to *ABL* exon 3 *(92)*.

by cytogenetics ($n = 81$; $p < 0.0001$), and (3) the BCR ratio determined by Southern blot analysis ($n = 122$; $p < 0.0001$) *(92)* (**Fig. 15**).

Leukemia-Specific Rearrangements

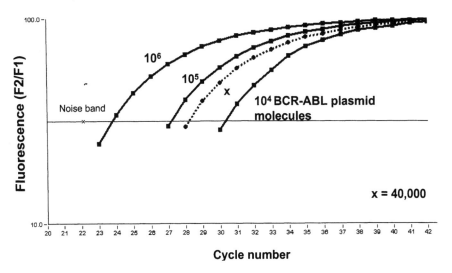

Fig. 13. Example of real-time PCR. Three standard dilutions of plasmid pGD210 (b3a2$^{BCR-ABL}$) were compared with a patient's sample of unknown BCR-ABL concentration. Each point represents the fluorescence intensity (F2/F1) measured after each PCR cycle. Plotting the cycle threshold of the unknown sample on the standard curve revealed that 40,000 BCR-ABL transcripts were present at the start of the reaction.

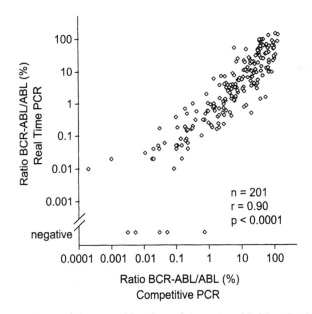

Fig. 14. Comparison of the quantification of the ratio of BCR-ABL/ABL with real-time PCR vs competitive PCR. In five samples positive with competitive PCR, no BCR-ABL transcripts were detected by real-time PCR. The ratios derived by both methods correlate with $r = 0.90$, $p < 0.0001$ *(92)*.

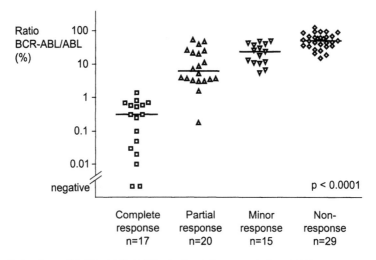

Fig. 15. Ratios of BCR-ABL/ABL derived from real-time PCR according to contemporaneous cytogenetic response. The ratios of BCR-ABL/ABL are significantly different among complete, partial, minor, and nonresponders ($p < 0.0001$) *(92)*.

Real-time PCR approaches with TaqMan or hybridization probes are reliable and sensitive methods to monitor CML patients after therapy. The major advantages of the methodology are that amplification and product analysis are performed in the same reaction vessel, avoiding the risk of contamination, and that the results are standardized by the quantification of housekeeping genes.

1.2.6. Other Methods

Several alternative techniques have also been employed. They are mostly too cumbersome, inexact, or underdeveloped for routine assessment of residual leukemia. Some examples are as follows:

1. *Chimerism analysis.* This method distinguishes between genomic DNA or cells from different individuals and can be used in patients after allogeneic BMT to calculate the proportion of host to donor cells. Typically, PCR is used to amplify polymorphic markers *(93–95)*. Chimerism analysis does not distinguish between malignant or normal cells and, therefore, cannot be used directly to detect residual leukemia.
2. *RNAse protection assays.* These can be used to quantify levels of BCR-ABL mRNA *(96,97)*.
3. *Pulsfield gel electrophoresis.* This method enables resolution of much larger DNA fragments than is possible on standard gels. Combined with Southern blotting, it can be used to detect rearrangements outside the M-bcr and also within the *ABL* gene *(98–100)*.

Leukemia-Specific Rearrangements

4. In situ *PCR*. This method used on single cells can specifically identify cells with BCR-ABL transcripts. Its results are concordant with those of karyotyping and RT-PCR. Because of its limited sensitivity and specificity, however, it appears to have limited value in the analysis of MRD *(101)*. Positive cells are enumerated by low cytometry or fluorescent microscopy *(102)*.

Thus, there are a number of methods available to detect BCR-ABL rearrangements/fusion products. Described herein is a protocol to quantify BCR-ABL transcripts using real time PCR with fluorescent hybridization probes.

2. Materials
2.1. RNA Extraction, cDNA Synthesis

1. RNA extraction kit: RNeasy (Qiagen, Hilden, Germany) or High Pure (Roche Diagnostics,).
2. RT-PCR kit including random hexamer primers and Molony murine leukemia virus (MMLV) RT.

2.2. Quantitative Real-Time PCR

1. LightCycler instrument.
2. Microcentrifuge.
3. Vortex.
4. LightCycler-DNA Master Hybridization Probes (Roche Molecular Biochemicals, Mannheim, Germany).
5. dNTPplus (dATP, dUTP, dGTP, dCTP) (Roche Molecular Biochemicals).
6. Heat-labile uracil DNA glycosylase (UDG) (Roche Molecular Biochemicals).
7. Amplification primers (MWG, Ebersberg, Germany).
8. Hybridization probes (TIB MOLBIOL, Berlin, Germany).

3. Methods
3.1. RNA Extraction, cDNA Synthesis

1. Extract total leukocyte RNA from 10–20 mL of peripheral blood (PB) and/or from 1 to 5 mL of bone marrow (BM) aspirate after lysis of red blood cells *(103)*.
2. Process the samples as soon as possible after aspiration, although some may spend 1–3 d in transit.
3. Perform RNA extraction by CsCl gradient centrifugation *(103)* or by commercially available extraction kits.
4. Reverse-transcribe RNA using random hexamer priming and MMLV RT as described *(103)*.
5. Store the cDNA samples at –20°C.

3.2. Quantitative Real-Time PCR

1. Perform PCR using 2 µL of master mix ([LightCycler™ DNA Master Hybridization Probes; Roche Diagnostics] containing buffer, dATP, dCTP, dGTP, dUTP,

Table 3
Oligonucleotides Used in Real-Time PCR Assay for BCR-ABL Transcripts

Primers	Sequence[a]	Mapping
B2A	5' TTCAGAAGCTTCTCCCTGACAT	*BCR* exon b2 (*54*)
A2N	5' CCCAACCTTTTCGTTGCACTGT	*ABL* exon 2 (*103*)
PE1+	5' CAGATCTGGCCCAACGATGG	*BCR* exon e1 (*92*)
NA4-	5' CGGCTCTCGGAGGAGACGTAGA	*ABL* exon 4 (*104*)
Hybridization probes		
a3-3'HP	5' LC Red 640-AATGGGGAATGGTGTGAAGCCCAAA-P	*ABL* exon 3 (*92*)
a3-5'HP	5' TGAAAAGCTCCGGGTCTTAGGCTATAATCA-F	*ABL* exon 3 (*92*)

[a]F, fluorescein; P, phosphate; LC Red 640, LightCycler fluorescence dye 640.

and *Taq* polymerase), 4 mM MgCl$_2$, 0.25 μM of each 3' and 5' fluorescent hybridization probes (TIB MolBiol, Berlin, Germany), 0.5 μM of each 3' and 5' oligonucleotide primer (highly purified salt-free grade; MWG) (**Table 3**), 1 U of heat-labile UDG (Roche Diagnostics), 2 μL of cDNA, and water to a final volume of 20 μL.

2. Prior to amplification, incubate the mixes for 5 min at room temperature to allow degradation of specific contaminating PCR products from previous amplifications by UDG. To improve reliability of the assay, prepare master mixes for 35 samples (**Table 4**).

3. Deactivate heat-labile UDG by an initial denaturation step of 1 min at 95°C.

4. Amplify in a three-step cycle procedure (denaturation at 95°C, 1 s, ramp rate 20°C/s; annealing at 64°C, 10s, ramp rate 20°C/s; and extension at 72°C, 26 s, ramp rate 2°C/s) for 45 cycles (**Table 5**). The following primers were used for amplification: b2a2, b3a2, b2a3, or b3a3 BCR-ABL, primers B2A and NA4–; e1a2 BCR-ABL, primers PE1+ and NA4–; ABL, primers A2N and NA4– (**Fig. 12, Table 3**).

5. Perform amplification, fluorescence detection, and postprocessing calculations using the LightCycler apparatus (Roche Diagnostics).

5' Hybridization probes are labeled with fluorescein, 3' probes with LC Red640. Fluorescence is measured after each annealing step and expressed as the ratio between fluorescence at 640 nm (designated F2) and at 530 nm (background, designated F1).

The fluorescence signal is plotted against the cycle number for all samples and external standards. These standards consist of serial dilutions (10^1–10^7 molecules per reaction) of plasmids pGD210 (b3a2[BCR-ABL]) and pB190 (e1a2[BCR-ABL]). Initially, the crossover point is determined for each standard dilution, i.e., the point at which the signal rose above the background level. The higher the initial number of starting molecules, the earlier the signal

Leukemia-Specific Rearrangements

Table 4
Reaction Mix for BCR-ABL, ABL, and G6PD Transcript Quantification[a]

	Stock concentration	Final concentration	Volume (35 samples) (μL)	Volume (n samples) (μL)
LightCycler DNA Master Hybridization Probes			70	$(n + 1) \times 2$
MgCl$_2$	25 mM	3 mM	84	$(n + 1) \times 2.4$
3' and 5' fluorescent hybridization probe mix	10 μM	0.25 μM	17.5	$(n + 1) \times 0.5$
3' oligonucleotide primer	100 μM	0.5 μM	3.5	$(n + 1) \times 0.1$
5' oligonucleotide primer	100 μM	0.5 μM	3.5	$(n + 1) \times 0.1$
Uracil DNA glycosylase	1 U/μL	1 U	35	$(n + 1) \times 1$
cDNA			70	$(n + 1) \times 2$
dH$_2$O			416.5	$(n + 1) \times 11.9$
Total volume			700	$(n + 1) \times 20$

[a]Mix for 35 samples.

Table 5
Temperature Profile of the PCR Cycles

Parameter	Value		
Cycles	45		
Temperature target	Segment 1	Segment 2	Segment 3
Target temperature (°C)	95	64	72
Incubation time (s)	1	10	26
Temperatur transition rate (°C/s)	20	20	2
Acquisition mode	None	None	Single

appears above the background (**Fig. 13**). A standard curve for each run is constructed by plotting the crossover point against the log (number of standard molecules). The number of target molecules in each sample is then calculated automatically by reference to this curve. Results were expressed initially as the number of target molecules/2 μL of cDNA. Normalized levels of disease are calculated as the ratios (expressed as percentage) between *BCR-ABL* and *ABL* transcripts in 2 μL of cDNA.

3.3. Conclusion

Quantitative data on MRD may be achieved by various methods. However, no standard technique is used. Interlaboratory reproducibility needs a standardization of the method and of the interpretation of the results. The efficiency of this technology needs to be confirmed in large clinical trials. Recommendations of the European Investigators on CML group for the clinical use of quantitative PCR monitoring in CML have been published *(105)*. The new real-time RT-PCR procedures promise to greatly simplify the cumbersome protocols that are currently in use. They also offer a unique opportunity to standardize the assay and to develop rigorous standards and controls. Quantitative real-time PCR soon will become a routine and robust basis for clinical decision making in leukemias with specific molecular markers.

References

1. Carlo Stella, C., Mangoni, L., Dotti, G. P., and Rizzoli, V. (1995) Techniques for detection of minimal residual disease. *Leuk. Lymphoma* **18(Supp. 1),** 75–80.
2. van Dongen, J. J., Szczepanski, T., de Bruijn, M. A. C., van de Beemd, M. W. M., de Bruin-Versteeg, S., Wijkhuijs, J. M., et al. (1996) Detection of minimal residual disease in acute leukemia patients. *Cytokines Mol. Ther.* **2,** 121–133.
3. Campana, D. and Pui, C. H. (1995) Detection of minimal residual disease in acute leukemia: methodological advances and clinical significance. *Blood* **85,** 1416–1434.
4. Reiter, A., Sohal, J., Kulkarni, S., Chase, A., Macdonald, D. H. C., Aguiar, R. C. T., et al. (1998) Consistent fusion of ZNF198 to the fibroblast growth factor receptor1 in the t(8;13)(p11;q12) myeloproliferative syndrome. *Blood* **92,** 1735–1742.
5. Sawyers, C. L. (1999) Chronic myeloid leukemia. *N. Engl. J. Med.* **340,** 1330–1340.
6. Virchow, R. (1845) Weisses Blut. *Frorieps Notizen* **36,** 151–156.
7. Nowell, P. C. and Hungerford, D. A. (1960) A minute chromosome in human chronic granulocytic leukemia. *Science* **132,** 1497–1501.
8. Rowley, J. D. (1973) A new consistent chromosome abnormality in chronic myelogenous leukaemia detected by quinacrine fluorescence and Giemsa staining. *Nature* **243,** 290–293.
9. Groffen, J., Stephenson, J. R., Heisterkamp, N., de Klein, A., Bartram, C. R., and Grosveld, G. (1984) Philadelphia chromosomal breakpoints are clustered within a limited region, bcr, on chromosome 22. *Cell* **36,** 93–99.
10. Stam, K., Heisterkamp, N., Grosveld, G., de Klein, A., Verma, R. S., Coleman, M., et al. (1985) Evidence of a new chimeric bcr/c-abl mRNA in patients with chronic myelocytic leukemia and the Philadelphia chromosome. *N. Engl. J. Med.* **313,** 1429–1433.
11. Daley, G. Q., van Etten, R. A., and Baltimore, D. (1990) Induction of chronic myelogenous leukemia in mice by the P210bcr/abl gene of the Philadelphia chromosome. *Science* **247,** 824–830.

Leukemia-Specific Rearrangements

12. Heisterkamp, N., Jenster, G., ten Hoeve, J., Zovich, D., Pattengale, P. K., and Groffen, J. (1990) Acute leukaemia in bcr/abl transgenic mice. *Nature* **344**, 251–253.

13. Melo, J. V., Gordon, D. E., Cross, N. C. P., and Goldman, J. M. (1993) The ABL-BCR fusion gene is expressed in chronic myeloid leukemia. *Blood* **81**, 158–165.

14. Lion, T. (1996) Monitoring of residual disease in chronic myelogenous leukemia: methodological approaches and clincal aspects. *Leukemia* **10**, 896–906.

15. Kantarjian, H. M., Smith, T. L., O'Brien, S., Beran, M., Pierce, S., Talpaz, M., and and the Leukemia Service (1995) Prolonged survival in chronic myelogenous leukemia after cytogenetic response to interferon-α therapy. *Ann. Intern. Med.* **122**, 254–261.

16. Hook, E. B. (1977) Exclusion of chromosomal mosaicism: tables of 90%, 95%, and 99% confidence limits and comments on use. *Am. J. Hum. Genet.* **29**, 94–97.

17. Cortes, J., Talpaz, M., O'Brien, S., Rios, M. B., Majlis, A., Keating, M., Freireich, E. J., and Kantarjian, H. (1998) Suppression on cytogenetic clonal evolution with interferon alfa therapy in patients with Philadelphia chromosome-positive chronic myelogenous leukemia. *J. Clin. Oncol.* **16**, 3279–3285.

18. Kantarjian, H. M., Dixon, D., Keating, M. J., Talpaz, M., Walters, R. S., McCredie, K. B., and Freireich, E. J. (1988) Characteristics of accelerated disease in chronic myelogenous leukemia. *Cancer* **61**, 1441–1446.

19. Tkachuk, D. C., Westbrook, C. A., Andreeff, M., Donlon, T. A., Cleary, M. L., Suryanarayan, K., et al. (1990) Detection of bcr-abl fusion in chronic myelogeneous leukemia by in situ hybridization. *Science* **250**, 559–562.

20. Nacheva, E., Holloway, T., Brown, K., Bloxham, D., and Green, A. R. (1994) Philadelphia-negative chronic myeloid leukaemia: detection by FISH of BCR-ABL fusion gene localized either to chromosome 9 or chromosome 22. *Br. J. Haematol.* **87**, 409–412.

21. Hochhaus, A., Reiter, A., Skladny, H., Melo, J. V., Sick, C., Berger, U., et al. (1996) A novel BCR-ABL fusion gene (e6a2) in a patient with Philadelphia chromosome negative chronic myelogenous leukemia. *Blood* **88**, 2236–2240.

22. Melo, J. V. (1996) The diversity of BCR-ABL fusion proteins and their relationship to leukemia phenotype. *Blood* **88**, 2375–2384.

23. Weber-Matthiesen, K., Winkemann, M., Müller-Hermelink, A., Schlegelberger, B., and Grote, W. (1992) Simultaneous fluorescence immunophenotyping and interphase cytogenetics: a contribution to characterization of tumor cells. *J. Histochem. Cytochem.* **40**, 171–175.

24. Haferlach, T., Winkemann, M., Nickenig, C., Meeder, M., Ramm-Petersen, L., Schoch, R., et al. (1997) Which compartments are involved in Philadelphia-chromosome positive chronic myeloid leukaemia? An answer at the single cell level by combining May-Grünwald-Giemsa staining and fluorescence *in situ* hybridization techniques. *Br. J. Haematol.* **97**, 99–106.

25. Bentz, M., Cabot, G., Moos, M., Speicher, M. R., Ganser, A., Lichter, P., and Döhner, H. (1994) Detection of chimeric BCR-ABL genes on bone marrow

samples and blood smears in chronic myeloid and acute lymphoblastic leukemia by in situ hybridization. *Blood* **83,** 1922–1928.

26. Garcia-Isidoro, M., Tabernero, M. D., Garcia, J. L., Najera, M. L., Hernandez, J. M., Wiegant, J., et al. (1997) Detection of the Mbcr/abl translocation in chronic myeloid leukemia by fluorescence in situ hybridization: comparison with conventional cytogenetics and implications for minimal residual disease detection. *Hum. Pathol.* **28,** 154–159.

27. Chase, A., Grand, F., Zhang, J. G., Blackett, N., Goldman, J., and Gordon, M. (1997) Factors influencing the false positive and negative rates of *BCR-ABL* fluorescence in-situ hybridization. *Genes Chromosomes Cancer* **18,** 246–253.

28. Cox Froncillo, M. C., Cantonetti, M., Masi, M., Lentini, R., Giudiceandrea, P., Maffei, L., et al. (1995) Cytogenetic analysis is non-informative for assessing the remission rate in chronic myeloid leukemia (CML) patients on interferon-alpha (IFN-alpha) therapy. *Cancer Genet. Cytogenet.* **84,** 15–18.

29. Mühlmann, J., Thaler, J., Hilbe, W., Bechter, O., Erdel, M., Utermann, G., and Duba, H. C. (1998) Fluorescence in situ hybridization (FISH) on peripheral blood smears for monitoring Philadelphia chromosome-positive chronic myeloid leukemia (CML) during interferon treatment: a new strategy for remission asssessment. *Genes Chromosomes Cancer* **21,** 90–100.

30. Cox Froncillo, M. C., Maffei, L., Cantonetti, M., Del Poeta, G., Lentini, R., Bruno, A., et al. (1996) FISH analysis for CML monitoring? *Ann. Hematol.* **73,** 113–119.

31. Tchirkov, A., Giollant, M., Tavernier, F., Briancon, G., Tournilhac, O., Kwiatkowski, F., et al. (1998) Interphase cytogenetics and competitive RT-PCR for residual disease monitoring in patients with chronic myeloid leukaemia during interferon-α therapy. *Br. J. Haematol.* **101,** 552–557.

32. Verfaillie, C., Bhatia, R., Miller, W., Mortari, F., Roy, V., Burger, S., et al. (1996) BCR/ABL-negative primitive progenitors suitable for transplantation can be selected from the marrow of most early-chronic phase but not accelerated-phase chronic myelogenous leukemia patients. *Blood* **87,** 4770–4779.

33. Kirk, J. A., Reems, J. A., Roecklein, B. A., Van Devanter, D. R., Bryant, E. M., Radich, J., et al. (1995) Benign marrow progenitors are enriched in the CD34+/HLA-DRlo population but not in the CD34+/CD38lo population in chronic myeloid leukemia: an analysis using interphase fluorescence in situ hybridization. *Blood* **86,** 737–743.

34. Sinclair, P. B., Green, A. R., Grace, C., and Nacheva, E. P. (1997) Improved sensitivity of BCR-ABL detection: a triple-probe three-color fluorescence in situ hybridization system. *Blood* **90,** 1395–1402.

35. Buno, I., Wyatt, W. A., Zinsmeister, A. R., Dietz-Band, J., Silver, R. T., and Dewald, G. W. (1998) A special fluorescent in situ hybridization technique to study peripheral blood and assess the effectiveness of interferon therapy in chronic myeloid leukemia. *Blood* **92,** 2315–2321.

36. Dewald, G. W., Wyatt, W. A., Juneau, A. L., Carlson, R. O., Zinsmeister, A. R., Jalal, S. M., et al. (1998) Highly sensitive fluorescence in situ hybridization

Leukemia-Specific Rearrangements

method to detect double BCR/ABL fusion and monitor response to therapy in chronic myeloid leukemia. *Blood* **91,** 3357–3365.

37. El Rifai, W., Ruutu, T., Vettentanta, K., Temtamy, S., and Knuutila, S. (1996) Minimal residual disease after allogeneic bone marrow transplantation for chronic myeloid leukaemia: a metaphase-FISH study. *Br. J. Haematol.* **92,** 365–369.

38. Seong, D. C., Kantarjian, H. M., Ro, J. Y., Talpaz, M., Xu, J., Robinson, J. R., Deisseroth, A. B., et al. (1995) Hypermetaphase fluorescence in situ hybridization for quantitative monitoring of Philadelphia chromosome-positive cells in patients with chronic myelogenous leukemia during treatment. *Blood* **86,** 2343–2349.

39. Seong, D., Giralt, S., Fischer, H., Hayes, K., Glassman, A., Arlinghaus, R., et al. (1997) Usefulness of detection of minimal residual disease by 'hypermetaphase' fluorescent *in situ* hybridization after allogeneic BMT for chronic myelogenous leukemia. *Bone Marrow Transplant.* **19,** 565–570.

40. Reiter, A., Skladny, H., Hochhaus, A., Seifarth, W., Heimpel, H., Bartram, C. R., et al. (1997) Molecular response of CML patients treated with interferon-α monitored by quantitative Southern blot analysis. *Br. J. Haematol.* **97,** 86–93.

41. Fishleder, A. J., Shadrach, B., and Tuttle, C. (1989) *bcr* rearrangement: Potential false positive secondary to an EcoRI restriction fragment length polymorphism. *Leukemia* **3,** 746–748.

42. Grossman, A., Mathew, A., O'Connell, M. P., Tiso, P., Distenfeld, A., and Benn, P. (1990) Multiple restriction enzyme digests are required to rule out polymorphism in the molecular diagnosis of chronic myeloid leukemia. *Leukemia* **4,** 63–64.

43. Popenoe, D. W., Schaefer Rego, K., Mears, J. G., Bank, A., and Leibowitz, D. (1986) Frequent and extensive deletion during the 9;22 translocation in CML. *Blood* **68,** 1123–1128.

44. Bartram, C. R., Bross Bach, U., Schmidt, H., and Waller, H. D. (1987) Philadelphia-positive chronic myelogenous leukemia with breakpoint 5' of the breakpoint cluster region but within the bcr gene. *Blut.* **55,** 505–511.

45. Saglio, G., Guerrasio, A., Rosso, C., Zaccaria, A., Tassinari, A., Serra, A., et al. (1990) New type of Bcr/Abl junction in Philadelphia chromosome-positive chronic myelogenous leukemia. *Blood* **76,** 1819–1824.

46. Stock, W., Westbrook, C. A., Peterson, B., Arthur, D. C., Szatrowski, T. P., Silver, R. T., et al. (1997) Value of molecular monitoring during treatment of chronic myeloid leukemia: A Cancer and Leukemia Group B Study. *J. Clin. Oncol.* **15,** 26–36.

47. Verschraegen, C. F., Talpaz, M., Hirsch Ginsberg, C. F., Pherwani, R., Rios, M. B., Stass, S. A., and Kantarjian, H. M. (1995) Quantification of the breakpoint cluster region rearrangement for clinical monitoring in Philadelphia chromosome-positive chronic myeloid leukemia. *Blood* **85,** 2705–2710.

48. Steegmann, J. L., Requena, M. J., Casado, L. F., Pico, M., Panarrubia, M. J., Ferro, M. T., et al. (1996) Southern technique and cytogenetics are comple-

mentary and must be used together in the evaluation of Ph1, M-BCR positive chronic myeloid leukemia (CML) patients treated with alpha interferon (IFN-ALPHA). *Am. J. Hematol.* **53,** 169–174.

49. Yoffe, G., Blick, M., Kantarjian, H., Spitzer, G., Gutterman, J., and Talpaz, M. (1987) Molecular analysis of interferon-induced suppression of Philadelphia chromosome in patients with chronic myeloid leukemia. *Blood* **69,** 961–963.

50. Guo, J. Q., Lian, J. Y., Xian, Y. M., Lee, M. S., Deisseroth, A. B., Stass, S. A., et al. (1994) BCR-ABL protein expression in peripheral blood cells of chronic myelogenous leukemia patients undergoing therapy. *Blood* **83,** 3629–3637.

51. Guo, J. Q., Lian, J., Glassman, A., Talpaz, M., Kantarjian, H., Deisseroth, A. B., and Arlinghaus, R. B. (1996) Comparison of *bcr-abl* protein expression and Philadelphia chromosome analyses in chronic myelogenous leukemia patients. *Am. J. Clin. Pathol.* **106,** 442–448.

52. Morgan, G. J., Hughes, T., Janssen, J. W., Gow, J., Guo, A. P., Goldman, J. M., et al. (1989) Polymerase chain reaction for detection of residual leukaemia. *Lancet* **1,** 928,929.

53. Hughes, T., Martiat, P., Morgan, G., Sawyers, C., Witte, O. N., and Goldman, J. M. (1990) Significance of residual leukaemia transcripts after bone marrow transplant for CML. *Lancet* **335,** 50.

54. Hughes, T., Janssen, J. W. G., Morgan, G., Martiat, P., Saglio, G., Pignon, J. M., et al. (1990) False-positive results with PCR to detect leukaemia-specific transcript. *Lancet* **335,** 1037,1038.

55. Hughes, T. and Goldman, J. M. (1990) Improved results with PCR for chronic myeloid leukaemia. *Lancet* **336,** 812.

56. Cross, N. C. P., Feng, L., Chase, A., Bungey, J., Hughes, T. P., and Goldman, J. M. (1993) Competitive polymerase chain reaction to estimate the number of BCR-ABL transcripts in chronic myeloid leukemia patients after bone marrow transplantation. *Blood* **82,** 1929–1936.

57. Lion, T., Henn, T., Gaiger, A., Kalhs, P., and Gadner, H. (1993) Early detection of relapse after bone marrow transplantation in patients with chronic myelogenous leukaemia. *Lancet* **341,** 275,276.

58. Malinge, M. C., Mahon, F. X., Delfau, M. H., Daheron, L., Kitzis, A., Guilhot, F., et al. (1992) Quantitative determination of the hybrid Bcr-Abl RNA in patients with chronic myelogenous leukaemia under interferon therapy. *Br. J. Haematol.* **82,** 701–707.

59. Hochhaus, A., Lin, F., Reiter, A., Skladny, H., Mason, P. J., van Rhee, F., et al. (1996) Quantification of residual disease in chronic myelogenous leukemia patients on interferon-α therapy by competitive polymerase chain reaction. *Blood* **87,** 1549–1555.

60. Cross, N. C. P., Melo, J. V., Feng, L., and Goldman, J. M. (1994) An optimized multiplex polymerase chain reaction (PCR) for detection of BCR-ABL fusion mRNAs in haematological disorders. *Leukemia* **8,** 186–189.

61. Melo, J. V., Myint, H., Galton, D. A., and Goldman, J. M. (1994) P190BCR-ABL chronic myeloid leukaemia: the missing link with chronic myelomonocytic leukaemia? *Leukemia* **8,** 208–211.

Leukemia-Specific Rearrangements

62. Clarkson, B. and Strife, A. (1993) Linkage of proliferative and maturational abnormalities in chronic myelogenous leukemia and relevance to treatment. *Leukemia* **7,** 1683–1721.

63. Morley, A. (1998) Quantifying leukemia. *N. Engl. J. Med.* **339,** 627–629.

64. Cross, N. C. P. (1997) Assessing residual leukaemia. *Baillieres Clin. Haematol.* **10,** 389–403.

65. Cross, N. C. P., Feng, L., Zhang, J. G., and Goldman, J. M. (1994) Competitive PCR to monitor residual disease after bone marrow transplantation for chronic myeloid leukaemia, in *Molecular Diagnosis and Monitoring of Leukaemia and Lymphoma* (Borden, E. C., Goldman, J. M., and Grignani, F., eds.), Ares-Serono Symposia Publications, Ares-Serono, Rome, pp. 119–126.

66. Potter, M. N., Cross, N. C. P., van Dongen, J. J., Saglio, G., Oakhill, A., Bartram, C. R., and Goldman, J. M. (1993) Molecular evidence of minimal residual disease after treatment for leukaemia and lymphoma: an updated meeting report and review. *Leukemia* **7,** 1302–1314.

67. Zhang, J. G., Lin, F., Chase, A., Goldman, J. M., and Cross, N. C. P. (1996) Comparison of genomic DNA and cDNA for detection of residual disease after treatment of chronic myeloid leukemia with allogeneic bone marrow transplantation. *Blood* **87,** 2588–2593.

68. Hochhaus, A., Lin, F., Reiter, A., Skladny, H., van Rhee, F., Shepherd, P. C. A., et al. (1995) Variable numbers of BCR-ABL transcripts persist in CML patients who achieve complete cytogenetic remission with interferon-α. *Br. J. Haematol.* **91,** 126–131.

69. Biernaux, C., Loos, M., Sels, A., Huez, G., and Stryckmans, P. (1995) Detection of major bcr-abl gene expression at a very low level in blood cells of some healthy individuals. *Blood* **88,** 3118–3122.

70. Bose, S., Deininger, M., Gora-Tybor, J., Goldman, J. M., and Melo, J. V. (1998) The presence of typical and atypical BCR-ABL fusion genes in leukocytes of normal individuals: biological significance and implications for the assessment of minimal residual disease. *Blood* **92,** 3362–3367.

71. Melo, J. V. (1996) The molecular biology of chronic myeloid leukaemia. *Leukemia* **10,** 751–756.

72. Lion, T., Izraeli, S., Henn, T., Gaiger, A., Mor, W., and Gadner, H. (1992) Monitoring of residual disease in chronic myelogenous leukemia by quantitative polymerase chain reaction. *Leukemia* **6,** 495–499.

73. Thompson, J. D., Brodsky, I., and Yunis, J. J. (1992) Molecular quantification of residual disease in chronic myelogenous leukemia after bone marrow transplantation. *Blood* **79,** 1629–1635.

74. Nagel, S., Schmidt, M., Thiede, C., Huhn, D., and Neubauer, A. (1996) Quantification of Bcr-Abl transcripts in chronic myelogenous leukemia (CML) using standardized, internally controlled, competitive differential PCR (CD-PCR). *Nucleic Acids Res.* **24,** 4102,4103.

75. Lin, F., van Rhee, F., Goldman, J. M., and Cross, N. C. P. (1996) Kinetics of increasing BCR-ABL transcript numbers in chronic myeloid leukemia patients who relapse after bone marrow transplantation. *Blood* **87,** 4473–4478.

76. Delage, R., Soiffer, R. J., Dear, K., and Ritz, J. (1991) Clinical significance of *bcr-abl* gene rearrangement detected by polymerase chain reaction after allogeneic bone marrow transplantation in chronic myelogenous leukemia. *Blood* **78,** 2759–2767.

77. Lin, F., Kirkland, M. A., van Rhee, F., Chase, A., Coulthard, S., Bungey, J., et al. (1996) Molecular analysis of transient cytogenetic relapse after allogeneic bone marrow transplantation for chronic myeloid leukaemia. *Bone Marrow Transplant.* **18,** 1147–1152.

78. van Rhee, F., Lin, F., Cullis, J. O., Spencer, A., Cross, N. C. P., Chase, A., et al. (1994) Relapse of chronic myeloid leukemia after allogeneic bone marrow transplant: the case for giving donor leukocyte transfusions before the onset of hematologic relapse. *Blood* **83,** 3377–3383.

79. Raanani, P., Dazzi, F., Sohal, J., Szydlo, R., van Rhee, F., Reiter, A., et al. (1997) The rate and kinetics of molecular response to donor leucocyte transfusions in chronic myeloid leukaemia patients treated for relapse after allogeneic bone marrow transplantation. *Br. J. Haematol.* **99,** 945–950.

80. Corsetti, M. T., Lerma, E., Dejana, A., Basta, P., Ferrara, R., Benvenuto, F., et al. (1999) Quantitative competitive reverse transcriptase-polymerase chain reaction for BCR-ABL on Philadelphia-negative leukaphereses allows the selection of low-contaminated peripheral blood progenitor cells for autografting in chronic myelogenous leukemia. *Leukemia* **13,** 999–1008.

81. Hochhaus, A., Reiter, A., Saussele, S., Reichert, A., Emig, M., Kaeda, J., et al. (2000) Molecular heterogeneity in complete cytogenetic responders after interferon-α therapy for chronic myelogenous leukemia: Low levels of minimal residual disease are associated with continuing remission. *Blood* **95,** 62–66.

82. Reiter, A., Marley, S. B., Hochhaus, A., Sohal, J., Raanani, P., Hehlmann, R., et al. (1998) BCR-ABL positive progenitors in chronic myeloid leukaemia patients in complete cytogenetic remission after treatment with interferon-α. *Br. J. Haematol.* **102,** 1271–1278.

83. Kurzrock, R., Estrov, Z., Kantarjian, H., and Talpaz, M. (1998) Conversion of interferon-induced, long-term cytogenetic remissions in chronic myelogenous leukemia to polymerase chain reaction negativity. *J. Clin. Oncol.* **16,** 1526–1531.

84. Gaiger, A., Henn, T., Horth, E., Geissler, K., Mitterbauer, G., Maier Dobersberger, T., et al. (1995) Increase of bcr-abl chimeric mRNA expression in tumor cells of patients with chronic myeloid leukemia precedes disease progression. *Blood* **86,** 2371–2378.

85. van Rhee, F., Hochhaus, A., Lin, F., Melo, J. V., Goldman, J. M., and Cross, N. C. P. (1996) p190 BCR-ABL mRNA is expressed at low levels in p210-positive chronic myeloid and acute lymphoblastic leukemias. *Blood* **87,** 5213–5217.

86. Saglio, G., Pane, F., Gottardi, E., Frigeri, F., Buonaiuto, M. R., Guerrasio, A., de Micheli, D., et al. (1996) Consistent amounts of acute leukemia-associated P190BCR/ABL transcripts are expressed by chronic myelogenous leukemia patients at diagnosis. *Blood* **87,** 1075–1080.

87. Mensink, E., van de Locht, A., Schattenberg, A., Linders, E., Schaap, N., Guerts van Kessel, A., and de Witte, T. (1998) Quantitation of minimal residual

Leukemia-Specific Rearrangements

disease in Philadelphia chromosome positive chronic myeloid leukaemia patients using real-time quantitative RT-PCR. *Br. J. Haematol.* **102,** 768–774.

88. Preudhomme, C., Révillion, F., Merlat, A., Hornez, L., Roumier, C., Duflos-Grardel, N., et al. (1999) Detection of BCR-ABL transcripts in chronic myeloid leukemia (CML) using a 'real time' quantitative RT-PCR assay. *Leukemia* **13,** 957–964.

89. Heid, C. A., Stevens, J., Livak, K. J., and Williams, P. M. (1996) Real time quantitative PCR. *Genome Res.* **6,** 986–994.

90. Wittwer, C. T., Herrmann, M. G., Moss, A. A., and Rasmussen, R. P. (1997) Continuous fluorescence monitoring of rapid cycle DNA amplification. *Biotechniques* **22,** 130–138.

91. Wittwer, C. T., Ririe, K. M., Andrew, R. V., David, D. A., Gundry, R. A., and Balis, U. J. (1997) The LightCycler™: a microvolume multisample fluorimeter with rapid temperature control. *Biotechniques* **22,** 176–181.

92. Emig, M., Saussele, S., Wittor, H., Weisser, A., Reiter, A., Willer, A., et al. (1999) Accurate and rapid analysis of residual disaese in patients with CML using specific fluorescent hybridization probes for real time quantitative RT-PCR. *Leukemia* **13,** 1825–1832.

93. Lawler, M., Humphries, P., and Mccann, S. R. (1991) Evaluation of mixed chimerism by in vitro amplification of dinucleotide repeat sequences using the polymerase chain reaction. *Blood* **77,** 2504–2514.

94. Rapanotti, M. C., Arcese, W., Buffolino, S., Iori, A. P., Mengarelli, A., De Cuia, M. R., et al. (1997) Sequential molecular monitoring of chimerism in chronic myeloid leukemia patients receiving donor lymphocyte transfusion for relapse after bone marrow transplantation. *Bone Marrow Transplant.* **19,** 703–707.

95. Gardiner, N., Lawler, M., O'Riordan, J. M., Duggan, C., De Arce, M., and Mccann, S. R. (1998) Monitoring of lineage-specific chimaerism allows early prediction of response following donor lymphocyte infusions for relapsed chronic myeloid leukaemia. *Bone Marrow Transplant.* **21,** 711–719.

96. Shtivelman, E., Gale, R. P., Dreazen, O., Berrebi, A., Zaizov, R., Kubonishi, I., et al. (1987) *bcr-abl* RNA in patients with chronic myelogenous leukemia. *Blood* **69,** 971–973.

97. Dhingra, K., Talpaz, M., Riggs, M. G., Eastman, P. S., Zipf, T., Ku, S., and Kurzrock, R. (1991) Hybridization protection assay: a rapid, sensitive, and specific method for detection of Philadelphia chromosome-positive leukemias. *Blood* **77,** 238–242.

98. Westbrook, C. A., Rubin, C. M., Carrino, J. J., Le Beau, M. M., Bernards, A., and Rowley, J. D. (1988) Long-range mapping of the Philadelphia chromosome by pulsed-field gel electrophoresis. *Blood* **71,** 697–702.

99. Jiang, X. Y., Trujillo, J. M., Dao, D., and Liang, J. C. (1989) Studies of BCR and ABL gene rearrangements in chronic myelogenous leukemia patients by conventional and pulsed-field gel electrophoresis using gel inserts. *Cancer Genet. Cytogenet.* **42,** 287–294.

100. Min, G. L., Martiat, P., Pu, G. A., and Goldman, J. (1990) Use of pulsed field gel electrophoresis to characterize BCR gene involvement in CML patients lacking M-BCR rearrangement. *Leukemia* **4,** 650–656.
101. Preudhomme, C., Chams-Eddine, L., Roumier, C., Duflos-Grardel, N., Denis, C., Cosson, A., and Fenaux, P. (1999) Detection of BCR-ABL transcripts in chronic myeloid leukemia (CML) using an *in situ* RT-PCR assay. *Leukemia* **13,** 818–823.
102. Testoni, N., Martinelli, G., Farabegoli, P., Zaccaria, A., Amabile, M., Raspadori, D., et al. (1996) A new method of "in-cell reverse transcriptase-polymerase chain reaction" for the detection of BCR/ABL transcripts in chronic myeloid leukemia patients. *Blood* **87,** 3822–3827.
103. Cross, N. C. P., Hughes, T. P., Feng, L., O'Shea, P., Bungey, J., Marks, D. I., et al. (1993) Minimal residual disease after allogeneic bone marrow transplantation for chronic myeloid leukaemia in first chronic phase: correlations with acute graft-versus-host disease and relapse. *Br. J. Haematol.* **84,** 67–74.
104. Slade, M. J., Smith, B. M., Sinnett, H. D., Cross, N. C. P., and Coombes, R. C. (1999) Quantitative polymerase chain reaction for the detection of micrometastases in patients with breast cancer. *J. Clin. Oncol.* **17,** 870–879.
105. Lion, T. (1994) Clinical implications of qualitative and quantitative polymerase chain reaction analysis in the monitoring of patients with chronic myelogenous leukemia. The European Investigators on Chronic Myeloid Leukemia Group. *Bone Marrow Transplant.* **14,** 505–509.

7

Detection of t(2;5)(p23;q35) Translocation by Long-Range PCR of Genomic DNA

Yunfang Jiang, L. Jeffrey Medeiros, and Andreas H. Sarris

1. Introduction

Many types of human leukemias and lymphomas are associated with specific chromosomal translocations that correlate with specific histologic and immunologic phenotypes (1). Anaplastic large-cell lymphoma (ALCL) of T-cell or null-cell lineage is a clinically aggressive non-Hogkins lymphoma of which a large subset of cases carry the t(2;5)(p23;q35) translocation. Molecular cloning of the breakpoints has revealed that this translocation fuses the nucleophosmin (*NPM*) gene on chromosome 5q35 with a protein kinase gene (anaplastic lymphoma kinase [*ALK*]) on chromosome 2p23. This results in the formation of a fusion protein with the N-terminal sequence derived from the *NPM* gene and the C-terminal cytoplasmic sequences from the *ALK* gene, including the consensus protein tyrosine kinase residues (2). Studies of the t(2;5) in ALCL using restriction fragment length analysis demonstrated clustering of the breakpoints. More detailed analysis revealed that the translocation occurs on variable locations in both chromosomes. These are located within the same introns of both genes in essentially all patients (3). Consequently, the translocation does not alter the reading frames of both derivative chromosomes, and the fusion mRNAs and proteins are identical in most translocations.

Reverse transcriptase polymerase chain reaction (RT-PCR) has detected the NPM-ALK translocation in up to 50% of ALCL cases. A long-range genomic PCR assay (3) has been developed that utilizes genomic DNAs as templates, 5'-primers derived from the *NPM* gene, and 3'-primers derived from the *ALK* gene. There are two advantages of this PCR assay over RT-PCR. First, long-range genomic PCR generates unique amplicons for each patient, in contrast to RT-PCR, which generates identical amplicons for NPM-ALK fusion transcripts (4). Thus,

From: *Methods in Molecular Medicine, vol. 68: Molecular Analysis of Cancer*
Edited by: J. Boultwood and C. Fidler © Humana Press Inc., Totowa, NJ

RT-PCR cannot exclude false positive reactions arising from sample cross-contamination. Second, long-range genomic PCR allows one to avoid extra glassware, reagents, and procedures necessary for the preparation of RNA.

The long-range PCR of genomic DNA to detect t(2;5) uses several strategies: first, a nested technique with two sets of NPM and ALK primers; second, a pair of β-globin primers to amplify a 3016-bp fragment of the β-globin gene to verify the presence of large-size amplifiable DNA; third, Southern blot hybridization with a radioactive-labeled NPM-ALK junction probe to verify the specificity of PCR products; fourth, DNA sequencing to confirm the difference in size between amplicons and the uniqueness of their breakpoint sequences. From our studies on primary ALCL tumors and t(2;5)-positive cell lines derived from tumor tissues *(5–9)*, we have demostrated that the long-range genomic PCR generates NPM-ALK amplicons varying from a few hundred base pairs to more than 2000 bp that are unique to each patient and each cell line. The sensitivity of the method has been determined by a serial dilution $(10^{-1}–10^{-5})$ of t(2;5)-positive cell line DNA into normal genomic DNA followed by nested PCR plus Southern hybridization. From our observation, 100% or 20% positive signals were generated in the dilutions of 10^{-4} (6–8 genomes/reaction) or 10^{-5} (0.6–0.8 genomes/reaction), and Southern signal is at least 10-fold stronger than that of ethidium bromide staining. Direct DNA sequencing has mapped the breakpoints in unique positive t(2;5) cell lines and patients *(9)*.

2. Materials

2.1. Computer Resources

A computer with an Internet connection running World Wide Web software, such as Netscape or Internet Explorer, is necessary for sequence blast and primer design.

2.2. Cells and Patient Samples

1. SUP-M2, SU-DHL-1, and UCONN-L2 carrying the t(2;5)(p23;q35) translocation were used as positive controls and were obtained from Dr. Stephen Morris at St. Jude Children's Research Hospital *(2,10,11)*.
2. Human DNA obtained from nonneoplastic tissue was used as a negative control and was used to serially dilute the t(2;5) cell line DNA in order to keep the amount of total DNA at 0.5 µg in every reaction.
3. Fresh or frozen samples of ALCL tumors for DNA extraction from M. D. Anderson Cancer Center.

2.3. Preparation of Genomic DNA, PCR Reagents, and Equipment

1. Primers (*see* **Note 1**): Two pairs of specific primers are used for detection of the *NPM-ALK* fusion: the 5'-end primers (outer and inner) derived from the *NPM*

Long-Range PCR for t(2;5)

Table 1
Oligonucleotide Primers Used in Amplification of Genomic DNA and Southern Blots (*see* Note 2)

Name	Sequence	Locus	Ref.
NPM-A	5'-TCC CTT GGG GGC TTT GAA ATA ACA CC-3'	NPM (outer)	*(2)*
ALK-A	5'-CGA GGT GCG GAG CTT GCT CAG C-3'	ALK (outer)	*(2)*
NPM-B	5'-ACC AGT GGT CTT AAG GTT GA-3'	NPM (inner)	*(3)*
ALK-B	5'-TTG TAC TCA GGG CTC TGC A-3'	ALK (inner)	*(3)*
5'-Globin	5'-GAA GAG CCA AGG ACA GGT AC-3'	β-Globin	*(5)*
3'-Globin	5'-GTT TGA TGT AGC CTC ACT TC-3'	β-Globin	*(5)*
NPM probe	5'-AGT GTG GTT CAG GGC CAG TG-3'	NPM	
ALK probe	5'-GCT CCA TCT GCA TGG CTT GC-3'	ALK	

gene and the 3'-end primers (outer and inner) from the *ALK* gene *(3)* (*see* **Table 1**). The primers from the β-globin locus are used in separate tubes as a control for the presence of adequate DNA. *NPM* or *ALK* probe is labeled with radioactive P[32] and is used in Southern blot hybridization.

2. Wizard genomic DNA purification kit for genomic DNA extraction (Promega, Madison, WI).
3. PCR tubes (0.5-mL thin-walled) (Perkin-Elmer Applied Biosystems, Foster City, CA).
4. AmpliTaq DNA polymerase, 10X PCR buffer (10 m*M* Tris-HCl, pH 8.3, 50 m*M* KCl), 25 m*M* magnesium, 10 m*M* of each dNTP (Perkin-Elmer). Store at –20°C.
5. Spectrophotometer for DNA quantitation (Beckman, Fullerton, CA).
6. Model 392 Applied Biosystems DNA/RNA Synthesizer for synthesis of all oligonucleotide primers synthesis (Perkin-Elmer). Primers are stored at –20°C.
7. 9600 Thermal cycler (Perkin-Elmer).
8. Model 373A automated DNA sequencer, Amplitaq cycle sequencing kit, and fluorescence-labeled dideoxy termination (Perkin-Elmer).

2.4. Gel Electrophoresis

1. Agarose, ultrapure (Life Technologies, Gaithersburg, MD).
2. 50X TAE buffer: 40 m*M* Tris-acetate, 1 m*M* EDTA (Fisher, Pittsburgh, PA).
3. 10X DNA loading buffer: 20% Ficoll-400, 100 m*M* EDTA (pH 8.0), 1% sodium dodecyl sulfate (SDS), 0.25% bromophenol blue, and 0.25% xylene cyanol.
4. *Hae*III-digested φX174 DNA molecular weight markers (Life Technologies).

2.5. Radioactive Southern Blots

1. 2.5 *M* HCl: stock solution.
2. 4 *M* NaOH: stock solution.
3. 20X SSPE buffer: 150 m*M* NaCl, 10 m*M* NaH$_2$PO$_4$, 1 m*M* EDTA, pH 7.4. This may be purchased (Fisher).

100   *Jiang et al.*

4. 10% (w/v) SDS (ultrapure) (Life Technologies): stock solution.
5. Sonicated salmon sperm DNA (10 mg/mL) (Life Technologies).
6. 50X Denhardt's solution: 2% (w/v) bovine serum albumin, 2% (w/v) Ficoll™, 2% (w/v) polyvinylpyrrolidone: stock solution.
7. Hybridization solution: 5X SSPE, 5X Denhardt's solution, 0.5% SDS, and 50 µg/mL sonicated salmon sperm DNA.
8. $[\gamma\text{-}^{32}\text{P}]$ATP (10 µCi/µL, 3000 Ci/mM) (Amersham Pharmacia Biotech, Piscataway, NJ).
9. T4 polynucleotide kinase (Life Technologies).
10. Hybond-N+ membrane (Amersham Pharmacia Biotech).
11. Whatman 3MM filter paper (Fisher).
12. Glass hybridization tubes (Fisher).
13. Rolling bottle hybridization oven (Fisher).
14. Saran Wrap (Fisher).
15. X-Ray film (X-OMAT™AR) (Eastman Kodak, Rochester, NY).
16. Film cassette (Eastman Kodak).

3. Methods

3.1. DNA Preparation

1. Genomic DNAs from human tissue or peripheral blood or bone marrow are extracted by using genomic DNA purification kit (*see* **Note 3**).
2. Quantitate genomic DNAs with a spectophotometer at 260 nm (1 A_{260} unit of double-stranded DNA = 50 µg/mL).
3. Dilute each concentrated DNA template to a final working concentration of 0.1 µg/µL. We assume that 1 µg of DNA = 120,000–160,000 cells *(5)*.

3.2. Serial Dilution of t(2;5) Cell Line DNA

Normal human genomic DNA is extracted from peripheral blood mononuclear cells of normal donors. The t(2;5) translocation in normal DNA is not detectable by long-range PCR *(7)*. Genomic DNA from the t(2;5)-positive cell line (SUP-M2) is diluted into normal genomic DNA in a range of 10^{-1}–10^{-5}, and a constant amount of 0.5 µg of total DNA is used for PCR amplification to determine the sensitivity of the method.

3.3. Long-Range Genomic DNA PCR

The long-range genomic DNA PCR takes place in two rounds to ensure maximum yield of specific and full-length fragments (*see* **Note 4**). In each round of reaction, blank PCR reactions without the addition of DNA templates, negative human DNA obtained from nonneoplastic tissue, DNA from t(2;5)(p23;q35)-positive cell lines, and a separate control tube for DNA integrity (β-globin, *see* **Note 5**) are simultaneously run to exclude cross-contamination and the presence of amplifiable long templates.

Long-Range PCR for t(2;5)

3.3.1. First-Round PCR

The outer NPM-A and ALK-A primers (*see* **Note 6**) are used in the first-round PCR.

1. Make a set of 0.5-mL thin-walled PCR tubes with first-round PCR date and numbers (*see* **Note 7**).
2. Carry out the PCR reaction in a final volume of 50 µL containing 0.5 µg of genomic DNA, 1X PCR buffer, 1.5 mM MgCl$_2$, 250 µM dNTP, and 50 ng of each primer.
3. Transfer the reaction tubes to the thermal cycler preheated to 80°C and incubate for 5 min (*see* **Note 8**).
4. Add in each tube 1.5 U of AmpliTaq DNA polymerase (*see* **Note 9**) and mix well.
5. After hot starting with the enzyme, run the continuous cycling as follows: 92°C for 1 min; 35 cycles of 92°C for 40 s, 64°C for 1 min, and 72°C for 4 min; 72°C for 10 min.
6. Once PCR is completed, store the PCR products at 4°C.

3.3.2. Second-Round PCR

The inner NPM-B and ALK-B primers are used for amplification in the second round of PCR (nested PCR) as follows:

1. Make a set of 0.5-mL thin-walled PCR tubes with the nested PCR date and numbers that correspond to the numbers of first-round PCR.
2. Carry out the PCR reaction in a final volume of 50 µL containing 1 µL of initial PCR product, 1X PCR buffer, 1.5 mM MgCl$_2$, 250 µM dNTP, and 50 ng of each primer.
3. Transfer the reaction tubes to a thermal cycler preheated to 80°C and incubate for 5 min.
4. Add in each tube 1.5 U of AmpliTaq DNA polymerase and mix well.
5. Run the nested PCR cycling as follows: 92°C for 1 min; 20 cycles of 92°C for 40 s, 54°C for 1 min, 72°C for 3 min; 72°C for 10 min.
6. Store the PCR products at 4°C for further analysis.

3.4. Exclusion of Artifacts

To exclude the possibilities of false annealing of primers or cross-contamination, gel electrophoresis and Southern blot hybridization are performed as follows:

3.4.1. Gel Electrophoresis

Eighteen microliters of amplified PCR products, including positive and negative cell lines, β-globin, and ALCL DNA-amplified products, as well as 0.5 µg of *Hae*III-digested φX174 DNA marker are size-fractionated on 0.8% TAE-agarose gel containing 0.1 µg/mL of ethidium bromide and photographed under ultraviolet (UV) light.

3.4.2. Radioactive Southern Blot Hybridization (see **Note 10**)

3.4.2.1. DNA TRANSFER TO MEMBRANE

1. After photography, incubate the gel in 0.25 M HCl for 10 min, and then briefly rinse in distilled water.
2. Denature the gel with 0.4 M NaOH for 15 min, and transfer directly with the same solution onto a Hybond-N+ membrane overnight.
3. Neutralize the membrane in 6X SSPE for 5 min, and then air-dry.

3.4.2.2. PROBE LABELING (*SEE* **NOTE 11**)

1. Carry out the labeling reaction in a total volume of 25 µL of containing 5 pmol of oligonucleotide, 1X forward reaction buffer, 10 U T4 polynucleotide kinase, and 25 µCi [γ-^{32}P]ATP.
2. Incubate the mixture at 37°C for 30 min.
3. Stop the reaction by heating at 65°C for 10 min.

3.4.2.3. DNA HYBRIDIZATION

Prehybridization, hybridization, and washes are performed in glass tubes in a rolling bottle hybridization oven.

1. Prehybridize the membrane in 10 mL of hybridization solution at 42°C for at least 1 h.
2. Pour off the prehybridization solution, add T4 kinase-labeled NPM-ALK junction probe into 5 mL of fresh hybridization solution, mix well, and hybridize the membrane at 42ºC overnight.
3. Following hybridization, wash the membrane two times in 2X SSPE, 0.1% SDS at 37°C for 10 min.
4. Replace the solution with 0.1X SSPE, 0.1% SDS for 10 min × 2 at room temperature.
5. Air-dry the membranes, wrap in plastic wrap, place in a film cassette with an intensifying screen, and expose to an X-ray film (*see* **Note 12**) at –70°C for 30 min or longer for optimal signals.

3.4.3. DNA Sequencing

Positive PCR amplicons can be directly sequenced for determination of breakpoints by using the amplification primers (*see* **Note 13**) with an automated DNA sequencer.

4. Notes

1. Several Web-based softwares are available for primer design, such as Oligo analyzer 2.0 from Integrated DNA Technologies (www.idtdna.com), PrimerExpress 1.0 from Perkin-Elmer (www.appliedbiosystems.com), Primer3 (www.genome.wi.mit.edu).
2. Error correction: Primer names and sequences fir ALK-S (5'-ACC AGT GTT CTT AAG GTT GA-3', ALK) and NPM-B (5'-CGA GGT GCG GAG CTT GCT CAG C-3', NPM) are switched owing to typographical errors in the publications of Sarris et al. *(5,6)*. They have been corrected in this chapter (**Table 1**).

Long-Range PCR for t(2;5) 103

3. For DNA extraction from fresh tumors, it is recommended that the tissue be kept on ice between the time of excision and the time of extraction. Since ALCL often involves the lymph node sinuses only focally, the extraction should use as much tissue as possible.

4. Watch closely for cross-contamination: sample to sample or PCR product to template, or PCR product to reagents or template to reagents. Physically separate the individual parts of the DNA extraction from the pre-PCR preparation, and from the post-PCR analysis. Also separate the PCR area from the molecular cloning area. Use UV light in all types of contamination. Always include blank and negative controls alongside each set of PCR reactions.

5. β-globin primers have been introduced into long-range genomic DNA PCR as a size control for DNA templates tested in separate reaction tubes. They can also serve as internal control for template quality and quantity in the same reaction tube with the NPM and ALK primers (multiplex PCR) to exclude false negatives owing to reaction failure in a particular tube. However, as more primer pairs are included, additional adjustments of the PCR conditions are needed. For example, primer positions, primer sequences, primer concentrations, relative size of the amplicons, and reaction kinetics need to be adjusted to maintain maximum sensitivity.

6. Basic purification with desalting for primers, which removes organic salts, residual synthesis reagents, and very short oligonucleotide truncation products, is sufficient for routine PCR. However, simple desalting does not remove all impurities. Some amount of truncated oligonucleotides is always present, and the relative proportion of undesired truncated material increases as oligonucleotide length increases. It is recommended that for oligonucleotides >40 bases in length be further purified. Methods to accomplish this include denaturing acrylamide/urea gels (polyacrylamide gel electrophoresis), or high-performance liquid chromatography purification. For maximum sensitivity, we recommend that all primers be purified.

7. Make a master mixture for PCR reagents to avoid tube-to-tube variation. To avoid cross-contamination, add the master mix first and then the templates into reaction tubes in the following order: blank, negative controls, patient samples, to positive controls. For sensitivity assays, the order of adding templates should be from lower to higher concentrations.

8. An alternative hot-start method is suggested to simplify PCR preparation. *Taq* enzyme can be added into a master mixture at the beginning, prepare all reactions on ice ready to run. Preheat the themal cycler to 90°C and hold, then load the reaction tubes, and start the PCR cycles. This technique can reduce nonspecific amplification and avoid variation of the amount of *Taq* added to each reaction tube. The use of a master mixture can save time in the preparation of a large number of PCR reactions.

9. In our experiments, AmpliTaq DNA polymerase is sufficient to amplify fragments as large as 2.5 kb. For longer templates, other enzymes are available, such as rthDNA polymerase, XL (Perkin-Elmer) or Expand Long Template PCR system (Boehringer Mannheim).

10. Alternatively, one can use the nonradioactive Southern analysis system, the Gene Images AlkPhos generation and detection system (Amersham Pharmacia Biotech) with high sensitivity (10^{-5} μg of DNA; Jiang, Y. F., personal communication) and specificity. The use of this system will avoid the need of a special area and conditions for radioactive labeling and detection.
11. The *NPM-ALK* junction probe (5'-AGC ACT TAG TAG TGT ACC GCC GGA-3') used initially by us *(5)* for Southern blot hybridization was designed for detection of fusion transcripts after RT-PCR and contains coding sequences from both NPM and ALK loci. However, it may not be optimal for detection of all genomic fusion amplicons because the translocation point is in a noncoding region of both genes *(3)*. New NPM and ALK probes have been designed and are given in this chapter to detect genomic DNA PCR products. Their sequences are located downstream of NPM-B and ALK-B, respectively, and are designated as NPM and ALK probes, respectively (**Table 1**).
12. An alternative to traditional autoradiography with X-ray film is Gel Doc 2000 Gel Documentation System (Bio-Rad, Hercules, CA). This system uses a CCD camera to capture and store images electronically. These data subsequently can be handed with image analysis software, such as Adobe Photoshop#5.5 (Adobe Systems, San Jose, CA) to prepare figures for publication and presentation.
13. The PCR amplification primers can be used as sequencing primers. For longer amplicons (>800 bp), additional internal primers can be designed on the basis of the deduced sequences.

References

1. Rowley, J. D. (1984) Biological implications of consistent chromosome rearrangements in leukemia and lymphoma. *Cancer Res.* **44,** 3159–3168.
2. Morris, S. W., Kirstein, M. N., Valentine, M. B., Dittmer, K. G., Shapiro, D. N., and Saltman, D. L. (1994), Look AT: fusion of a kinase gene, ALK, to a nuclear protein gene, NPM, in non-Hodgkin's lymphoma. *Science* **263,** 1281–1284.
3. Waggott, W., Lo, Y. M., Bastard, C., Gatter, K. C., Leroux, D., Mason, D. Y., et al. (1995) Detection of NPM-ALK DNA rearrangement in CD30 positive anaplastic large cell lymphoma. *Br. J. Haematol.* **89,** 905–907.
4. Downing, J. R., Shurtleff, S. A., Zielenska, M., Curcio-Brint, A. M., Behm, F. G., Head, D. R., et al. (1995) Molecular detection of the (2;5) translocation of non-Hodgkin's lymphoma by reverse transcriptase-polymerase chain reaction. *Blood* **15,** 3416–3422.
5. Sarris, A. H., Luthra, R., Papadimitracopoulou, V., Waasdorp, M., Dimopoulos, M. A., McBride, J. A., et al. (1996) Amplification of genomic DNA demonstrates the presence of the t(2;5) (p23;q35) in anaplastic large cell lymphoma, but not in other non-Hodgkin's lymphomas, Hodgkin's disease, or lymphomatoid papulosis. *Blood* **1,** 1771–1779.
6. Sarris, A. H., Luthra, R., Papadimitracopoulou, V., Waasdorp, M., Dimopoulos, M. A., McBride, J. A., et al. (1997) Long-range amplification of genomic DNA detects the t(2;5)(p23;q35) in anaplastic large-cell lymphoma, but not in other non-

Hodgkin's lymphomas, Hodgkin's disease, or lymphomatoid papulosis. *Ann. Oncol.* **8(Suppl. 2),** 59–63.

7. Sarris, A. H., Luthra, R., Kliche, K. O., McBride, J. A., Andreeff, M., and Cabanillas, F. (1997) The t(2;5)(p23;q35) is not detectable in normal donor peripheral blood mononuclear cells by polymerase chain reaction amplification (PCR) of genomic DNA. *Blood* **90(Suppl. 1),** 335a.

8. Sarris, A. H., Luthra, R., Cabanillas, F., Morris, S. W., and Pugh, W. C. (1998) Genomic DNA amplification and the detection of t(2;5)(p23;q35) in lymphoid neoplasms. *Leuk. Lymphoma* **29,** 507–514.

9. Luthra, R., Pugh, W. C., Waasdorp, M., Morris, W., Cabanillas, F., Chan, P. K., and Sarris, A. H. (1998) Mapping of genomic t(2;5)(p23;q35) breakpoints in patients with anaplastic large cell lymphoma by sequencing long-range PCR products. *Hematopathol. Mol. Hematol.* **11,** 173–183.

10. Morgan, R., Smith, S. D., Hecht, B. K., Christy, V., Mellentin, J. D., Warnke, R., and Cleary, M. L. (1989) Lack of involvement of the c-fms and N-myc genes by chromosomal translocation t(2;5)(p23;q35) common to malignancies with features of so-called malignant histiocytosis. *Blood* **73,** 2155–2164.

11. Fischer, P., Nacheva, E., Mason, D. Y., Sherrington, P. D., Hoyle, C., Hayhoe, F. G., and Karpas, A. (1988) A Ki-1 (CD30)-positive human cell line (Karpas 299) established from a high-grade non-Hodgkin's lymphoma, showing a 2;5 translocation and rearrangement of the T-cell receptor beta-chain gene. *Blood* **72,** 234–240.

8

Use of DNA Fingerprinting to Detect Genetic Rearrangements in Human Cancer

Vorapan Sirivatanauksorn, Yongyut Sirivatanauksorn, Arthur B. McKie, and Nicholas R. Lemoine

1. Introduction

The polymerase chain reaction (PCR) has revolutionized the isolation and analysis of nucleic acid fragments from a wide variety of sources. PCR-based methods for nucleic acid detection and fingerprinting have become vital to modern molecular genetics, whether for the analysis of populations of organisms to determine population structure of an ecosystem, sampling a set of DNA sequences to infer evolutionary history, sampling genetic loci to build a map, or sampling differentially expressed genes to identify phenotypic markers. PCR can be used to generate high resolution genetic maps of human and comparative genomes. Compared with Southern blot analysis, which detects restriction fragment length polymorphisms (RFLPs) and hypervariable minisatellite loci, PCR is faster, less labor-intensive, less expensive, and requires relatively small amounts of DNA. Additionally, PCR may be a more practical approach for large-scale mapping projects.

The classic approach to DNA fingerprinting utilizes variable number tandem repeat (VNTR) polymorphism in which alleles differ by a variable number of tandem repeats. Although the term *VNTR* could, in theory, encompass a wide range of repeat lengths, in practice the term is usually reserved for moderately large arrays of a repeat unit that is typically in the 5- to 64-bp region. If the VNTR locus is a member of a repeated DNA family, the use of a VNTR probe will produce a complex polymorphic band pattern on hybridization. The hybridizing bands appear on the filter as a ladder of bands, referred to as the *DNA fingerprint*, which visually resembles the bar-codes used by stores to identify and price merchandise.

From: *Methods in Molecular Medicine, vol. 68: Molecular Analysis of Cancer*
Edited by: J. Boultwood and C. Fidler © Humana Press Inc., Totowa, NJ

1.1. Arbitrarily Primed PCR

The arbitrary primer-based DNA amplification technique recently has been proposed as an alternative targeting tool for genetic typing and mapping. This strategy uses randomly generated primers to initiate amplification of discrete but arbitrary portions of the genome. It has been called by a plethora of terms such as random amplified polymorphic DNA *(1)*, DNA amplification fingerprinting *(2)*, multiple arbitrarily amplicon profiling *(3)*, and arbitrarily primed PCR (AP-PCR) *(4)*.

AP-PCR is one of the fingerprinting techniques described by Welsh and McClelland in 1990 *(4)*. It was originally used to distinguish strains of *Staphylococcus* sp. and *Streptococcus* sp. by comparing polymorphisms in AP-PCR genomic fingerprints using PCR-length primers (18–32 nucleotides). This technique is a modification of PCR, a method that is widely used to copy sections of DNA for identifying gene structure or matching tissue specimens. PCR conventionally uses two primers whose complementary sequences flank the desired sequence to amplify a region of DNA. The primers usually have specific nucleotide sequences that bind to previously identified segments of DNA. They bind to specific sites on opposing strands of the double-stranded DNA and, with successive cycles of PCR, make millions of copies of the intervening stretch of DNA. Normally, the primers are annealed to the template DNA at relatively high stringency. High stringency during the primer-annealing step ensures that the primers do not interact with the template DNA at positions where they do not match completely.

By contrast, AP-PCR allows the detection of polymorphisms without prior knowledge of nucleotide sequence. It is based on the selective amplification of genomic sequences that, by chance, are flanked by adequate matches to an arbitrarily chosen primer. The method utilizes short primers of arbitrary nucleotide sequence (10–20 bases) that are annealed in the first few cycles of PCR at low stringency. The low stringency of the early cycles ensures the generation of products by allowing priming with fortuitous matches or near matches between primers and template. This approach results in a high number of products having the original primer sequence at both ends. After a few low-stringency cycles, the annealing temperature is raised and the reaction is allowed to continue under standard, high-stringency PCR conditions. This step will amplify a discrete number of sequences among those initially targeted and permits the unbiased analysis of the cell genome. Alternatively, an intermediate stringency primer-annealing step may be used throughout the PCR to achieve the same outcome. AP-PCR products are resolved on polyacrylamide gels and detected by autoradiography. If two template genomic DNA sequences are different, their AP-PCR products display different banding patterns. Such differ-

DNA Fingerprinting in Human Cancer

109

ences can be exploited in ways largely analogous to the uses of RFLP, including genetic mapping, taxonomy, phylogenetics, and the detection of mutations.

AP-PCR has three advantages when compared with classic DNA fingerprinting. First, minor amounts of template DNA are sufficient for analysis (50 ng of genomic DNA for AP-PCR vs 5–10 µg for Southern blotting). Second, somatic mutations detected in tumor fingerprints can, by chance, directly reflect a mutation in a coding sequence. Third, the possibility of reamplification, cloning, and sequencing of polymorphic bands enables the rapid identification of the sequences probably linked to tumor progression.

1.2. The Applications of AP-PCR

Because no laborious cloning, nucleotide sequencing, or Southern blot hybridization is required, AP-PCR permits the rapid and cost-effective detection of polymorphisms and genetic markers in a variety of plants and animals. The most frequent use of AP-PCR has been for the detection of dominant polymorphic markers in genetic mapping experiments (1). Welsh and McClelland (5) applied the technique of AP-PCR to genetic mapping in the mouse. They noted that AP-PCR is, in many respects, dramatically easier and faster than established methods for genetic mapping. Polymorphisms detected by AP-PCR also can be used as taxonomic markers in population studies of a wide variety of organisms (6). It has been applied extensively in plant breeding studies and in the differentiation of the strains of microorganisms (7). DNA fingerprinting of different strains has shown polymorphic sequences that can be used to identify the different genomes.

The reproducible and semiquantitative amplification of multiple sequences provides a powerful tool to study somatic genetic alterations in tumorigenesis. Peinado et al. (8) showed the ability of AP-PCR to detect both qualitatively and quantitatively and to isolate, in a single step, DNA sequences representing two of the genetic alterations that underlie the aneuploidy of colorectal cancer cells: losses of heterozygosity and chromosomal gains. Moreover, they confirmed that AP-PCR could yield information on the overall chromosomal composition of the cell. The intensities of the bands derived from single-copy sequences were proportional to the concentration of the target sequences. The outstanding result using AP-PCR fingerprinting in the field of cancer research was the discovery of the microsatellite mutator phenotype mechanism for carcinogenesis in sporadic and hereditary colon cancers (9). AP-PCR is also useful for the detection and isolation of DNA sequences to levels well below the minimum levels required by other available methods (10), and the products can be used to clone or hybridize back to digested genomic DNA (11). In addition, AP-PCR can be applied to RNA to detect differentially expressed genes in a technique called RNA-AP-PCR (12).

1.3. Interspersed Repetitive Element PCR (Alu-PCR) DNA Fingerprinting

A major limitation of the standard PCR regime is that it allows amplification of a DNA sequence flanked between two convergent primers, each of which primes DNA chain extension in the direction of the other primer. Often, however, it is desirable to be able to access uncharacterized DNA sequences flanking a region for which sequence information is available. Interspersed repetitive element (IRE)-based PCR strategies have been used as a tool since 1989 *(13)*, and, they have had a major impact on human genome research.

Developed mainly around the primate-specific, simple-interspersed, nuclear-repeat element Alu, IRE-PCR has made it possible to amplify human genomic sequences from complex mixtures such as that encountered with a monochromosomal somatic cell hybrid. This application has now encompassed analysis and screening of large cloned DNA fragments such as yeast artificial chromosomes and bacterial atificial chromosomes.

Employing primers specific for the Alu repeat element was seen as an alternative to using arbitrarily designed 10-mers. The mammalian genome contains approx 10^6 copies of the Alu repeat element representing 7% of the total DNA per cell. The highly ubiquitous distribution of the Alu repeat means that the coverage of the genome afforded by Alu sequence-primed amplification could potentially be of high resolution. Additionally, rearrangements of genes at translocation breakpoints and recombination "hot spots" often have been often attributable to interspersed DNA elements.

By using the restriction enzymes to predigest the genomic template in this approach, it is analogous to the preparation of "representations" of the tester DNA by PCR in representational difference analysis. Both approaches are necessary to define a subpopulation of fragments that may be more readily analyzed. Additionally, varying the restriction enzyme used in the predigestion defined the spectrum of band sizes obtained in subsequent amplifications with the same Alu-specific primer. Therefore, we have two variable parameters to achieve multiple fingerprint profiles from the same DNA samples if we also apply primers specific to different regions of the Alu repeat element.

Our group applied the Alu-PCR fingerprinting technique to DNA from pancreatic cancer and paired normal samples to isolate and identify fragments of genomic DNA rearranged in malignant cells *(14)*. Abnormalities were detectable in about 8.5% of the genomic fragments sampled in this analysis. Clearly, only a fraction of the genome is sampled in each Alu primer/restriction digest combination, and some are more useful than others. Because the digests use a single primer in the PCR reaction, only sequences lying between repeats in inverted orientation to one another will be amplified, and because their orientation is essentially random, this could result in about 30% of the inter-Alu sequences being potential templates in each case. Like the alternative genome-scanning technique of respresentational difference analysis, there is a bias toward the generation of smaller fragments, partly owing to the predigestion of the template DNA and partly because of the kinetics of PCR amplification. However, these are tags that enable the subsequent isolation of larger rearranged fragments by hybridization.

1.4. Alu-PCR: Advantageous in Screening for Tumor-Specific Lesions

Because Alu repeats contain runs of deoxyadenosine residues, they are often involved as targets for such ubiquitous somatic mutations, so that about one-third have deletion mutations in replication error phenotype (RER^+) cancers *(9)*. Interestingly, Alu repeats can even be involved in the genesis of inactivating mutations; for instance, one of the most common germline mutations in the DNA mismatch repair gene *MLH1* is a 3.5-kb genomic deletion that appears to result from Alu-mediated recombination *(15)*. Alu elements are also involved in the production of oncogenes as a result of chromosomal translocation events joining the *BCR* and *ABL* loci and the *LCK* and *TCRB* loci *(16,17)*. Hence, the approach of using Alu sequences as the priming sites for the amplification of fingerprints from genomic DNA may have an advantage compared to AP-PCR if such regions are particularly affected by the cancer-associated rearrangements. However, it is likely that most rearrangements at repeat sequences are not significant to tumorigenesis. It may be possible to exploit other high-abundance repetitive elements in the human genome to similar ends, such as the L1 and MER families *(18,19)*.

In conclusion, the Alu-specific PCR genomic fingerprinting technique allows the scanning of the human genome for genetic rearrangements associated with a cancer phenotype. With the generation of sequence tags for these rearrangements, their use as molecular probes may facilitate the isolation of gene sequences involved. Further analysis of such genes associated with these rearrangements may lead to the mutational mechanism and its contribution to the molecular pathology of cancers.

2. Materials

2.1. Arbitrarily Primed PCR

1. Thermocycler (e.g., Peltier Thermal Cycler, model PTC-100™).
2. Sequencing gel electrophoresis apparatus (40 cm long, 30 cm wide, 0.4 mm thick).
3. Gel dryer.
4. X-Ray film and exposure cassette.
5. Stocks of all four dNTPs (5 mM).

112 Sirivatanauksorn et al.

6. Stock of arbitrary primer (100 μM).
7. Radioisotope ([α-^{32}P] or [γ-^{33}P]) dATP (>2500 Ci/mmol).
8. *Taq* polymerase (5 U/μL).
9. Formamide dye solution: 96% formamide, 0.1% bromophenol blue, 0.1% xylene cyanol, 10 mM EDTA.
10. 10X Tris-borate-EDTA (TBE) buffer: 90 mM Tris-borate, 20 mM Na$_2$EDTA, pH 8.3.
11. Acrylamide stock solution (40% acrylamide:*bis*-acrylamide [29:1]).

2.2. Alu-Polymerase Chain Reaction

1. Thermocycler (e.g., Peltier Thermal Cycler, model PTC-100™).
2. Sequencing gel electrophoresis apparatus (40 cm long, 30 cm wide, 0.4 mm thick).
3. Gel dryer.
4. X-Ray film and exposure cassette.
5. Stocks of all four dNTPs (5 mM).
6. Stock of Alu primer (100 μM).
7. (α-^{32}P) dATP (3000 Ci/mmol).
8. Restriction enzyme *Alu*I (8 U/μL).
9. *Taq* polymerase (5 U/μL).
10. Formamide dye solution: 96% formamide, 0.1% bromophenol blue, 0.1% xylene cyanol, 10 mM EDTA.
11. 10X TBE buffer: 90 mM Tris-borate, 20 mM Na$_2$EDTA, pH 8.3.
12. Acrylamide stock solution (40% acrylamide:*bis*-acrylamide [29:1]).

3. Methods
3.1. Arbitrarily Primed PCR

1. Mix template DNA (100–200 ng) with reaction mixture for a 25-μL final reaction containing arbitrary primer, 1 to 2 Ci of [α-^{32}P]dATP or [γ-^{33}P]dATP, 0.2 mM of each dNTP, 10 mM Tris-HCl, pH 9.2, 3.5 mM MgCl$_2$, 75 mM KCl, and 0.5 U of *Taq* polymerase in a final volume of 25 μL.
2. Perform thermocycling using 5 cycles of 94°C for 1 min, 45°C for 5 min, and 72°C for 5 min; then 35 cycles of 94°C for 1 min, 60°C for 1 min, 72°C for 2 min. Add a final chase cycle of 72°C for 5 min to allow complete elongation of all products.
3. Mix amplification products with 5 μL of formamide dye solution, denature at 95°C for 3 min, and load 5 μL onto a 8% nondenaturing acrylamide gel mix prepared in 1X TBE buffer. Perform electrophoresis using a sequencing apparatus at 12 W overnight.
4. After electrophoresis, transfer the gel to Whatman 3MM paper, and dry under vacuum.
5. Autoradiograph the dried gel using an X-ray film at room temperature for 12 h.

3.2. Alu Polymerase Chain Reaction

1. Perform restriction digests of DNA samples at 37°C overnight. Use 10 U of restriction enzyme *Alu*I in a 20-μL reaction volume containing 1–5 μg of DNA.

DNA Fingerprinting in Human Cancer

2. Standardize the conditions for PCR amplification as follows: 50 mM KCl, 10 mM Tris-HCl, pH 8.3, 1.5 mM MgCl$_2$, 0.1% Triton X-100, 0.2 mM dNTPs, 1 U of *Taq* polymerase in a 50-μL reaction volume. The Alu primer concentration is a little higher (at 2 μM) than normally used in an attempt to favor annealing of the primer to the repeat elements by displacing any rapidly forming duplexes in the template by virtue of this high concentration.

3. Perform thermocycling using 94°C for 3 min; then 10–15 cycles of 57°C for 30 s, 72°C for 1 min, 94°C for 45 s. Add a final chase cycle of 72°C for 5 min to allow complete elongation of all products.

4. Achieve radioactive labeling of PCR products by the addition of 1 to 2 Ci of [α-^{32}P]ATP (and the reduction of the unlabeled dATP in the buffer to 0.01 mM) followed by 20 more cycles of the above parameters.

5. Mix amplification products with 5 μL of formamide dye solution, denature at 95°C for 3 min, and load 5 μL onto a 6% nondenaturing acrylamide gel mix prepared in 1X TBE buffer. Perform electrophoresis using a sequencing apparatus at 12 W overnight.

6. After electrophoresis, mount the gel wet on a piece of old X-ray film or Whatman 3MM paper covered with Saran wrap™, and then expose to an X-ray film within a cassette at –70°C overnight.

References

1. Williams, J. G., Kubelik, A. R., Livak, K. J., Rafalski, J. A., and Tingey, S. V. (1990) DNA polymorphisms amplified by arbitrary primers are useful as genetic markers. *Nucleic Acids Res.* **18,** 6531–6535.

2. Caetano-Anolles, G., Bassam, B. J., and Gresshoff, P. M. (1991) DNA amplification fingerprinting using very short arbitrary oligonucleotide primers. *Biotechnology (NY)* **9,** 553–557.

3. Caetano-Anolles, G., Bassam, B. J., and Gresshoff, P. M. (1992) DNA fingerprinting: MAAPing out a RAPD redefinition? *Bio/Technology* **19,** 937.

4. Welsh, J. and McClelland, M. (1990) Fingerprinting genomes using PCR with arbitrary primers. *Nucleic Acids Res.* **18,** 7213–7218.

5. Welsh, J. and McClelland, M. (1991) Genomic fingerprinting using arbitrarily primed PCR and a matrix of pairwise combinations of primers. *Nucleic Acids Res.* **19,** 5275–5279.

6. Welsh, J., Pretzman, C., Postic, D., Saint Girons, I., Baranton, G., and McClelland, M. (1992) Genomic fingerprinting by arbitrarily primed polymerase chain reaction resolves Borrelia burgdorferi into three distinct phyletic groups. *Intl. J. Syst. Bacteriol.* **42,** 370–373.

7. Preus, H. R., Haraszthy, V. I., Zambon, J. J., and Genco, R. J. (1993) Differentiation of strains of Actinobacillus actinomycetemcomitans by arbitrarily primed polymerase chain reaction. *J. Clin. Microbiol.* **31,** 2773–2776.

8. Peinado, M. A., Malkhosyan, S., Velazquez, A., and Perucho, M. (1992) Isolation and characterisation of allelic losses and gains in colorectal tumors by arbitrarily primed polymerase chain reaction. *Proc. Natl. Acad. Sci. USA* **89,** 10,065–10,069.

9. Ionov, Y., Peinado, M. A., Malkhosyan, S., Shibata, D., and Perucho, M. (1993) Ubiquitous somatic mutations in simple repeated sequences reveal a new mechanism for colonic carcinogenesis. *Nature* **10,** 558–563.
10. Roninson, I. B., Chin, J. E., Choi, K. G., Gros, P., Housman, D. E., Fojo, A., et al. (1986) Isolation of human mdr DNA sequences amplified in multidrug-resistant KB carcinoma cells. *Proc. Natl. Acad. Sci. USA* **83,** 4538–4542.
11. Wesley, C. S., Ben, M., Kreitman, M., Hagag, N., and Eanes, W. F. (1990) Cloning regions of the Drosophila genome by microdissection of polytene chromosome DNA and PCR with nonspecific primer. *Nucleic Acids Res.* **18,** 599–603.
12. Welsh, J., Chada, K., Dalal, S. S., Cheng, R., Ralph, D., and McClelland, M. (1992) Arbitrarily primed PCR fingerprinting of RNA. *Nucleic Acids Res.* **20,** 4965–4970.
13. Nelson, D. L., Ledbetter, S. A., Corbo, L., Victoria, M. F., Ramirez-Solis, R., Webster, T. D., et al. (1989) Alu polymerase chain reaction: a method for rapid isolation of human-specific sequences from complex DNA sources. *Proc. Natl. Acad. Sci. USA* **86,** 6686–6690.
14. McKie, A. B., Iwamura, T., Leung, H. Y., Hollingsworth, M. A., and Lemoine, N. R. (1997) Alu-polymerase chain reaction genomic fingerprinting technique identifies multiple genetic loci associated with pancreatic tumourigenesis. *Genes Chrom. Cancer* **18,** 30–41.
15. Nystrom-Lahti, M., Kristo, P., Nicolaides, N. C., Chang, S. Y., Aaltonen, L.A., Moisio, A. L., et al. (1995) Founding mutations and Alu-mediated recombination in hereditary colon cancer. *Nat. Med.* **1,** 1203–1206.
16. Tycko, B., Smith, S. D., and Sklar, J. (1991) Chromosomal translocations joining LCK and TCRB loci in human T cell leukemia. *J. Exp. Med.* **174,** 867–873.
17. Chissoe, S. L., Bodenteich, A., Wang, Y. F., Wang, Y. P., Burian, D., Clifton, S. W., et al. (1995) Sequence and analysis of the human ABL gene, the BCR gene, and regions involved in the Philadelphia. *Genomics* **27,** 67–82.
18. Skowronski, J., Fanning, T. G., and Singer, M. F. (1988) Unit-length line-1 transcripts in human teratocarcinoma cells. *Mol. Cell. Biol.* **8,** 1385–1397.
19. Jurka, J. (1990) Novel families of interspersed repetitive elements from the human genome. *Nucleic Acids Res.* **18,** 137–141.

9

Mutation Analysis of Large Genomic Regions in Tumor DNA Using Single-Strand Conformation Polymorphism

Lessons from the ATM Gene

Igor Vorechovsky

1. Introduction

1.1. Detection of Point Mutations in Tumor DNA

In recent years, we have seen a dramatic improvement in our ability to detect nucleotide changes in tumor DNA using a number of techniques for mutation detection that have become routine instruments in many laboratories. The choice of a suitable method or methods of mutation analysis is governed by many factors, including the costs, experimental sensitivity, expected mutation pattern in the target sequence and its functional consequences, as well as staff expertise, personal experience, and preference. The primary selection criterion for such a method is the ability of a technique to search for the presence of unknown mutations in the analyzed regions (scanning methods) as opposed to looking for known mutations already characterized at the nucleotide level. Scanning procedures represent a cost-effective alternative to nucleotide sequencing (*see* Chapter 13), but usually at a price of an inferior detection rate. The former group of techniques includes procedures based on conformation polymorphism changes, denaturing gradient gel electrophoresis (*see* Chapter 10), constant denaturant capillary electrophoresis, and mismatch repair and RNase cleavage methods (*see* Chapter 11). The latter group, exemplified by techniques using sequence-specific oligonucleotides, oligonucleotide liagation assay, and ligase chain reaction (*1*), is less frequently used for analyzing molecular changes in tumor samples. A wise choice of most appropriate procedures is a

From: *Methods in Molecular Medicine, vol. 68: Molecular Analysis of Cancer*
Edited by: J. Boultwood and C. Fidler © Humana Press Inc., Totowa, NJ

115

crucial step for the identification of molecular changes underlying cancer development and for the correct interpretation of mutation screening.

1.2. Single-Strand Conformation Polymorphism Analysis

Single-strand conformation analysis (SSCP) *(2,3)* is one of the simplest scanning techniques for detecting unknown mutations. Sequence variants usually exhibit differences in mobility of single-stranded fragments under nondenaturing electrophoretic conditions. Mobility shifts of DNA fragments result from mutation-induced changes of the tertiary structure of DNA *(4)*. The principle of the technique is shown in **Fig. 1**. The term polymerase chain reaction (PCR)-SSCP refers to a PCR-amplified product analyzed by SSCP.

SSCP is particularly useful when searching for small deletions or insertions and single-base mutations and polymorphisms. Note that large insertions or deletions on the order of kilobases encompassing the amplified region are likely to go undetected.

2. Materials

2.1. Polymerase Chain Reaction

1. Template: high-molecular DNA or cDNA extracted from tumor/normal cells.
2. *Taq* polymerase.
3. PCR buffer.
4. dNTPs.
5. Tested oligonucleotide primers.
6. Double-distilled H_2O.
7. α-^{32}P-dCTP or α-^{33}P-dCTP for isotopic detection.
8. Suitable restriction endonucleases, if the fragment size is too large for sensitive detection.
9. Formamide buffer: 95% formamide, 0.05% bromophenol blue, 0.05% xylene cyanol, 50 mM NaOH.
10. Thermal cycler.

2.2. Gel Electrophoresis

1. Gel electrophoresis apparatus.
2. Power pack.
3. Gel plates.
4. Combs.
5. Plastic film (Saran Wrap).
6. Filter papers.
7. Optional: temperature control of gel plates (water jacket, fans).
8. Acrylamide/bisacrylamide
9. Ammonium sulfate.
10. TEMED.

PCR-SSCP Analysis of ATM Gene in Cancer

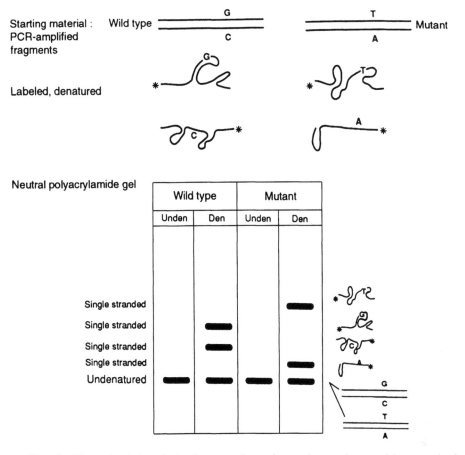

Fig. 1. The principle of single strand conformation polymorphism analysis. Reprinted from **ref. 26** with permission from Elsevier.

11. Glycerol.
12. 10X Tris-borate EDTA (TBE) buffer: 0.9 M Tris-borate, 20 mM EDTA.
13. For isotopic detection of labeled fragments: Kodak X-OMAT films, X-ray cassettes, developer.

3. Methods
3.1. Polymerase Chain Reaction

PCR usually involves the incorporation of a label, either directly into the product or via an isotopically or nonisotopically labeled oligonucleotide primer. Alternatively, DNA fragments can be labeled after electrophoresis (e.g., by silver staining). The PCR should be tested using an agarose gel before running SSCP gels to determine whether the product is clean. PCR products with spurious bands should be avoided. A meticulous computer-assisted oligo-nucleotide primer design will pay off here.

A typical 100-µL PCR setup for direct isotopic labeling includes 10 µL of 10X PCR buffer (containing 1.5 mM MgCl$_2$), 5 µL of dNTP (2.5 mM stock solution), 5 µL of primer mix (final concentration 0.1–1 µM), 5 × 5 µL of DNA (10–100 mg/µL), 0.5 µL of Taq polymerase (5 U/µL), approx 0.1–0.5 µL of α-^{32}P or α-^{33}P-dCTP (10 mCi/mL, 3000 Ci/mmol), and ddH$_2$O up to 100 µL. This amount is for at least five separate PCR reactions. A 20-µL reaction contains 5 µL of the template, which is convenient for dispensing multiple samples. The concentration of the labeled dNTPs depends on the sequence composition of the amplicon. After adding the enzyme-containing mixture to the template, thermal cycling should commence as soon as possible.

When using multiple samples, the amount of each template in the reaction tube should be the same. The usual amount of DNA per reaction is 50–100 ng. If the efficiency of PCR is markedly different from sample to sample (e.g., owing to the presence of enzyme inhibitors following DNA extraction from paraffin-embedded tissue), the template concentration should be further adjusted. However, loading different amounts of differentially labeled PCR products may result in altered mobilities of DNA fragments, and this may lead to difficulties in the interpretation of SSCP patterns. Different signal intensities from different samples are generally associated with a suboptimal detection rate, and every effort should be made to normalize the signal to allow the accurate evaluation of fragment mobility.

After completing the PCR, a restriction endonuclease digestion may help achieve a suitable fragment size for SSCP if the initial amplicon is too large. However, this extra step may be costly when analyzing multiple samples, and a subsequent complex SSCP pattern may be difficult to interpret.

Before running the electrophoresis, a formamide buffer is added in excess. No mixing is necessary before denaturing samples on a PCR cycler and loading onto an SSCP gel.

3.2. Gel Electrophoresis

1. Assemble glass plates for the gel.
2. In a beaker, mix the following components for a 100-mL gel solution: 5 mL of 10X TBE, 12 mL of 40% acrylamide/bisacrylamide (crosslinking 2.5%), 5 mL of glycerol, 1 mL of 10% ammonium persulfate, and ddH$_2$O up to 100 mL.
3. Add 50 µL of TEMED (Bio-Rad, Hercules, CA) and immediately pour into the gel plate assembly. Insert the comb and leave for at least 1.5 h to polymerize.
4. Remove the comb, clean the plates, assemble the gel, and fill the tank reservoir with 0.5X TBE. Check that there are no air bubbles in the gel, that the wells are undamaged, and that there is no leakage between the wells. Loading bromophenol dye to suspected wells is helpful for identifying leakages.

PCR-SSCP Analysis of ATM Gene in Cancer

5. Denature the PCR products at 95°C for 5 min and load the wells. If the gel is run at room temperature, the applied power should not lead to an increased temperature of the plates. A thermometer attached to the plate is useful for monitoring the electrophoresis.
6. After completing the electrophoresis, transfer the gel to a sheet of filter paper, cover with Saran Wrap, and dry using a gel dryer. Expose the dried gel to an X-ray film for a few hours to overnight. Several exposures may be required for the correct reading of the autoradiogram.

3.3. Sensitivity of PCR-SSCP

The sensitivity of the PCR-SSCP method has been subject to controversy. Although the technique is generally believed to be efficient with the detection rate of >85% in a single run for fragments shorter than 300 bp (5), some previous estimates were lower (6). The sensitivity of PCR-SSCP depends on several factors, including the mutation pattern in the target sequence.

Since the higher-order structure of nucleic acids is dependent on the entire sequence of the amplified fragment, the sensitivity of SSCP in detecting a given variation will vary from one fragment to another (5). Unlike, e.g., denaturing gradient gel electrophoresis (see Chapter 10), there is no adequate theoretical model for predicting the three-dimensional structure of single-stranded DNA under a given set of conditions (5). Can we still say how sensitive our SSCP analysis is for a sequence of interest?

Because the tertiary structure of single-stranded fragments depends on physical conditions such as pH, ionic strength, and temperature, these factors are likely to influence SSCP patterns and need to be controlled. Although not previously endorsed (7), adding glycerol to SSCP gels was found to improve detection rate by reducing the pH of the Tris-borate buffer by the reaction of glycerol and borate ion (8). Temperature is a particularly important variable. If not controlled, an excessive running power may generate heat, resulting in the disappearance of mobility shifts (7). Optimized crosslinking and polyacrylamide gel concentrations are generally recommended (5,7).

The analysis of globin, p53, and rhodopsin mutations suggested that the type of mutation (transition vs transversion) did not play a major role in determining whether a mutation was detected by SSCP analysis (9). Although the position of the base substitutions was found to be more important than the type of base substitution (9), it appears that the sequence flanking mutated residues plays an even more significant role (7).

Although the sensitivity was found to vary dramatically with the size of the DNA fragments analyzed, with the optimal size fragments for the detection of sensitive base substitution at about 150 bp (9), subsequent studies did not support such a steep decline in sensitivity (5,10). The blind quality control study of fragments larger than 450 bp reported a detection rate of 84% (10), an and even higher rate was found by running fragments between 300 and 800 bp in low-pH buffer systems *(8)*. Since a single base change contributes to the tertiary structure in a larger fragment less than in small one, the probability of detecting a base change in fragments larger than 300 bp is generally considered to be lower than for optimally sized fragments.

The fact that a shift of a mutated fragment is detected under certain physical conditions led the authors to suggest the use of varying running conditions *(5,11)*. This approach is warranted together with the use of complementary methods for mutation detection of single nucleotide changes, (*see* Chapters 10–13), if a high or 100% detection rate is desired. The most commonly changed variables are polyacrylamide and buffer concentrations, use of an alternative gel matrix such as the MDE gel (AT Biochem), and changing glycerol concentration in the gel.

In practice, however, the use of too thick gels, excessive amounts of loaded DNA (sometimes owing to insufficient labeling of fragments), inappropriate pH of the gel, a high voltage leading to gel overheating, and analyzing PCR products with spurious fragments are among the most common mistakes of inexperienced users. Each of these factors drastically affects the sensitivity of detection of conformational changes in single-strand fragments. These may have been reasons behind a controversy in the estimates of sensitivity *(5)*. The sensitivity is generally considered to be very high if SSCP is performed using optimal conditions.

3.4. Mutation Analysis of ATM Using PCR-SSCP

The ability of PCR-SSCP to detect mutations also reflects the size of analyzed region. The analysis of multiple PCR-amplified fragments from large genes or genomic regions may decrease the sensitivity to an unacceptably low level.

We have partially addressed this concern in the PCR-SSCP analysis of the human *ATM* gene *(12)*. *ATM* is deficient in patients with ataxia telangiectasia (A-T), a multisystem recessive condition with a high risk of developing lymphoreticular malignancies. The gene contains 66 small coding exons *(13–15)* of the average size of 253 bp spanning about 184 kb of genomic sequence *(16)*. Since the size of exons is suitable for SSCP analysis, all coding exons were individually amplified using oligonucleotides primed to the flanking intronic sequence. By analyzing cDNA prepared from A-T patients, the mutation pattern in patients' germlines was previously found to be dominated by small insertions, deletions, and point mutations, whereas most mutations were private *(17)*. Assuming that A-T patients had two mutated copies of *ATM* and all mutations were in the regions covered by the oligonucleotide primers, we could estimate the detection rate of our SSCP mutation assay at 70% *(13)*. This figure may be an underestimate, if the assumptions are not met. Such an estimate,

PCR-SSCP Analysis of ATM Gene in Cancer

however, applies to the whole gene represented by 65 amplicons. The probability of detecting a mutation in an average PCR segment (approx 1/65 of the screened region) would be $^{65}\sqrt{0.7} \cong 0.995$. Such a high detection rate is likely to reflect the mutation pattern found in the germline of A-T patients, dominated by small deletions, insertions, and point mutations, changes readily identified by SSCP. The detection rate is likely to be different when analyzing genes with a distinct mutation pattern.

As the majority of SSCP changes in the germline of A-T patients result in a premature termination of the ATM translation product, the protein truncation test (*see* Chapter 12), is an obvious method of choice for the identification of unknown A-T alleles in the germline *(18,19)*. However, this test may not be the most appropriate for analyzing the same gene in tumor cells. By using the SSCP analysis of tumor DNA extracted from presentation samples of patients with sporadic T-cell prolymphocytic leukemia (T-PLL), a malignancy exhibiting phenotypic similarities to a leukemia seen in A-T, *ATM* was found to be mutated in about one-half of T-PLL cases *(20,21)*. A variety of techniques for mutation detection have now indicated that the gene is likely to be inactivated or mutated in most, if not all, T-PLL patients *(20–23)*. The presence of loss-of-function mutations, frequent loss of the wild-type allele in tumor cells, and clustering of missense mutation in the highly conserved 3' part of the gene suggest that *ATM* functions as a tumor suppressor gene in the develoment of T-PLL. Although mutations have not been found in all cases, the detection rate using a single pass of SSCP was found similar to that in the germline of A-T patients *(20)*, suggesting that the inactivation or mutation of *ATM* is probably an essential step among genetic alterations leading to T-PLL. Although the possibility of a predisposing heterozygote change could not be excluded in T-PLL samples with mutations identical to those previously reported in the germline (normal cells were not available), the vast majority of T-PLL cases contained mutations not previously found in A-T, suggesting somatic changes *(20)*. The *ATM* mutation pattern in T-PLL was found to be markedly distinct from that found in the germline of A-T patients. While the frame-shift mutations predominate in the germline, most mutations in T-PLL tumor samples were missense mutations *(20)*, a characteristic type of mutation in tumor cells.

Thus, although the protein truncation test (PTT) appears to be a method of choice for analyzing the germline changes with reported sensitivity similar to that of SSCP *(18,19)*, PTT alone would be unlikely to detect missense mutations that characterize the somatic mutation pattern in the same gene in tumor cells. The PTT might even miss T-PLL alterations altogether. This case illustrates the need for employing a combination of wisely selected, preferably complementing techniques, particularly in the absence of our knowledge about the mutation pattern of the analyzed gene or genomic segment.

Negative results of PCR-SSCP mutation screening need a cautious interpretation. The absence of *ATM* mutations in a large number of breast cancer samples analyzed does not exclude the presence of mutations in this malignancy *(24)*. However, it is unlikely that the gene would be frequently altered in breast cancer, certainly not to an extent similar to that found in T-PLL. No somatic *ATM* mutations have been identified so far in tumor DNA isolated from breast cancer, but, given a high population prevalence of breast tumors as compared to T-PLL, it is possible that this may be the case in a small proportion of breast tumors. To address this area of question, large sets of samples will need to analyzed.

SSCP is also sensitive in detecting mutations in mixed populations of cells containing normal and mutated alleles. A study of the *p53* gene detected mutations against the background of 85–95% of the wild-type allele *(25)*, a figure sufficient to identify clonal changes in tumors containing a substantial proportion of normal cells.

In conclusion, PCR-SSCP is a rapid, simple, and cost-effective scanning method for mutation detection. It is particularly useful for the initial screening of optimally sized PCR-amplified fragments for point mutations, small deletions, and insertions. It serves well as an inexpensive method of choice for screening candidate cancer susceptibility genes and in situations in which the detection rate of mutation screening is not required to be absolute. If the expected mutation pattern is not known, a combination of suitable techniques discussed in this book should provide a more sensitive and specific tool for analyzing a growing number of cancer susceptibility genes and also more accurate estimates of cancer risk conferred by genetic alterations.

Acknowledgments

This work was supported by a grant from the European Community BIOMED programme (QLRT-1999-00786) and the International Young Investigator Award in Oncology from Bristol Myers Squibb.

References

1. Landegren, U. (ed.) (1996) *Laboratory Protocols for Mutation Setection.* Oxford University Press, NY, pp. 192.
2. Orita, M., Suzuki, Y., Sekiya, Y., and Hayashi, K. (1989) Rapid and sensitive detection of point mutations and DNA polymorphisms using the polymerase chain reaction. *Genomics* **5,** 874–879.
3. Orita, M., Iwahana, H., Kanazawa, H., and Sekiya, T. (1989) Detection of polymorphism of human DNA by gel electrophoresis as single strand conformation polymorphism. *Proc. Natl. Acad. Sci. USA* **86,** 2766–2770.
4. Hayashi, K. (1996) PCR-SSCP—single strand conformation polymorphism analysis of PCR products, in *Laboratory Protocols for Mutation Detection.* (Landegren, U., ed.), Oxford University Press, NY, pp. 14–22.

PCR-SSCP Analysis of ATM Gene in Cancer

5. Hayashi, K. and Yandell, D. W. (1993) How sensitive is PCR-SSCP? *Hum. Mutat.* **2,** 338–346.
6. Sarkar, G., Yoon, H.-S., and Sommer, S. S. (1992) Screening for mutations by RNA single strand conformation polymorphisms (rSSCP): comparison with DNA-SSCP. *Nucleic Acids Res.* **20,** 871–878.
7. Glavac, D. and Dean, M. (1993) Optimization of the single-strand conformation polymorphism (SSCP) technique for detection of point mutations. *Hum. Mutat.* **2,** 404–414.
8. Kukita, Y., Tahira, T., Sommer, S. S., and Hayashi, K. (1997) SSCP analysis of long DNA fragments in low pH gel. *Hum. Mutat.* **10,** 400–407.
9. Sheffield, V. C., Beck, J. S., Kwitek, A. E., Sandstrom, D. W., and Stone, E. M. (1993) The sensitivity of single-strand conformation polymorphism analysis for the detection of single base substitutions. *Genomics* **16,** 325–332.
10. Jordanova, A., Kalaydjieva, L., Savov, A., Claustres, M., Schwarz, M., Estivill, X., et al. (1997) SSCP analysis: a blind sensitivity trial. *Hum. Mutat.* **10,** 65–70.
11. Leren, T. P., Solberg, K., Rodningen, O. K., Ose, L., Tonstad, S., and Berg, K. (1993) Evaluation of running conditions for SSCP analysis: application of SSCP for detection of point mutations in the LDL receptor gene. *PCR Methods Appl.* **3,** 159–162.
12. Savitsky, K., Bar-Shira, A., Gilad, S., Rotman, G., Ziv, Y., Vanagaite, L., et al. (1995) A single ataxia telangiectasia gene with a product similar to PI-3 kinase. *Science* **268,** 1749–1753.
13. Vorechovsky, I., Luo, L., Prudente, S., Chessa, L., Russo, G., Kanariou, M., et al. (1996) Exon-scanning mutation analysis of the ATM gene in patients with ataxia-telangiectasia. *Eur. J. Hum. Genet.* **4,** 352–355.
14. Rasio, D., Negrini, M., and Croce, C. M. (1995) Genomic organization of the ATM locus involved in ataxia-telangiectasia. *Cancer Res.* **55,** 6053–6057.
15. Uziel, T., Savitsky, K., Platzer, M., Ziv, Y., Helbitz, T., Nehls, M., et al. (1996) Genomic Organization of the ATM gene. *Genomics* **33,** 317–320.
16. Platzer, M., Rotman, G., Bauer, D., Uziel, T., Savitsky, K., Bar-Shira, A., et al. (1997) Ataxia-telangiectasia locus: sequence analysis of 184 kb of human genomic DNA containing the entire ATM gene. *Genome Res.* **7,** 592–605.
17. Gilad, S., Khosravi, R., Shkedy, D., Uziel, T., Ziv, Y., Savitsky, K., et al. (1996) Predominance of null mutations in ataxia-telangiectasia. *Hum. Mol. Genet.* **5,** 433–439.
18. Telatar, M., Wang, Z., Udar, N., Liang, T., Bernatowska-Matuszkiewicz, E., Lavin, M., et al. (1996) Ataxia-telangiectasia: mutations in ATM cDNA detected by protein-truncation screening. *Am. J. Hum. Genet.* **59,** 40–44.
19. Telatar, M., Teraoka, S., Wang, Z., Chun, H. H., Liang, T., Castellvi-Bel, S., et al. (1998) Ataxia-telangiectasia: identification and detection of founder-effect mutations in the ATM gene in ethnic populations. *Am. J. Hum. Genet.* **62,** 86–97.
20. Vorechovsky, I., Luo, L., Dyer, M. J., Catovsky, D., Amlot, P. L., Yaxley, J. C., et al. (1997) Clustering of missense mutations in the ataxia-telangiectasia gene in a sporadic T-cell leukaemia. *Nat. Genet.* **17,** 96–99.
21. Yuille, M. A., Coignet, L. J., Abraham, S. M., Yaqub, F., Luo, L., Matutes, E., et al. (1998) *ATM* is usually rearranged in T-cell prolymphocytic leukaemia. *Oncogene* **16,** 789–796.

22. Stilgenbauer, S., Schaffner, C., Litterst, A., Liebisch, P., Gilad, S., Bar-Shira, A., et al. (1997) Biallelic mutations in the ATM gene in T-prolymphocytic leukemia. *Nat. Med.* **3,** 1155–1159.
23. Stoppa-Lyonnet, D., Soulier, J., Lauge, A., Dastot, H., Garand, R., Sigaux, F., and Stern, M. H. (1998) Inactivation of the *ATM* gene in T-cell prolymphocytic leukemias. *Blood* **91,** 3920–3926.
24. Vorechovsky, I., Rasio, D., Luo, L., Monaco, C., Hammarstrom, L., Webster, A. D., et al. (1996) The *ATM* gene and susceptibility to breast cancer: analysis of 38 breast tumors reveals no evidence for mutation. *Cancer Res.* **56,** 2726–2732.
25. Wu, J. K., Ye, Z., and Darras, B. T. (1993) Sensitivity of single-strand conformation polymorphism (SSCP) analysis in detecting p53 point mutations in tumors with mixed cell populations. *Am. J. Hum. Genet.* **52,** 1273–1275.
26. Prosser, J. (1993) Detecting single-base mutations. *Trends Biotechnol.* **11,** 238–246.

10

Mutational Analysis of Oncogenes and Tumor Suppressor Genes in Human Cancer Using Denaturing Gradient Gel Electrophoresis

Per Guldberg, Kirsten Grønbæk, Jesper Worm, Per thor Straten, and Jesper Zeuthen

1. Introduction

Denaturing gradient gel electrophoresis (DGGE) was introduced 20 years ago *(1)* as a gel system to separate DNA fragments. The seminal principle of this methodologic conquest was that DNA molecules were not separated according to size, as in conventional electrophoresis, but rather, according to base composition and sequence-related properties. Since then, the technology has been developed into a powerful, yet still challenging, method for detection of single base changes. In combination with polymerase chain reaction (PCR), it has been widely used by research and diagnostic laboratories in the analysis of cancer and inherited disease. The principles and potential applications of DGGE have been described in detail in a number of excellent reviews *(2–4)* and are outlined only briefly in the following sections.

1.1. Overview

Why use DGGE at all instead of sequencing or more simple and straightforward mutation detection methods, in particular single-strand conformation polymorphism analysis? DGGE is advantageous for several reasons. First, DGGE has a very high mutation detection rate, close to 100%, provided that the experiment has been correctly designed. Second, the behavior of DNA molecules in denaturing gradient gels can be accurately modeled by computer, which may drastically reduce the need for empirical optimization. Third, the sensitivity of DGGE is high, allowing detection of a mutant DNA species present in a low proportion in a background of wild-type DNA (down to the

From: *Methods in Molecular Medicine, vol. 68: Molecular Analysis of Cancer*
Edited by: J. Boultwood and C. Fidler © Humana Press Inc., Totowa, NJ

5% level by conventional ethidium bromide staining). Fourth, owing to the resulting physical separation between mutant and wild-type DNA, DGGE provides a simple means of enriching the mutant DNA for further analysis. Fifth, DGGE is highly flexible, meaning that multiple PCR products with different thermal properties can be analyzed simultaneously in the same gel. This is particularly useful in diagnostic settings in which one or a few DNA samples must be scanned for mutations in an entire gene.

Despite the obvious advantages of DGGE, two matters are important to consider before deciding whether DGGE is an appropriate method for a given application: (1) the design of PCR primers to generate amplification products that are suitable for DGGE analysis may be a cumbersome process that requires computer modeling and a certain degree of personal experience; and (2) once PCR primers have been properly designed, the method is simple to perform with a relatively high throughput. Hence, generally speaking, DGGE may be considered the method of choice when primers have already been designed, or when the number of samples to be analyzed is so high that it outweighs the work involved in the phase of establishment.

1.2. Principle of DGGE

1.2.1. DNA Melting Theory

In aqueous solutions kept at a temperature below 60°C, DNA takes a double-stranded, helical conformation maintained by hydrogen bonds between base pairs on opposite strands and stacking interactions between neighboring bases on the same strand. When the temperature is raised abruptly, the two strands come apart and take a single-stranded, random coil conformation. This helix–to–random chain transition is termed *DNA melting* and may also be induced by chemical denaturants. Because the forces holding a DNA helix include both base pairing and stacking interactions, the melting temperature (T_m) of a DNA molecule is determined by the overall sequence, not just the GC content.

When a DNA molecule is subjected to gradual heating, it melts in a series of steps in which each step represents the melting of a discrete segment, termed a *melting domain (2,4)*. A DNA molecule may contain several melting domains, each consisting of 25–300 contiguous base pairs, with T_m values in the range of 60–85°C. The domain that melts at the lowest temperature is referred to as the lowest-melting domain; the most stable domain is the highest-melting domain. A base substitution or other type of mutation may change the T_m of the domain in which it resides up to 1°C.

1.2.2. The Experimental System

The DGGE system elegantly uses the melting properties of DNA and the changes that mutations impose on these properties. A standard denaturing

Mutational Analysis by DGGE

gradient gel contains a uniform concentration of polyacrylamide and an increasing gradient of denaturants, usually a combination of urea and formamide. An increase in denaturant concentration has been shown to be equivalent to a rise in temperature, and a gradient of denaturants hence simulates a temperature gradient within the gel. Because the concentrations of denaturant alone are not sufficient to provide DNA melting, the gel is immersed in a bath of electrophoresis buffer kept at a temperature just below incipient DNA melting, usually at 56–60°C.

When a DNA molecule with two or more melting domains is electrophoresed through a denaturing gradient gel, it initially moves with a constant velocity determined by its size. At a certain point in the gel, a level of denaturant will be reached that exactly matches the melting temperature of the lowest-melting domain. This domain will be destabilized, resulting in the abrupt formation of a partially melted, three-armed intermediate that moves with a very low velocity. Small shifts in the T_m of this domain induced by the introduction of base substitutions will cause the domain to unwind at different concentrations of denaturant and, accordingly, at different positions in the gel, providing the basis for physical separation between wild-type and mutant species (*5*).

When the highest-melting domain of a DNA fragment melts, the fragment undergoes complete strand dissociation, and the resolving power of the gel is lost. To overcome this limitation, a modification was designed that involves the attachment of a GC-rich sequence, usually called a GC-clamp, to one of the ends of the DNA fragment. The GC-clamp introduces a new highest-melting domain and works as a "handle" to keep the strands together. A GC-clamp is easily added by PCR using primers, one of which has been extended by a 30- to 60-bp GC-rich sequence at its 5' end (*6*). **Figure 1** outlines the whole procedure of GC-clamping and resolution by DGGE.

In rare cases in which a mutation does not affect thermostability and, therefore, cannot be visualized as a mobility shift in a denaturing gradient gel, increased resolution may be achieved by analyzing heteroduplexes, i.e., hybrids formed between wild-type and mutant DNA molecules (**Fig. 2**). Under appropriate conditions, heteroduplexes are formed when wild-type and mutant DNA fragments are mixed, heated to separate the strands, and then reannealed to allow a reassortment of the single-stranded species with their complements. Four different species are expected from such reassortment: wild-type homoduplexes, mutant homoduplexes, and two different heteroduplexes composed of one wild-type strand and one mutant strand. The formation of heteroduplexes is initiated during late cycles of PCR and can be driven to completion by subsequent heating and reannealing of the PCR product. Heteroduplexes are retarded in a denaturing gradient gel at a lower concentration of denaturant than the corresponding homoduplexes, presumably as a result of the instability caused by the presence of a non-Watson-Crick base pair (mismatch) (**Fig. 2**).

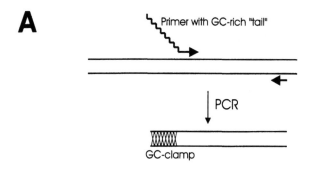

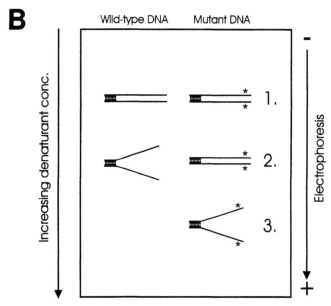

Fig. 1. Schematic representation of the principles of GC-clamping and resolution of mutations by DGGE. (**A**) PCR-mediated addition of a GC-clamp. The GC-rich primer tail gets incorporated and copied during PCR, providing a double-stranded GC-rich region at one end of the PCR product. (**B**) Resolution of mutations by DGGE. The concentration of denaturant at which branching and band focusing occur is strongly sequence dependent, forming the basis for physical separation between wild-type and mutant DNA molecules. In this example, mutant DNA melts at a higher concentration of denaturant than the corresponding wild-type DNA and, consequently, is retarded at a lower position in the gel.

1.3. Modes of Analysis

The principle of studying melting behaviors of DNA fragments in a denaturing environment for the purpose of identifying mutations has been taken into

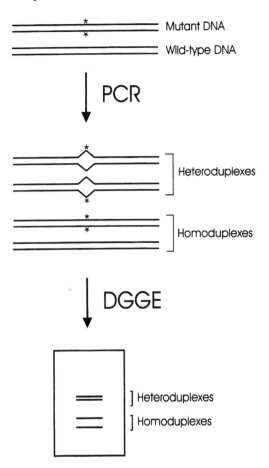

Fig. 2. Diagrammatic representation of heteroduplex analysis by DGGE. PCR amplification of a target sequence from a specimen containing both mutant and wild-type DNA results in the formation of four double-stranded species: mutant homoduplexes, wild-type homoduplexes, and two heteroduplexes. Owing to the presence of destabilizing mismatches, the heteroduplex molecules melt at a lower denaturant concentration and usually produce more-pronounced band shifts than the corresponding homoduplex molecules.

several methodologic variants. These variants include temperature gradient gel electrophoresis, in which a temperature gradient is maintained along the separation space (7), two-dimensional gene scanning, which is based on multiplex PCR followed by size separation in combination with DGGE (8); bisulfite-DGGE, for detection of mutations and aberrant methylation patterns in very GC-rich DNA (9); and a variety of capillary formats. This chapter is confined to the use of chemical denaturants in standard slab gel operations.

1.3.1. Parallel DGGE

The most commonly used configuration of DGGE is one in which the gel contains a linear gradient of denaturants in the same direction as the applied electric field (**Fig. 1**). In this configuration, a DNA molecule travels through an ascending denaturant concentration until it reaches a gradient level where its continued migration is severely retarded because of partial melting of the double helix. Loading in adjacent lanes allows analysis and comparison of multiple samples.

1.3.2. Perpendicular DGGE

Perpendicular gels contain a linear gradient of denaturant perpendicular to the direction of electrophoresis, and the sample is loaded in a single well spanning the entire width of the gel. In this configuration, a DNA molecule travels through a particular, unchanging denaturant concentration. The final pattern usually shows a single or multiphasic S-shaped curve, of which each steep part represents the melting of a domain.

Perpendicular DGGE provides an experimental system to examine the melting properties of a DNA molecule. Although this may be valuable in the analysis of DNA fragments of unknown sequence, computer modeling is a simpler and more accurate approach to designing DGGE conditions for genes of known sequence.

1.3.3. Constant Denaturant Gel Electrophoresis

Constant denaturant gels contain a uniform denaturant concentration corresponding to one of the steep parts of the profile observed by analysis of a DNA molecule in a perpendicular denaturing gradient gel *(10)*. Electrophoresis at this concentration provides the optimal conditions for separation between fragments differing in nucleotide sequence in the corresponding melting domain.

1.3.4. Double-Gradient DGGE

In double-gardient DGGE (DG-DGGE) analysis, the gel contains two colinear gradients: one of denaturant concentration and one of polyacrylamide concentration *(11)*. The porosity gradient provides recompacting of homo- and heteroduplex bands, resulting in a considerable improvement in band focusing. **Figure 3** provides an example of DG-DGGE.

1.3.5. Broad-Range DGGE

In broad-range DGGE, the gradient is typically 0–80% to accommodate different DNA fragments with a broad spectrum of melting temperatures *(12)*. This approach results in considerable savings when looking for mutations in a

Mutational Analysis by DGGE

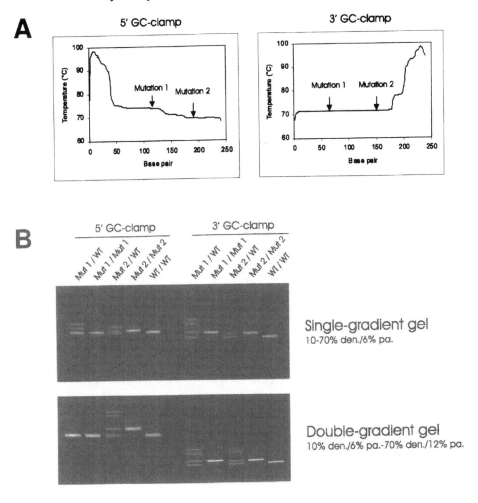

Fig. 3. Melting maps (**A**) and effect of GC-clamp positioning in conventional (single-gradient) and DG-DGGE (**B**). Attachment of a GC-clamp to the 5' end of the target sequence results in a fragment with three lower-melting domains. While conventional DGGE provides resolution of heterozygous mutations in both the lower and higher of these domains, the overall resolution is modest, and homoduplexes of the mutation in the higher-melting domain do not separate from wild-type homoduplexes. By contrast, a GC-clamp at the 3' end of the target sequence results in a single, flat lower-melting domain and clear resolution of both mutations in the heterozygous and homozygous constellations. With DG-DGGE, resolution of mutations is completely prevented in the higher-melting domain of the product carrying a 5' end GC-clamp. As with single-gradient DGGE, mutations are easily detected in the single-domain product, and band focusing is significantly improved. den., denaturant; pa., polyacrylamide.

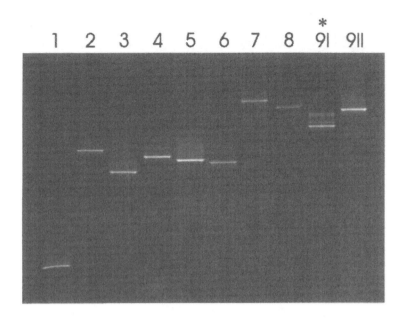

Fig. 4. One-step DGGE analysis of 10 GC-clamped PCR products covering the entire coding sequence of the *Fas* gene. Genomic DNA from a non-Hodgkin lymphoma was used as the template for 10 separate PCRs, and the products were subjected to broad-range DGGE (0–80% denaturant at 160 V and 56°C for 4.5 h). Four bands are observed in the 5' end of exon 9 (9I, denoted by an asterisk), indicating the presence of a mutation.

particular gene in only one sample, but it depends on careful considerations when designing the experiment. In our laboratory, we have established DGGE conditions for whole-gene analysis for several oncogenes and tumor suppressor genes, including the *ras* genes *(13)*, *p53* *(14)*, *PTEN* *(15)*, *Fas* *(16)*, and *CDK4* *(17)*. **Figure 4** provides an example of broad-range DGGE for scanning of one tumor specimen in an entire gene.

2. Materials

2.1. Computer Programs

MELT87 or MELT94, written in the laboratory of Lerman *(18)*, can be used. These programs calculate the theoretical melting map of a known DNA sequence using the Fixman-Friere modification of Poland's algorithm for DNA melting. A modified version, MacMELT™, is commercially available from Bio-Rad (Hercules, CA).

Mutational Analysis by DGGE

2.2. PCR Reagents

1. Standard PCR reagents.
2. *Taq* polymerase (*see* **Note 1**).
3. 5X PCR-compatible loading buffer: 0.04% cresol red, 60% sucrose.
4. Oligonucleotide primers, one GC-clamped (*see* **Notes 2** and **3**).

2.3. Solutions (see Note 4)

1. 50X TAE electrophoresis buffer: 2.0 *M* Tris-acetate, 0.05 *M* EDTA, pH 8.0.
2. Denaturant stock solution (0% denaturant): 6% acrylamide (acrylamide:bis = 19:1) in 1X TAE.
3. Denaturant stock solution (80% denaturant): 5.6 *M* urea, 32% (v/v) formamide, 6% acrylamide in 1X TAE.
4. Denaturant stock solution for DG-DGGE (70% denaturant): 4.9 *M* urea, 28% (v/v) formamide, 12% acrylamide in 1X TAE.
5. Photo-flo 600 solution (Kodak).
6. 20% Ammonium persulfate.
7. TEMED.
8. Ethidium bromide (2 µg/mL) in 1X TAE buffer.

2.4. Gel Equipment and Thermoregulation (see Note 5)

Gel systems can be commercially acquired from CBC Scientific or Bio-Rad, or they may be built from components from various sources. The system described next is routinely used in our laboratory and is based on a standard slab gel system.

1. PROTEAN II xi Cell (Bio-Rad). Modify the central cooling core by cutting out the central portion. This modification ensures uniform temperature in the gel when the electrophoresis cell is immersed in a temperature-controlled buffer bath (*see* **Note 5**).
2. Glass plates: 16×20 cm (inner plate) and 18.3×20 cm (outer plate).
3. Spacers and combs (1 mm).
4. Glass or acrylic tank: approx $45 \times 30 \times 30$ cm (length × width × height).
5. Immersion circulator that combines heating, thermoregulation, and stirring.
6. Two-chamber gradient maker and magnetic stirrer.
7. Power supply.
8. Polypropylene spheres.

3. Methods

3.1. Fragment Design

The requirement for detailed theoretical considerations prior to PCR and DGGE analysis is at the same time the great advantage and a potential hindrance for routine use. Primer pairs have to be designed for both optimal PCR amplification and optimal melting behavior. To ensure appropriate melting temperatures of the primers, and to minimize self-complementarity and cross homologies, we recommend the use of a primer designer program. For simulation and modulation of melting profiles, the use of the MELT programs is invaluable. Although there are no strict rules that should be followed when designing experiments, and although mutations may be detected even under suboptimal conditions, we recommend the following guidelines for optimal performance:

1. Aim at a fragment size of 150–350 bp (including GC-clamp) (*see* **Note 6**).
2. Ensure that the entire sequence to be analyzed is contained within one lower-melting domain (*see* **Subheading 3.1.1.** and **Fig. 3**).
3. Avoid internal melting domains deviating by more than 0.2°C from the average domain temperature (*19*).
4. Ensure that the temperature of strand dissociation is higher than the melting temperature of the lower-melting domain of interest (*see* **Subheading 3.1.2.**).

3.1.1. Melting Profiles

The MELT programs generate the melting map for a known DNA sequence, i.e., a plot of the midpoint temperature at which each base pair of the sequence is in 50:50 equilibrium between the helical and melted configurations (*18*). Each melting domain of the DNA fragment appears as a horizontal line and is usually clearly demarcated from the adjacent domains on either side.

To determine the optimal position of the GC-clamp, add 40 bp of GC-rich sequence to either end of the fragment and recalculate the melting maps (**Fig. 3**). The addition of a GC-clamp may have quite a dramatic impact on the melting properties of a DNA fragment, and it is not always possible to predict the optimal position of the GC-clamp solely on the basis of the melting map of the native DNA. If the unclamped end of the fragment has a lower melting temperature than the remainder of the lower-melting domain, include a short GC-clamp at this end to make the entire sequence behave as a single melting domain.

3.1.2. Length of GC-Clamp (see **Note 7**)

1. Using the MELT program, calculate for the 40-bp GC-clamped PCR product the temperature at which strand dissociation becomes significant, in practice the temperature at which log dissociation constant (Kd) is –5.
2. Increase the length of the GC-clamp until the temperature of strand dissociation is 0.5–1°C higher than the melting temperature of the domain of interest.

3.2. Polymerase Chain Reaction

As with other PCR applications, it is important that the PCR be optimized (e.g., by varying the annealing temperature and the concentrations of $MgCl_2$

Mutational Analysis by DGGE

and dimethyl sulfoxide). The inclusion of a GC-clamp does not appear to interfere significantly with the amplification process. Because only the GC-clamp remains double-stranded after electrophoresis, and because ethidium bromide stains single-stranded DNA only weakly, a considerable product yield is required. Unspecific bands must be avoided because they may be misinterpreted as evidence for the presence of a mutation.

3.2.1. Generation of Heteroduplexes (see **Subheading 1.2.2.** and **Note 8**)

Using a thermal cycler, subject the sample to a denaturation/reannealing program consisting of 95°C for 10 min, 65°C for 60 min, and 37°C for 60 min.

3.3. DGGE Analysis

3.3.1. Preparation of Gel (see **Note 9**)

1. Clean glass plates carefully with ethanol and cover them with a thin layer of Photo-flo 600 solution to reduce surface tension. Assemble the gel sandwich according to the supplier's instructions.
2. From the stock solutions of acrylamide and denaturants, prepare two solutions of 14 mL each (for a 28-mL gel), corresponding to the two end points of the desired denaturant concentration range.
3. Add 50 µL of 20% ammonium persulfate and 6 µL of TEMED to each solution and mix by gently swirling.
4. Pour the two gel solutions into the gradient maker, ensuring that the solution of higher denaturant is poured into the mixing chamber (the chamber with the outlet and the magnetic stirrer). Avoid the introduction of bubbles by too vigorous mixing.
5. Open the valve interconnecting the two chambers and let some solution pass between the chambers to ensure that the connecting pipe is not blocked by air bubbles.
6. Open the outlet and introduce the gradient into the gel sandwich from the top by gravity flow or with a peristaltic pump.
7. Insert the comb gently and at an angle and let the gel polymerize for 30–45 min.
8. Remove the comb and immediately flush the wells carefully with 1X TAE buffer to remove unpolymerized acrylamide (*see* **Note 10**).

3.3.2. Running and Staining the Gel (see **Notes 11 and 12**)

1. Attach the gel sandwich to the central cooling core, fill the upper buffer chamber with 1X TAE buffer, and load the samples. Immediately immerse the gel assembly into the temperature-controlled tank filled with 1X TAE buffer, and cover the buffer surface with polypropylene spheres to minimize evaporation. Apply the required voltage.
2. After electrophoresis, stain the gel in 1X TAE buffer containing ethidium bromide (2 µg/mL) for 10 min. Destain the gel in 1X TAE buffer if required. Photograph the gel on an ultraviolet transilluminator.

3.3.3. Enrichment of Mutant DNA for Sequence Analysis (see **Note 13**)

1. Localize the mutant homoduplex band or one of the heteroduplex bands, and excise it from the gel with a clean scalpel.
2. Incubate the gel slice in 100 μL of H_2O overnight (or longer) at 4°C.
3. Dilute the eluate 100-fold and 10,000-fold, and use 1 μL of the original eluate and 1 μL of each of the two dilutions as templates in three separate PCRs.
4. Analyze the amplification products by agarose gel electrophoresis, and use the product from the highest dilution (for which amplification was successful) as the template for the sequencing reaction.

4. Notes

1. In DGGE analysis of PCR products, polymerase-induced errors result in the production of mutant sequences that are physically separated from the correctly amplified sequences. Because the PCR-induced mutations are scattered randomly in the target sequence, the mutant amplicons will migrate to different positions in the denaturing gradient gel and result in a background smear. For detection of mutations present in a low proportion, the use of polymerases with low error rates may significantly reduce the background and improve resolution.
2. A considerable fraction of oligonucleotides synthesized by standard methods may be of incorrect length or contain nucleotide misincorporations that will be resolved in a denaturing gradient gel and result in a background smear. The number of errors increases with the length of the primer. Generally, we recommend that primers longer than 60 bp be ordered high-performance liquid chromatography-purified to be of the correct length.
3. When designing GC-clamps, avoid guanosine stretches and include a thymidine for every 20–25 bp.
4. Zero percent denaturant stock is acrylamide in 1X TAE buffer; one hundred percent denaturant is an arbitrary standard defined as 7 M urea (42 g/100 mL) and 40% (v/v) formamide.
5. Successful DGGE analysis depends on accurate temperature control within the gel. While the bath temperature may be set anywhere between 50°C and 60°C (depending on the melting temperature of the DNA fragment), the temperature must remain constant during the run. To avoid local temperature differences, it is important that the glass plates of the gel sandwich be in direct contact with the heated buffer on both sides, and that the buffer be constantly circulated by means of a stirring device.
6. We generally recommend that the maximum fragment length be set at 350 bp. Although DGGE has the potential to detect mutations in even longer fragments, the resolution of some mutations may be poor, the required running time may be inconveniently long, and the number of bases to be sequenced to finally identify the mutation may be inconveniently high. The fragment size must be more carefully considered when analyzing multiple different PCR products in the same gel.
7. The usefulness of DGGE for detection of mutations may be limited by the eventual occurrence of strand dissociation. The rate of strand dissociation (bimolecu-

Mutational Analysis by DGGE

lar melting) is determined by the equilibrium constant of dissociation at the temperature of migration arrest, which may be estimated by using the MELT program (not a facility of the commercially available MacMELT program). Detection of mutations is completely hindered if complete strand dissociation occurs at a temperature below that at which partial melting of the molecule takes place. The temperature of strand dissociation may be elevated by increasing the length of the GC-clamp. For most DNA regions with melting temperatures in the range of 60–75°C, a 40-bp GC-clamp (or even shorter) will be sufficient to prevent strand dissociation. For some sequences, however, the GC content is so high that strand dissociation cannot be prevented by means of GC-clamping. The use of a psoralen derivative (ChemiClamp) to covalently link the strands may be a useful alternative for DGGE analysis of such GC-rich DNA regions *(20)*.

8. Tumor specimens usually contain a mixture of cancerous cells and stromal tissue, implying that heteroduplexes will automatically be formed during PCR amplification of the target sequence. For analysis of tumor cell lines that often harbor mutations in the hemizygous constellation, it is recommended that cell line DNA be mixed with normal control DNA prior to PCR to ensure detection of all types of mutation.

9. The concentration of denaturant, x, at which a melting domain melts can be estimated by $x = (T_m - T_b)/0.3$, where T_m is the melting temperature of the domain, as determined by MELT, and T_b is the bath temperature. The choice of gradient range depends on the separation required; the narrower the gradient, the higher the resolution. Typically, a top-to-bottom difference of 30–40% denaturant centred above x gives satisfactory resolution.

10. Gels may be prepared the day before use and stored at room temperature or at 4°C.

11. The running time required for resolution of mutations may be determined by time travel experiments, preferably aided by the inclusion of control mutations. When the fragment has reached the position in the gel at which it partially melts, there will be a very small increment in migration depth, and bands will be well focused. For analysis of multiple different PCR products in the same gel, the running time is determined as the time it takes for all products to reach the positions in the gel at which they are retarded. For PCR products of 250–300 bp in length, typical running conditions in a 16-cm gel containing 6% polyacrylamide are 5 h at 160 V. For DG-DGGE, the running times are generally somewhat longer but much more flexible, allowing overnight runs (typically at 90–100 V) without loss of band focusing.

12. It is generally recommended that the buffer be recirculated from the tank to the cathode chamber of the gel apparatus to avoid changes in pH during the run. However, it is our experience that changes in pH do not reduce the quality of DGGE analyses in standard 5-h runs (at 160 V) or overnight runs (at 90 V).

13. If the proportion of mutated cells in a tumor specimen is very low, all mutant sequence will be used up in the formation of heteroduplexes during PCR (*see* **Subheading 1.2.2.**). Therefore, the heteroduplexes must be recovered, in which the mutant DNA is present in a 50:50 ratio with wild-type DNA. If heteroduplex

DNA is eluted from the excized gel slice, reamplified (*see* **Subheading 3.3.3.**), and then subjected to another round of DGGE, all four duplexes appear, allowing recovery of the mutant DNA in a more or less pure form. For most sequencing purposes, this extra round of enrichment can be omitted because sequence analysis of heteroduplexes will be sufficient to identify the mutation.

References

1. Fischer, S. G. and Lerman, L. S. (1979) Length-independent separation of DNA restriction. *Cell* **16,** 191–200.
2. Myers, R. M., Maniatis, T., and Lerman, L. S. (1987) Detection and localization of single base changes by denaturing gradient gel electrophoresis. *Methods Enzymol.* **155,** 501–527.
3. Fodde, R. and Losekoot, M. (1994) Mutation detection by denaturing gradient gel electrophoresis (DGGE). *Hum. Mutat.* **3,** 83–94.
4. Abrams, E. S. and Stanton, V. P. (1992) Use of denaturing gradient gel electrophoresis to study conformational transitions in nucleic acids. *Methods Enzymol.* **212,** 71–104.
5. Fischer, S. G. and Lerman, L. S. (1983) DNA fragments differing by single basepair substitutions are separated in denaturing gradient gels: correspondence with melting theory. *Proc. Natl. Acad. Sci. USA* **80,** 1579–1583.
6. Sheffield, V. C., Cox, D. R., Lerman, L. S., and Myers, R. M. (1989) Attachment of a 40-base-pair G+C-rich sequence (GC-clamp) to genomic DNA fragments by the polymerase chain reaction in improved detection of single-base changes. *Proc. Natl. Acad. Sci. USA* **86,** 232–236.
7. Wartell, R. M., Hosseini, S., Powell, S., and Zhu, J. (1998) Detecting single base substitutions, mismatches and bulges in DNA by temperature gradient gel electrophoresis and related methods. *J. Chromatogr. A.* **806,** 169–185.
8. Van Orsouw, N. J., Li, D., van der Vlies, P., Scheffer, H., Eng, C., Buys, C. H. C. M., Li, F. P., and Vijg, J. (1996) Mutational scanning of large genes by extensive PCR multiplexing and two-dimensional electrophoresis: application to the RB1 gene. *Hum. Mol. Genet.* **5,** 755–761.
9. Guldberg, P., Grønbæk, K., Aggerholm, A., Platz, A., thor Straten, P., Ahrenkiel, V., Hokland, P., and Zeuthen, J. (1998) Detection of mutations in GC-rich DNA by bisulphite denaturing gradient gel electrophoresis. *Nucleic Acids Res.* **26,** 1548,1549.
10. Hovig, E., Smith-Sørensen, B., Brøgger, A., and Børresen, A. L. (1991) Constant denaturant gel electrophoresis, a modification of denaturing gradient gel electrophoresis, in mutation detection. *Mutat. Res.* **262,** 63–71.
11. Cremonesi, L., Firpo, S., Ferrari, M., Righetti, P. G., and Gelfi, C. (1997) Doublegradient DGGE for optimized detection of DNA point mutations. *Biotechniques* **22,** 326–330.
12. Guldberg, P. and Güttler, F. (1994) 'Broad-range' DGGE for single-step mutation scanning of entire genes: application to human phenylalanine hydroxylase gene. *Nucleic Acids Res.* **22,** 880,881.

Mutational Analysis by DGGE

13. Nedergaard, T., Guldberg, P., Ralfkiaer, E., and Zeuthen, J. (1997) A one-step DGGE scanning method for detection of mutations in the K-, N-, and H-ras oncogenes: mutations at codons 12, 13 and 61 are rare in B- cell non-Hodgkin's lymphoma. *Intl. J. Cancer* **71**, 364–369.

14. Guldberg, P., Nedergaard, T., Nielsen, H. J., Olsen, A. C., Ahrenkiel, V., and Zeuthen, J. (1997) Single-step DGGE-based mutation scanning of the p53 gene: application to genetic diagnosis of colorectal cancer. *Hum. Mutat.* **9**, 348–355.

15. Guldberg, P., thor Straten, P., Birck, A., Ahrenkiel, V., Kirkin, A. F., and Zeuthen, J. (1997) Disruption of the *MMAC1/PTEN* gene by deletion or mutation is a frequent event in malignant melanoma. *Cancer Res.* **57**, 3660–3663.

16. Grønbæk, K., thor Straten, P., Ralfkiaer, E., Ahrenkiel, V., Andersen, M. K., Hansen, N.E., Zeuthen, J., Hou-Jensen, K., and Guldberg, P. (1998) Somatic *Fas* mutations in non-Hodgkin's lymphoma: association with extranodal disease and autoimmunity. *Blood* **92**, 3018–3024.

17. Guldberg, P., Kirkin, A. F., Grønbæk, K., thor Straten, P., Ahrenkiel, V. and Zeuthen, J. (1997) Complete scanning of the CDK4 gene by denaturing gradient gel electrophoresis: a novel missense mutation but low overall frequency of mutations in sporadic metastatic malignant melanoma. *Intl. J. Cancer* **72**, 780–783.

18. Lerman, L. S. and Silverstein, K. (1987) Computational simulation of DNA melting and its application to denaturing gradient gel electrophoresis. *Methods Enzymol.* **155**, 482–501.

19. Abrams, E. S., Murdaugh, S. E., and Lerman, L. S. (1996) Intramolecular DNA melting between stable helical segments: melting theory and metastable states. *Nucleic Acids Res.* **23**, 2775–2783.

20. Costes, B., Girodon, E., Ghanem, N., Chassignol, M., Thuong, N. T., Dupret, D., and Goossens, M. (1993) Psoralen-modified oligonucleotide primers improve detection of mutations by denaturing gradient gel electrophoresis and provide an alternative to GC-clamping. *Hum. Mol. Genet.* **2**, 393–397.

11

Detection of Mutations in Human Cancer Using Nonisotopic RNase Cleavage Assay

Marianna Goldrick and James Prescott

1. Introduction

Nonisotopic RNase cleavage assay (NIRCA) is an RNase-cleavage-based method for mutation scanning that detects mutations as double-stranded cleavage products in duplex RNA targets. A central requirement for NIRCA is the ability to produce large amounts of double-stranded target RNA by in vitro transcription of PCR products containing opposable T7 phage promoters. The target regions are amplified from genomic DNA or cDNA using forward and reverse primers with T7 promoters added to their 5' ends. The crude polymerase chain reaction (PCR) products are then converted into double-stranded RNA by in vitro transcription with T7 polymerase, in reactions containing high concentrations of all four ribonucleotide triphosphates. Transcription typically results in a further amplification of the target region of at least 20-fold (*see* **Fig. 1**). After transcription, the reactions are heated and cooled to permit denaturation and hybridization of the complementary strands; mutations in the target region result in base pair mismatches in the duplex RNA, from hybridization of complementary wild-type and mutant transcripts. For heterozygous samples, the endogenous wild-type allele provides the reference strand needed to create the mismatch. For homozygous samples, wild-type and experimental PCR products are mixed before transcription to create the mismatches. After hybridization, the duplex RNA targets are treated with single-strand-specific ribonucleases to cleave mismatches on both strands. The reaction products are separated by electrophoresis on native agarose gels and detected by ethidium staining. Experimental samples are scored positive for mutations if they contain smaller fragments that are not present in a no-mismatch control.

From: *Methods in Molecular Medicine, vol. 68: Molecular Analysis of Cancer*
Edited by: J. Boultwood and C. Fidler © Humana Press Inc., Totowa, NJ

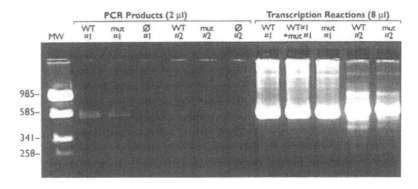

Fig. 1. Assessing efficiency of the transcription reaction. Target regions of approx 600 bp from the human *p53* tumor suppressor gene (samples #1) and from the *Factor IX* clotting factor gene (samples #2) were amplified with incorporation of opposable T7 promoters as described in the text. Left-hand side of gel shows 2 µL of each PCR product from indicated samples. Lanes marked Ø are no-template PCR controls. The right-hand side of the gel shows 8 µL the corresponding transcription reactions from each PCR product. The transcription reactions contained 2 µL of PCR product as template. Note the increase in ethidium-staining material seen after transcription. The ethidium-staining material trailing upward toward the wells in lanes containing transcription reactions may be owing to aberrant migration caused by the 3' overhangs in the duplex RNA (since transcription starts at the eighteenth base and runs off after transcribing the complement of the promoter at the opposite end), or may be due to excess of transcript derived from one strand. *Lane MW* contains molecular size markers, Sau3A restriction fragments of pUC 19 plasmid, with sizes in base pairs indicated.

In the protocol described below, the assay is carried out by the sequential addition of reagents for transcription, hybridization, and RNase cleavage to a single tube containing the crude PCR product; no intermediate purification of the reaction products is required. Once the PCR step is complete, the turnaround time for obtaining the assay results is approx 3 h. Many recent reports describe the use of NIRCA for mutational analysis of genes involved in human cancer and other genetic disorders (e.g., *see* **refs.** *1–23*).

1.1. Mismatch Cleavage by RNases

Historically, RNase A from bovine pancreas was used for mutation analysis *(24,25)*, but this enzyme is not ideal since it fails to cleave many mismatches and tends to generate a high background of nonspecific cleavage products *(26)*. More recently, a bacterial ribonuclease (RNase 1 from *Escherichia coli*) and a fungal ribonuclease (RNase T1 from aspergillus) have been found to be supe-

Use of NIRCA to Detect Mutations in Human Cancer

rior to RNase A for mismatch cleavage *(27)*. The mutation detection rate in NIRCA is maximized by treating the duplex RNA targets with a mixture of these two ribonucleases, which detect distinct but overlapping sets of mutations. The ability of RNase 1 and RNase T1 to cleave mismatches is dramatically increased by the use of a nonstandard reaction buffer containing intercalators and other components, which probably act on the substrate to increase the mismatch-induced helical distortion. A proprietary commercially available reaction buffer has been optimized for use with RNase 1 and RNase T1 (available from Ambion RNA Diagnostics, Austin, TX).

1.2. Sensitivity of NIRCA for Detecting Unknown Mutations

1.2.1. General Considerations

Generation of detectable cleavage products using NIRCA requires cleavage of both strands of the duplex RNA target. The extent of cleavage of a given mismatch depends not only on its sequence but also on the context in which it occurs. Since any point mutation results in a change of two nucleotides (a base pair), each mutation generates two reciprocal mismatches, from hybridization of the wild-type sense strand to the mutant antisense strand, and from hybridization of the wild-type antisense strand to the mutant sense strand. In the basic NIRCA protocol described below, the two reciprocal mismatches are generated in a single transcription reaction, from heterozygous PCR products with opposable T7 promoters. The duplex RNA samples comprise 25% of each reciprocal mismatch and 50% of duplex RNA with no mismatch. Mutations can be detected as long as one of the reciprocal mismatches is cleaved to detectable levels. If one of the reciprocal mismatches is refractory to cleavage, the observed extent of cleavage in the mixture will be reduced. The likelihood of cleaving both reciprocal mismatches is increased by using a mixture of RNases with distinct cleavage properties (i.e., RNase 1 and RNase T1). In some cases, however, both of the reciprocal mismatches are refractory to cleavage, and these mutations will not be detected. Most microinsertion/deletion mutations are detected, but very long insertion/deletion mutations may be cleaved less efficiently, probably owing to failure to cleave the shorter strand.

1.2.2. Assessing the Reciprocal Mismatches in Separate Reactions

In cases in which one reciprocal mismatch is not cleaved as well as the other, the assay can be made more sensitive, but also more laborious, by assessing the reciprocal mismatches in separate reactions. In this case, each mismatch comprises 50% of the sample. To assess the mismatches in separate reactions, the two strands of the unknown sample must be separately transcribed; however, each strand of the unknown sample may be cotranscribed with the complementary wild-type strand. To cotranscribe only one strand of the unknown sample along with the complementary wild-type strand, experimental PCR products containing a T7 promoter on one or the other end are mixed with wild-type PCR products having the T7 promoter on the opposite end. The wild-type and unknown target regions are amplified in separate reactions, using appropriate primer pairs, where only one of the primers contains a T7 promoter.

1.2.3. Sensitivity for Detecting Mutations in Mixed Populations of Normal and Mutant Cells

Patient samples obtained by routine methods frequently consist of tumor cells contaminated with normal cells such as lymphocytes, fibroblasts, and other stromal cells. The ability of NIRCA to detect mutations against a background of normal alleles has been assessed in a model system (*see* **Fig. 2**). In this system, a PCR product derived from a construct containing a 561-bp genomic fragment of the human *p53* tumor suppressor gene with a C > G transversion mutation was mixed with a wild-type *p53* PCR product in varying ratios, keeping the total amount of PCR product constant. These targets were assessed according to the standard NIRCA protocol, using a mixture of RNase 1 and RNase T1 for mismatch cleavage. Cleavage products resulting from the point mutation were detected when present at the level of 3% of the sample, i.e., when 97% of the sample consisted of the wild-type sequence. NIRCA has also been used to screen for *p53* mutations in bladder wash samples from patients diagnosed with bladder cancer. These samples typically consist of a mixture of tumor cells and normal cells sloughed off from the lumen of the bladder. Target regions of 561 bp (exons 5 + 6) and 765 bp (exons 7 + 8), which together account for 89% of all *p53* mutations reported in bladder cancer *(28)*, were amplified and screened from each patient. **Figure 3** shows representative cleavage products that were detected in several patient samples.

2. Materials

Store all reagents at –20°C unless otherwise noted. Enzymes should be stored in a nonfrost-free freezer.

2.1. PCR

1. 10X PCR buffer: 50 mM KCl, 10 mM Tris-HCl, pH 8.3, 1.5 mM MgCl$_2$.
2. dNTP stock solution: Mixture containing 2.5 mM of the sodium salts of each of the four deoxyribonucleotide triphosphates (dATP, dCTP, dGTP, TTP) in 10 mM Tris-HCl, pH 7.0.
3. Outer PCR primers: Mixture containing 5 µM of forward and reverse primers for preamplification of the target region to be screened (*see* **Note 1**).
4. PCR primers with T7 promoters: mixture containing 5 µM of forward and reverse primers, with the T7 bacteriophage promoter sequence added to the 5' end of each primer. The binding sites for these primers should lie within the region

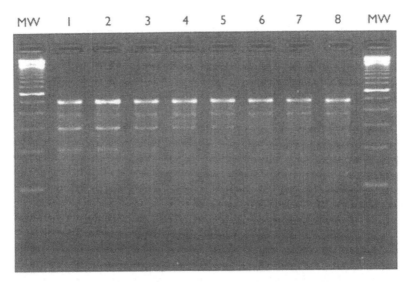

Fig. 2. Sensitivity of NIRCA for detecting mutations in mixed populations of normal and mutant cells. Target regions (561 bp of human *p53* genomic sequence spanning exons 5–6) were amplified by PCR from a sample with a C > G mutation at position 13172 (accession no. X54156) and from a normal control. The PCR products were quantitated and mixed in known ratios prior to the transcription step of the assay, keeping the total amount of PCR product constant in each reaction. Following transcription and hybridization, samples were treated with a mixture of RNase 1 + RNase T1 for cleavage of the mismatches as described in the text. The cleavage products (approx 325 and 225 bp) were resolved from the full-length product on a 3% agarose gel. *Lanes MW* contain molecular size markers (100-bp ladder; Life Technologies). The percentage of mutant PCR product used in each assay ranges from 50 to 3.1%, as follows: *lane 1*, 50%; *lane 2*, 25%; *lane 3*, 12.5%; *lane 4*, 8.3%; *lane 5*, 6.25%; *lane 6*, 4.2%; *lane 7*, 3.1%. *Lane 8* has the wild-type (no-mismatch) control sample. The larger cleavage product is detected down to the level of 3.1%. The sensitivity for detection of the smaller cleavage product is lower because less ethidium is bound to it (the amount of ethidium bound is proportional to the size of the fragment). The band migrating just below the full-length product is nonspecific.

amplified by the outer PCR primers in **item 3**, if a nested PCR strategy is used (*see* **Note 1**).
5. Thermostable polymerase.
6. Distilled deionized water.

2.2. Transcription of the PCR Product to Make Duplex RNA

1. 10X Transcription buffer: 400 mM Tris-HCl, pH 8.0, 60 mM MgCl$_2$, 20 mM spermidine HCl, 250 mM NaCl, 50 mM dithiothreitol.

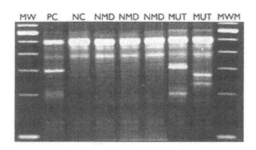

Fig. 3. Detection of *p53* mutations in bladder wash samples from cancer patients. Genomic DNA isolated from cell pellets recovered from bladder wash specimens of patients diagnosed with bladder cancer was used as template for amplifying *p53* target regions as described in the text. Targets consist of 561 bp (exons 5 + 6). Samples were transcribed, hybridized, and treated with a mixture of RNase 1 + RNase T1 for cleavage of mismatches as described in the text. Lanes marked MW contain molecular size markers as described in **Fig. 2** legend. *Lane PC* contains a positive control with a known mutation, and *lane NC* contains normal control sample. Patient samples scored as positive are indicated as MUT, while patient samples scored as NMD had no mutation detected.

2. rNTP stock solution: Mixture containing 2.5 m*M* of the sodium salts of each of the four ribonucleotide triphosphates (ATP, CTP, GTP, UTP) in 10 m*M* Tris-HCl, pH 7.0.
3. RNase-free distilled deionized water.
4. T7 RNA polymerase, 20 U/µL.
5. Hybridization solution: 50% deionized formamide, 25 m*M* NaCl, 5 m*M* disodium EDTA, pH 8.0.

2.3. RNase Cleavage of Mismatches

1. RNase digestion buffer (this reagent may be stored at room temperature).
   a. Recommended: RNase digestion buffer (pn no. 8527G; Ambion RNA Diagnostics). This buffer contains components required for optimal mismatch cleavage by RNase 1 and RNase T1.
   b. Alternative: 50 m*M* NaCl, 1 m*M* disodium EDTA, pH 8.0, 10 m*M* Tris-HCl, pH 7.5. This buffer is mainly useful with RNase A.
2. 100X RNase 1 Stock Solution: 16.5 U/µL recombinent RNase 1 from *E. coli*. Recommended, RNase 1 Stock Solution (pn no. 2283G; Ambion RNA Diagnostics).
3. 100X RNase T1 Stock Solution: 20,000 U/µL recombinent RNase T1 from aspergillus. Recommended, RNase T1 Stock Solution (pn no. 2284G; Ambion RNA Diagnostics).
4. (Optional) 100X RNase A Stock Solution: 0.165 mg/mL of RNase A from bovine pancreas (cat. no. R-5250; Sigma, St. Louis, MO) (approx 104 Kunitz units/mg protein), in 20 m*M* Tris-HCl, pH 7.5

Use of NIRCA to Detect Mutations in Human Cancer 147

2.4. Agarose Gel Analysis

1. Gel-loading solution: 3 M NaCl, 10 mM Tris-HCl, pH 7.5, 0.05% bromophenol blue, 10 µg/mL of ethidium bromide, 33% glycerol. Alternatively, High Resolution Gel Loading Solution (cat. no. 8542G; Ambion) may be used. This reagent may be stored at room temperature.
2. High-resolution agarose.
3. 10X Tris-borate EDTA (TBE): 0.9 M Tris-borate, 20 mM EDTA. Store at room temperature.
4. (Optional) Ethidium bromide stock solution: 10 mg/mL of ethidium bromide in distilled water. This solution may be stored at room temperature.

2.5. Equipment and Supplies

1. Equipment for preparing and running agarose gels:
   a. Horizontal electrophoresis box. Short, wide gel-boxes are most practical.
   b. Power source capable of at least 80 V.
2. Ultraviolet (UV) transilluminator.
3. Gel documentation system. A digital charge-coupled device camera is recommended. Alternatively, results may be recorded on Polaroid film.

3. Methods

3.1. Amplification of Target Region

Amplify the target region, typically ranging in size from 0.5 to 1 kb, from unknown and wild-type control samples and incorporate T7 phage promoters at each end of the amplified products (*see* **Note 1**). The use of software for computer-aided primer design is strongly recommended for choosing the PCR primers. Reaction volumes can be scaled according to user preference; two microliters of PCR product is needed for each sample in **Subheading 3.2.**

For a 50-µL PCR, combine the following components and amplify the target with 25–30 cycles according to standard protocols *(29)*: genomic DNA or first-strand cDNA, 5 µL of 10X PCR buffer, 2.5 µL of mixture of forward and reverse primers, 2.5 µL of dNTP stock solution, water to final volume of 50 µL, and 1 to 2 U of thermostable DNA polymerase.

3.2. In Vitro Transcription of Amplified Target Region

Transcribe the experimental and wild-type PCR products to make duplex RNA targets for RNase cleavage. Purification of the PCR products before transcription is not necessary, since the T7 promoter sequence in unincorporated PCR primers is single stranded, and therefore will not be recognized by T7 polymerase.

1. Prepare a transcription reaction master mix containing (by volume) 40% nuclease-free water, 15% 10X transcription buffer, 30% rNTP mix, and 15% T7

RNA polymerase. For each sample, 4 µL of transcription reaction master mix is needed. Mix thoroughly by repeated pipetting or by gently flicking the reaction vessel. Do not mix by vigorous vortexing. Spin briefly if desired.

2. Add 4 µL of transcription reaction master mix to 2 µL of each PCR product containing opposable T7 promoters (*see* **Note 2**). Mix gently but thoroughly.
3. Incubate for 1 h at 37°C.
4. Add 2 µL of hybridization solution to each reaction and mix briefly.
5. Heat reactions in a heat block at 95–105°C for 3–5 min. Remove the reactions and cool to room temperature (~5 min). Spin briefly if desired. This step permits complementary strands of wild-type and mutant transcripts to denature and reanneal to create the mismatches. Hybridization of the transcripts is very rapid owing to the high concentrations of the complementary transcripts and the low complexity of the reaction. If desired, the efficiency of the transcription reaction may be assessed at this point (*see* **Note 3**). Reactions may be stored at –20°C.

3.3. Treatment of Hybridized Samples with RNases

1. Prepare working solution containing RNase stock solution(s) diluted in RNase digestion buffer (*see* **Note 4**). The standard volume of RNase solution used for each sample is 24 µL. Standard RNase dilutions are 1:100 for each RNase. RNase 1 and RNase T1 are generally mixed in a single solution. Use RNase A alone owing to its greater tendency to cause overdigestion/nonspecific cleavage. The diluted RNase solutions may be mixed by gentle vortexing.
2. Add 24 µL of diluted RNase solution to each 8-µL transcription reaction and mix thoroughly. To conserve RNase digestion reagents, the reactions may be scaled down; for example, 4-µL aliquots of each transcription reaction may be removed to separate vessels (96-well U-bottomed microtiter plates are suggested) and treated with 12 µL of RNase solution. Microtiter plates must be covered during incubation to prevent evaporation.
3. Incubate the reactions for 30 min at 37°C.
4. Add 6 µL of gel loading solution to each sample and mix briefly.

3.4. Analyzing RNase Cleavage Products on Agarose Gel

1. Prepare a 2.5% high-resolution agarose gel in 1X TBE (*see* **Note 5**). Well capacity should be approx 25–30 µL. If desired, ethidium may be added to the lower buffer chamber to a final concentration of 0.5 µg/mL to improve staining of very small fragments (free ethidium runs in the opposite direction from nucleic acid, i.e., toward the cathode).
2. Load the reactions into the wells of the gel and run it at an appropriate voltage such that the dye band migrates approx 3 to 4 cm in about 30–45 min. Typically, this is achieved by running the gel at about 5 V/cm of distance between the anode and cathode, or at 80–90 V for short gel boxes. In the standard one-tube assay, the nominal final reaction volume is 38 µL, so there will be some sample remaining after loading. It is acceptable for the gel and buffer to become slightly warm, but not hot, during the run. The exact voltage, temperature, and duration of elec-

Use of NIRCA to Detect Mutations in Human Cancer

trophoresis are not critical parameters. Restriction fragments of plasmid DNA (e.g., pUC19 cut with Sau3A) can be used as molecular size markers (the mobility of duplex DNA is very similar to that of duplex RNA on native agarose gels).

3. When the dye band has migrated about 2.5–3 cm from the well, transfer the gel to a UV transilluminator and examine it for the presence of cleavage products.
4. Replace the gel in the buffer and continue electrophoresis for about 10–15 min longer. Examine the gel again under UV light and record the results (*see* **Note 6**). Mutations in experimental lanes are indicated by the presence of smaller subfragments that are not seen in the no-mismatch (wild-type) control lane. When assessing results using a digital camera, the image may be electronically manipulated to aid interpretation of the data (*see* **Fig. 4** and **Note 7**).

4. Notes

1. This step is often accomplished using a two-step nested PCR strategy. The first-step PCR uses genomic DNA or first-strand cDNA as template and forward and reverse primers with no extra sequences. The second PCR step uses an aliquot of the first-step PCR as template, and forward and reverse primers containing T7 promoters. The primer-binding sites for the second-step primers (or at least their 3' ends) are nested within the product amplified in the first-step PCR. The 20-base consensus T7 promoter sequence is added to 5' end of both the forward and reverse primers used for the second-step (nested) PCR. The promoters are thus incorporated into the ends of the amplified target (this is analogous to adding restriction site sequences to the ends of PCR primers to yield amplified products flanked by desired restriction sites). The consensus T7 promoter is: 5' TAATACGACTCACTATAGGG. The last three bases of the T7 promoter (GGG) comprise the transcription initiation site, that is, these are the first three bases of the transcripts, and the 3' end of the T7 promoter may be overlapped with the 5' end of the nested primer binding site to reduce slightly the size of the nested primers. The size of the nested T7 primers is typically in the range of 35–40 bases. Keep in mind when designing primers that mismatches that occur very close to the ends of the targets may be difficult to detect, since the cleavage products will consist of one very small fragment and one large fragment very close in size to the full-length uncleaved target. For this reason, genomic targets are usually designed to contain a minimum of ~50 bp of intron sequence flanking the coding regions to be screened, and when large regions are screened as smaller contiguous subregions, the adjacent targets should overlap by at least 15% of their size. When screening long contiguous coding regions, a single pair of outer primers can sometimes be used to generate a product for several adjacent nested PCRs *(1)*. Target regions are generally between about 0.5 and 1 kb, but longer targets have been used successfully (*see* **Fig. 4** for an example of detection of mutations in target regions of 1.6 kb).

   It may not always be necessary to use the two-stage nested PCR procedure. In principle, a single PCR reaction can be done using primers containing the T7 promoter sequences. However, the two-step amplification strategy compensates

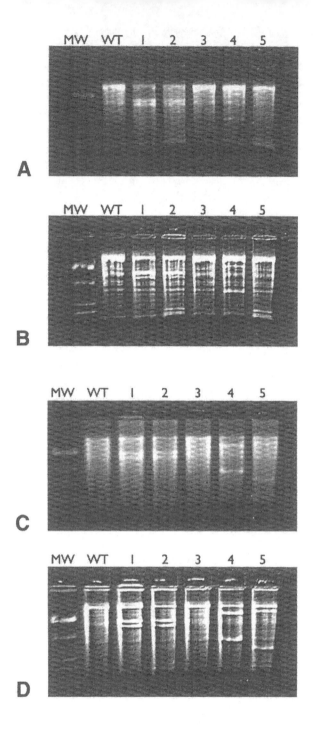

Fig. 4. Comparison of RNase A and RNase 1/RNase T1 mixture for detection of mutations in *APC* targets. Target regions spanning 1637 bp of coding sequence from the long exon of the adenomatous polyposis coli (*apc*) gene, associated with colorectal

Use of NIRCA to Detect Mutations in Human Cancer 151

for suboptimal yields owing to variation in the quality of the clinical/experimental samples and increases the specificity of the product when amplifying single-copy sequences from complex mixtures (genomic DNA or total RNA). When screening for mutations in plasmids, virus, bacteria, mitochondrial genes, existing PCR products, or other high copy number, low complexity samples, a single-step PCR step generally can be used.

2. If the experimental samples are known to be homozygous for the target region (e.g., when screening for mutations in X-linked genes from human males), 1 µL of the second-step experimental PCR product should be mixed with 1 µL of the second-step wild-type PCR product before transcription. When screening for somatic mutations in tumor samples, it is possible that mutations in autosomal genes may be homozygous owing to loss of the normal allele (loss of heterozygosity). However, in cases of loss of heterozygosity, it is likely that the wild-type sequence needed to create the mismatch will be provided by contaminating normal cells present in the sample.

3. To assess the efficiency of the transcription reaction, run all or some of the reaction after the hybridization step on a native agarose gel. As a control, also run the amount of PCR template that will be carried over in the transcription reaction (the amount of PCR product in the transcription reaction after hybridization is 25% of the total volume). The amount of ethidium-staining material in the transcription reaction should be at least 10-fold greater than the amount of PCR product used as template (*see* **Fig. 3**). Any excess of one strand produced in the transcription reaction will be degraded in the RNase step and have no detrimental effect on the assay.

4. Optimal concentrations of the RNases for particular targets may be determined empirically. The need to optimize RNase concentration for particular targets is generally greater for RNase A than for RNase 1 and RNase T1. For A+U-rich targets or targets containing short A+U-rich regions, a reduction in RNase A concentration is usually required to prevent overdigestion. RNase 1 concentrations may need to be reduced when yields of duplex RNA are low or when screening very long target regions (>1 kb).

Fig. 4. *(continued)* cancer, were screened using the standard NIRCA protocol. Transcription reactions were scaled up twofold, and equal aliquots were treated separately with either RNase A **(A,B)** or a mixture of RNase 1 + RNase T1 **(C,D)**, using the digestion buffers described in the text. Gels were imaged using a digital camera; (B,D) are the same gels shown in (A,C), respectively, but imaged using the contour filter option to enhance detection of faint cleavage products. Samples are shown in the same order for both gels. *Lane WT*, wild-type control; *lanes 1–5*, patient samples. Samples scored as positive are in *lanes 1, 2, 4*, and *5*. *Lane MW* contains molecular size markers as described in **Fig. 1** legend. Note that the samples treated with RNase A have more nonspecific cleavage products than the samples treated with RNases 1 + RNase T1.

To optimize the RNase cleavage step, a pilot experiment may be carried out on a small panel of samples containing a no-mismatch control and one or more samples with mutations. The samples should be treated with the RNase stock solutions separately and, if desired, with a mixture of RNase 1 and RNase T1. Use a range of RNase concentrations; for example, RNase stock solutions may be diluted 1:50, 1:100, and 1:300. Overdigestion is indicated by lack of all or most of the full-length duplex in the no-mismatch control, with samples running as diffuse smears. Overdigestion is more common with RNase A and RNase 1 than with RNase T1, especially if yields of duplex RNA target are low. Overdigestion with RNase A tends to generate discrete bands, whereas overdigestion with RNase 1 usually results in diffuse smears. Overdigestion with RNase T1 is rare. Some targets will show nonspecific cleavage products owing to cleavage at hypersensitive sites (e.g., A+U-rich regions). Nonspecific fragments are those seen in every sample, including the no-mismatch control, and their presence is not indicative of a mutation (*see* **Fig. 4**). Underdigestion is suggested if there is no difference between RNase-treated and untreated samples. Typically, there is a reduction in the total amount of duplex RNA as well as a detectable background of diffuse nonspecific digestion products in RNase-treated samples, compared with untreated samples. This difference may be more pronounced for longer targets. If transcription was suboptimal, there will be very little duplex RNA, and the ethidium-staining material remaining after RNase treatment may consist of residual PCR template, which can be mistaken for uncleaved target duplex. To determine whether this is a problem, run aliquots of the RNase-treated no-mismatch control duplex, along with the amount of PCR product carried over in the reaction as a control, as described in **Note 3**. If the band intensities are equal, there is no duplex RNA in the treated sample, owing to poor yield of transcript or to overdigestion.

5. Short gels are more practical than long ones because less agarose is required and samples can be easily run off the end of the gel, facilitating reuse of gels. For convenience, a single standard-length casting tray (~22 cm long) can be used to prepare several gels, by spacing multiple combs along the length of the tray at intervals of about 5 cm. Teflon combs are recommended. Chilling the gel at 4°C before removing the comb may help prevent the wells from tearing. Scrubbing the comb with hot tap water and a scouring sponge immediately after removing it from the solidified gel will minimize the tendency for it to cause agarose debris in the wells the next time it is used. Any shards of agarose or precipitated TBE present in the wells should be flushed out with running buffer before loading the samples. To minimize tearing of the wells, run the gel on an UV transparent tray that can be lifted out of the gel box and placed on the transilluminator for scoring samples. The agarose gels generally can be reused for analyzing multiple sets of samples. Run the fragments from the previous experiment off the bottom of the gel at low voltage prior to reuse. The TBE running buffer should be changed fairly frequently, after about 2 h of electrophoresis per liter of buffer. If the dye band becomes diffuse during electrophoresis, the buffer should be changed.

Use of NIRCA to Detect Mutations in Human Cancer   153

6. The following considerations should be kept in mind when scoring samples:
   a. Some targets will show nonspecific cleavage products owing to cleavage at hypersensitive sites, e.g., A+U-rich regions (this is more common with RNase A). Nonspecific fragments are those seen in every sample, including the no-mismatch control, and their presence is not indicative of a mutation.
   b. Occasionally, there may be nonspecific fragments that comigrate with mismatch-specific cleavage products in experimental lanes. This is more likely to be the case when RNase A is used for digestion (*see* **Fig. 4**). Experimental samples should be scored positive if they contain subfragments that show a significantly brighter fluorescent signal under UV light, compared with similar-sized, and usually less distinct, fragments in the no-mismatch control lane.
   c. The closer the mutation is to the end of the target region, the longer the gel must be run in order to detect it. To rule out cleavage products larger than ~90% of full length, gels must be run until the dye band has migrated ~4 cm (or has run off the bottom of a short gel) and carefully examined for the presence of a doublet running at the position of the full-length fragment in the no-mismatch control lane.
   d. Large cleavage products may be obscured when the amount of full-length duplex is very high. In cases of exceptionally high yields of RNA, large cleavage products may be more easily detected by running a reduced amount of the reaction.
   e. Cleavage products of the same size that are seen repeatedly in multiple samples may be owing to common sequence polymorphisms. Mutations in experimental samples which are also heterozygous for polymorphisms can generally still be detected by the altered mobility of one fragment.
   f. Samples containing faint or poorly resolved cleavage products, barely detectable over background, should be reanalyzed in a blinded test. If they are scored "plus-minus" a second time, they probably contain mutations.
7. To improve detection of faint cleavage products in samples assessed using digital gel documentation systems, the image can be manipulated electronically. For example, exposure times can be integrated over longer intervals, gray-scale settings can be adjusted, and various filter options such as contour imaging can be used to make faint cleavage products more pronounced (*see* **Fig. 4**). However, to avoid false positives when electronically manipulating the image, it is important always to compare cleavage patterns of experimental samples with that of the no-mismatch control.

References

1. Gibbons, R. J., Bachoo, S., Picketts, D. J., Aftimos, S., Asenbauer, B., Bergoffen, S. (1997) Mutations in transcriptional regulator ATRX establish the functional significance of a PHD-like domain. *Nat. Genet.* **17,** 146,147.
2. Firestein, G. S., Echeverri, F., Yeo, M., Zvaifler, N. J., and Green, D. R. (1997) Somatic mutations in the p53 tumor suppressor gene in rheumatoid athritis synovium. *Proc. Natl. Acad. Sci USA* **94,** 10,895–10,900.

3. Tsai, T., Davalath, S., Rankin, C., Radich, J. P., Head, D., Appelbaum, F. R., and Boldt, D. H. (1996) Tumor suppressor gene alteration in adult acute lymphoblastic leukemia (ALL). *Leukemia* **10**, 1901–1910.

4. Toyoshima, M., Hara, T., Zhang, H., Yamamoto, T., Akaboshi, S., Nanba, E., et al. (1998) Ataxia-telangiectasia without immunodeficiency: novel point mutations within and adjacent to the phosphatidylinositol 3-kinase-like domain. *Am. J. Med. Gene.* **75**, 141–144.

5. De Souza, A. T., Hankins, G. R., Washington, M. K., Orton, T. C., and Jirtle, R. L. (1995) M6P/IGF2R gene is mutated in human hepatocellular carcinomas with loss of heterozygosity. *Nat. Gene.* **11**, 447–449.

6. Faudoa, R., Xue, Z., Lee, F., Baser, M., and Hung, G. (2000) Detection of novel NF2 mutations by an RNA mismatch cleavage method. *Hum. Mutat.* **15**, 474–478.

7. Peral, B., Gamble, V., Strong, C., Ong, A. C., Sloane-Stanley, J., Zerres, K., et al. (1997) Identification of mutations in the duplicated region of the polycystic kidney disease gene (PKD1) by a novel approach. *Am. J. Hum. Gene.* **60**, 1399–1410.

8. Maslen, C., Babcock, D., Raghunath, M., and Steinman, B. (1997) A rare branch-point mutation is associated with missplicing of fibrillin-2 in a large family with congenital contractural arachnodactyly. *Am. J. Hum. Gene.* **60**, 1389–1398.

9. Janezic, S., Ziogas, A., Krumroy, L., Krasner, L., Plummer, S., Cohen, P., et al. (1999) Germline BRCA1 alterations in a population-based series of ovarian cancer patients. *Hum. Mol. Gene.* **8**, 889–897.

10. Macera, M., Godec, C., Sharma, N., and Verma, R. (1999) Loss of heterozygosity of the TP53 tumor suppressor gene and detection of point mutations by the non-isotopic RNase cleavage assay in prostate cancer. *Cancer Genet. Cytogenet.* **108**, 42–47.

11. Prescott, J., Patel, H., Tillman, S., McHugh, T., and Ralph, D. (1999) Cleavage of double-stranded copy RNA by RNase 1 and RNase T1 provides a robust means to dect p53 gene mutations in clinical specimens. *Electrophoresis* **20**, 1149–1161.

12. Moschese, V., Orlandi, P., Plebani, A., Arvanitidis, K., Fiorini, M., Speletas, M., et al. (Italian XLA Collaborative group) (2000) X-chromosome inactivation and mutation pattern in the Bruton's tyrosine kinase gene in patients with X-linked agammaglobulinemia. *Mol. Med.* **6**, 104–113.

13. Osato, M., Asou, N., Abdalla, E., Hoshino, K., Yamasaki, H., Okubo, T., et al. (1999) Biallelic and Heterozygous point mutations in the runt domain of the AML/PEBP2B gene associated with myeloblastic leukemias. *Blood* **93**, 1817–1824.

14. Orlandi, P., Ritis, K., Moschese, V., et al. (1999) Identification of nine novel mutations in the Bruton's tyrosine kinase gene in X-linked agammaglobulinemia patients. *Hum. Mutat.* (Mutation in Brief Online #285 http://journals.wiley.com/1059-7794).

15. Yoshihara, T., Yamamoto, M., Doyu, M., Mis, K. I., Hattori, N., Hasegawa, Y., et al. (2000) Mutations in the peripheral myelin protein zero and connexin 32 genes dected by non-isotopic Rnase cleavage assay and their phenotypes in Japenese patients with Charcot-Marie-Tooth disease. *Hum. Mutat.* **16**, 177,178.

16. Nakamura, M., Yamashita, T., Ando, Y., Tashima, K., Ohlsson, P., and Benson, M. (1999) Identification of a new transthyretin variant in familial amyloidotic poly-

neuropathy using electrospray ionization mass spectrometry and nonisotopic RNase cleavage assay. *Hum. Hered.* **49,** 186–189.

17. Hishinuma, A., Kasai, K., Masawa, N., Kanno, Y., Aimura, M., and Ieiri, T. (1998) Missense mutation (C1263R) in the thyroglobulin gene causes congenital goiter with mild hypothyroidism by impaired intracellular transport. *Endoc. J.* **45,** 315–327.

18. Gitomer, W., Reed, B., Ruml, L., Sakhaee, K., and Pak, C. (1998) Mutations in the genomic DNA for SLC3A1 patients with cystinuria. *J. Clin. Endocrinol. Metab.* **83,** 3688–3694.

19. Hung, G., Faudoa, R., Baser, M., Xue, Z., Kluwe, L., Slattery, W., et al. (2000) Neurofibromatosis 2 phenotypes and germ-line NF2 mutations determined by an RNA mismatch method and loss of heterozygosity analysis in NF2 Schwannomas. *Cancer Gentet. Cytogenet.* **118,** 167,168.

20. Giunta, C. and Steinmann, B. (2000) Compound heterozygosity for a disease-causing G1489D and disease-modifying G530S substitution in COL5A1 of a patient with the classical type of Ehlers-Danlos syndrome: an explanation of intrafamilial variability. *Am. J. Med. Gene.* **90,** 72–79.

21. Giunta, C. and Steinmann, B. (2000) Characterization of 11 new mutations in COL3A1 of individuals with Ehlers-Danlos syndrome Type IV: preliminary comparison of Rnase cleavage, EMC, and DHPLC assays. *Hum. Mutat.* **16,** 176,177.

22. Shen, D., Wu, Y., Subbarao, M., Bhat, H., Chillar, R., and Vadgama, J. (2000) Mutation analysis of BRCA1 gene in African American patients with breast cancer. *J. Natl. Med. Assoc.* **92,** 29–35.

23. Shen, D., Wu, Y., Chillar, R., and Vadgama, J. (2000) Missense alterations of BRCA1 gene detected in diverse cancer patients. *Anticancer Res.* **20,** 1129–1132.

24. Myers, R. M., Larin, Z., and Maniatis, T. (1985) Detection of single base substitutions by ribonuclease cleavage at mismatches in RNA:DNA duplexes. *Science* **230,** 1242–1246.

25. Winter, E., Yamamoto, F., Almoguera, C., and Perucho, M. (1985) A method to detect and characterize point mutations in transcribed genes. *Proc. Natl. Acad. Sci. USA* **82,** 7575–7579.

26. Theophilus, B. D. M., Latham, T., Grabowski, G. A., and Smith, F. I. (1989) Comparison of RNase A, a chemical cleavage and GC-clamped denaturing gradient gel electrophoresis for the detection of mutations in exon 9 of the human acid beta-glucosidase gene. *Nucleic Acids Res.* **17,** 7707–7722.

27. Goldrick, M. (1996) Detection of mutations by RNase cleavage (alternate protocol), in *Current Protocols in Human Genetics*, Suppl. 14 (Dracopoliu, N. C., Haines, J. L., and Korf, B. R., eds.), John Wiley & Sons, New York, pp. 7.2.5–7.2.17.

28. Hainaut, P., Hernandez, T., Robinson, A., Rodriguez-Tome, P., Flores, T., Hollstein, M., et al. (1998) *Nucleic Acids Res.* **26,** 205–213.

29. Innis, M. A., Gelfand, D. H., and Sninsky, J. J. (eds.) (1990) *PCR Protocols, A Guide to Methods and Applications.* Academic Press, San Diego, CA.

12

Mutational Analysis of the Neurofibromatosis Type 1 Gene in Childhood Myelodysplastic Syndromes Using a Protein Truncation Assay

Lucy Side

1. Introduction

Neurofibromatosis type 1 (NF1) is a common autosomal dominant condition affecting approx 1 in 3500 persons *(1)*. Individuals with NF1 have a small but significant risk of developing cancers, primarily derived from neural crest tissues, such as astrocytic brain tumors and malignant peripheral nerve sheath tumours *(1)*. In addition, children with NF1 are at increased risk of developing malignant myeloid disorders, particularly a form of myelodysplasia termed juvenile myelomonocytic leukemia (JMML) *(2–4)*. Thus, NF1 may be considered an heritable cancer syndrome, a group of disorders characterized by an increased risk of developing primary cancers.

The majority of heritable cancer syndromes are caused by an inherited mutation in a single copy of a tumor suppressor gene *(5–7)*. Tumor suppressor genes act to restrain cellular proliferation via several mechanisms including regulation of cell-cycle progression, signal transduction, and apoptosis. Classically, tumor suppressor genes behave in a recessive manner at the cellular level such that inactivation of both alleles is required for the development of a cancer *(5,6,8,9)*. This phenomenon, referred to as Knudson's two-hit hypothesis, was first described in relation to the childhood tumor retinoblastoma *(10)*. Here, a germline mutation of the retinoblastoma gene *(RB1)* confers a cancer predisposition and a subsequent "second hit" inactivates the other *RB1* allele, allowing the malignant clone to develop. Similarly, in NF1, individuals with a germline mutation of the neurofibromatosis type 1 gene *(NF1)* have a higher incidence of malignant neural crest tumors and JMML.

From: *Methods in Molecular Medicine, vol. 68: Molecular Analysis of Cancer*
Edited by: J. Boultwood and C. Fidler © Humana Press Inc., Totowa, NJ

157

The importance of tumor suppressor genes, however, is not restricted to a small number of individuals with familial cancer syndromes. Somatic mutations of these genes are often sustained in sporadic tumors. For instance, the *TP53* tumor suppressor gene is the most frequently mutated gene in human malignancy *(6)*. Other examples include the *APC* gene, inherited in familial adenomatous polyposis but frequently implicated in sporadic colon cancer *(11)*, and *RB1*, which is involved in the pathogenesis of many small-cell lung carcinomas *(6)*. Thus, the study of the genetics of heritable cancer syndromes has greatly enhanced our general understanding of the events resulting in tumor formation. This rationale led to our study of the *NF1* gene, in order to establish its role as a tumor suppressor gene in pediatric myelodysplasia in patients both with and without NF1 *(12,13)*.

In common with other tumor suppressor genes, *NF1* has proved a difficult target for mutational analysis. *NF1* is a large gene, comprising a 12 kb mRNA that encodes 59 exons and a 327 kDa protein *(14)*. Historically, conventional mutation detection methods including Southern blotting and single-strand conformation polymorphism analysis have proved relatively insensitive, detecting only 20% of *NF1* mutations in patients with an established clinical diagnosis of NF1 *(15)*. These problems are compounded by the fact that there does not appear to be a particular mutational "hot spot" in the *NF1* gene, and thus, it is necessary to analyze the entire coding sequence in the majority of patients with unknown mutations *(15)*. Approximately 80% of documented *NF1* gene alterations are nonsense or frameshift mutations and would be predicted to cause premature translation termination with consequent truncation of the protein *(15–17)*. For this reason, the in vitro transcription and translation technique (IVTT), also referred to as the protein truncation assay, has been successfully adapted for screening for mutations in *NF1* *(16,17)*.

The protein truncation assay has been shown to be sensitive, detecting 67–70% of germline *NF1* mutations, and has a specificity approaching 100% (Michael Luce, personal communication). Because only truncating mutations are detected, there is no need for extensive investigation of rare polymorphisms in order to determine whether they are pathogenic. In addition, because total cellular RNA is used as template, detailed knowledge of the genomic organization of a gene is not necessary. Thus, the protein truncation assay has proved an efficient method for analyzing candidate genes for mutations in human disease. This approach has been successful in establishing the role of a number of tumor suppressor genes including *DPC4/SMAD4* in pancreatic malignancies and *PTEN/MMAC1* in a variety of tumors including primary glioblastomas *(18,19)*.

The protein truncation assay was developed by two groups and originally was used for screening the dystrophin gene (*DMD*) in Duchenne muscular dys-

NF1 *Mutational Analysis by IVTT*

trophy and *APC* in patients with familial adenomatous polyposis *(20,21)*. Reverse transcriptase-polymerase chain reaction (RT-PCR) is used to amplify overlapping fragments of the coding sequence; in the case of *NF1*, we and others have found that RT-PCR products of approx 2 kb proved optimal for analysis *(12,17)*. The sense oligonucleotide primer is designed to encode a T7 RNA polymerase promoter sequence as well as a translation initiation sequence (*see* **Table 1**) *(12,17)*. Transcription and translation of the RT-PCR template can then be carried out as a coupled reaction, in a single tube, using a commercially available rabbit reticulocyte lysate mix (Promega, Madison, WI) to which a radiolabeled amino acid, such as ^{35}S-methionine, has been added. This enables in vitro synthesis of labeled polypeptides, which are then denatured and resolved by electrophoresis on a sodium dodecyl sulfate (SDS)-polyacrylamide gel. Truncated peptides generated from nonsense or frameshift mutations in the original coding sequence appear as additional smaller bands compared to the gene product of the normal allele. The size of the abnormal truncated protein may be estimated by comparison with a prestained protein marker; this allows the approximate position of the mutation in the coding sequence to be calculated.

RT-PCR product that gives rise to the truncated protein may then be cloned into a plasmid vector and dideoxy sequencing performed to confirm the putative mutation. However, a potential problem is that mRNAs harboring truncating mutations may be selectively degraded by various mechanisms such as exonucleolytic digestion *(22)*. Consequently, this RT-PCR product may be under-represented in the cloning reaction compared with that derived from the normal allele. Binnie et al. *(23)* have devised a strategy to circumvent this problem, which we have also used in our analysis of patients with *NF1* and myeloid disorders. Plasmid DNA is extracted from individual clones and subjected to a second round of IVTT. These polypeptides are analyzed by gel electrophoresis; only clones that are known to give rise to a truncated protein are then selected for sequencing. Because the position of the nucleotide alteration may be inferred from the size of the truncated peptide with reasonable accuracy (within approx 100 nt), appropriate primers can be designed, thus obviating the need to sequence the entire 2-kb RT-PCR product. We and others have found that this technique, termed second-stage IVTT, significantly reduces unnecessary sequencing of numerous plasmid clones that represent the normal allele *(12,23)*.

In our experience, therefore, the protein truncation assay has proved an efficient method of detecting mutations in a large gene such as *NF1* *(12,13)*. Obviously the quality of RNA extracted is crucial to the success of the assay, but we have used both fresh and frozen human blood and bone marrow mononuclear cells, as well as lymphoblastoid cell lines, with good results, despite the fact

Table 1
Oligonucleotide Primers for PCR Amplification of *NF1* Coding Sequence[a]

Segment	Nucleotides spanned[b]	Exons	Product size (bp)	Primer sequence[c,d]
1	1–1868	1–12b	1868	**1F**: ATG GTT ATA AGC GGC CTC ACT AC
				1R: TG ACA GGA ACT TCT ATC TGC CTG CTT A
2	1468–3583	10b–21	2115	**2F**: ATG GTG AAA CTA ATT CAT GCA GAT
				2R: T GTC AAA TTC TGT GCC TTG
3	3217–5256	19b–29	2039	**3F**: ATG GAA GCA GTA GTT TCA CTT
				3R: TAG GAC TTT TGT TCG CTC TGC TGA
4	4998–6987	28–38	1989	**4F**: ATG GAG TAC ACC AAG TAT CAT GAG
				4R: TAT ACG GAG ACT ATC TAA AGT ATG CAG
5	6574–8404	35–49	1830	**5F**: ATG GAG GCA TGC ATG AGA GAT ATT C
				5R: T CTG CAC TTG GCT TGC GGA T

[a]From **ref. *17*** with permission. bp, base pairs; F, forward primer; R, reverse primer.

[b]Numbering corresponds to cDNA sequence with base 1 representing the A of the initiating ATG.

[c]Forward primer should be tagged with the following T7 promoter sequence and eukaryotic translation initiation site at its 5' end: 5'-GGATCCTAATACGACTCACTATAGGGAGACCACC-3'.

[d]Forward and reverse primers should be tagged with appropriate sequences at the 5' end if the CloneAmp kit is to be used (*see* manufacturer's instructions).

NF1 *Mutational Analysis by IVTT* 161

that *NF1* is not expressed at high levels in these tissues. We have also successfully adapted the assay to analyze candidate tumor suppressor genes in other hematopoietic malignancies (L. Side, A. Banerjee, and K. M. Shannon, unpublished data).

2. Materials

2.1. Mononuclear Cell Separation

1. Culture medium: 90% RPMI 1640, 10% fetal bovine serum (Gibco-BRL, Gaithersburg, MD).
2. Density gradient: Histopaque™-1077 (Sigma, St. Louis, MO).

2.2. RNA Preparation

1. TRIzol™ reagent (Gibco-BRL).
2. Chloroform.
3. Isopropanol.
4. 75% Ethanol in RNase-free water.
5. RNase-free water (add 0.01% diethylpyrocarbonate to distilled water in glass bottles, allow to stand overnight, and autoclave).

2.3. First-Strand cDNA Synthesis

1. SuperScript™ II RNase H-Reverse Transcriptase (200 U/µL) (Gibco-BRL).
2. 5X First-strand buffer: 250 mM Tris-HCl, pH 8.3, 375 mM KCl, 15 mM MgCl$_2$, supplied with enzyme.
3. 0.1 M dithiothreitol (DTT) (supplied with enzyme).
4. 25 mM dNTPs (25 mM each of dATP, dCTP, dGTP, and dTTP) (Gibco-BRL).
5. RNasin (40 U/µL) (Promega, Madison, WI).
6. Random hexamer pd(N)$_6$ (1 mg/mL) (Pharmacia, Washington, DC).
7. Single-strand DNA-binding protein (US Biochemical, Cleveland, OH).
8. RNase-free water.

2.4. Polymerase Chain Reaction

1. 10X PCR buffer II (Perkin-Elmer, Foster City, CA).
2. 25 mM MgCl$_2$ (supplied with buffer).
3. 10 mM dNTPs (10 mM each of dATP, dCTP, dGTP, and dTTP).
4. AmpliTaq™ DNA polymerase (5 U/µL) (Perkin-Elmer).
5. Single-strand DNA-binding protein (US Biochemical).
6. Oligonucleotide primers (diluted to a concentration of 10 pmol/µL for each primer). Refer to **Table 1** for details of sequences.
7. AmpliWax™ PCR Gem 100 (Perkin-Elmer).
8. Sterile distilled water.
9. Perkin-Elmer 9600 thermocycling machine.

2.5. Agarose Gel Electrophoresis

1. 1X TAE buffer: 50X TAE buffer contains 242 g of Tris base, 57.1 mL of glacial acetic acid, and 100 mL of 0.5 M EDTA, pH 8.0; adjust to 1 L total volume with distilled water.

162   *Side*

2. Ethidium bromide (10 mg/mL stock solution).
3. DNA-grade agarose.
4. 10X Gel-loading dye: 0.25% bromophenol blue, 0.25% xylene cyanol, 15% Ficoll-400 (Pharmacia).
5. λHindIII DNA molecular marker (Gibco-BRL).
6. Distilled water.

2.6. IVTT Reaction

1. TNT T7 coupled reticulocyte lysate system (Promega).
2. RNasin (40 U/μL) (Promega).
3. EXPRE^{35}S^{35}S Translabel (Dupont NEN, Wilmington, DE).
4. PCR-amplified DNA template.

2.7. Sodium Dodecyl Sulfate Polyacrylamide Gel Electrophoresis

1. Reducing sample buffer: 10 mL of 1 M Tris-HCl, pH 6.8, 8 mL of 20% SDS, 4 mL of 2-β-mercaptoethanol, 8 mL of glycerol, 50 mL of sterile distilled water, 50 mL of 10% bromophenol blue.
2. 40% Acrylamide/bis solution (37.5:1) (Bio-Rad, Hercules, CA).
3. Stacking gel buffer stock: 0.5 M Tris-HCl, pH 6.8. Dissolve 6 g of Tris in 40 mL of distilled water, titrate to pH 6.8 with HCl, and adjust the volume to 100 mL with water and a filter.
4. Resolving gel buffer stock: 3 M Tris-HCl, pH 8.8. Dissolve 36.3 g of Tris in 50 mL of distilled water, titrate to pH 8.8 with HCl, and adjust volume to 100 mL with water and a filter.
5. 2% Ammonium persulfate solution: Add 0.2 g of solid ammonium persulfate to 10 mL of distilled water.
6. TEMED (Bio-Rad).
7. 10% SDS solution: Dissolve 10 g of SDS in 100 mL of distilled water.
8. Glass plates (20 × 20 cm) with 0.75 mm spacers (e.g., Protean II, Bio-Rad).
9. Running buffer (Tris:glycine:SDS, pH 8.3): For a 10X stock dissolve 30.3 g of Tris base, 144.0 g of glycine, and 10.0 g of SDS and adjust the volume to 1 L with sterile distilled water.
10. Prestained protein marker (e.g., Kaleidoscope prestained standards; Bio-Rad).

2.8. Fixation and Development

1. Fixative solution: 30% methanol, 10% glacial acetic acid (for 1 L add 600 mL of distilled water to 100 mL of glacial acetic acid and 300 mL of methanol).
2. (Optional) Entensify™, solutions A and B (DuPont).
3. Gel dryer (e.g., Model 583; Bio-Rad).

2.9. Cloning into Plasmid Vector/Dideoxy Sequencing

1. Low-melting-temperature DNA-grade agarose (e.g,. NuSieve GTG™; FMC Bioproducts, Rockland, ME).

NF1 *Mutational Analysis by IVTT*

2. 1X TAE buffer: 50X TAE buffer contains 242 g of Tris base, 57.1 mL of glacial acetic acid, and 100 mL of 0.5 M EDTA, pH 8.0, adjust to 1 L total volume with distilled water.
3. Ethidium bromide (10 mg/mL).
4. 10X Gel-loading dye: 0.25% bromophenol blue, 0.25% xylene cyanol, 15% Ficoll-400.
5. λ*Hind*III DNA molecular marker (Gibco-BRL).
6. Distilled water.
7. GENECLEAN™ kit (Bio 101, La Jolla, CA) or other appropriate reagents for agarose gel purification of PCR product.
8. CloneAmp™ kit (Gibco-BRL) or other suitable plasmid cloning reagents.
9. 10X Annealing buffer for CloneAmp kit: 0.2 M Tris-HCl, pH 8.4, 0.5 M KCl, 15 mM MgCl$_2$.
10. Subcloning efficiency DH5α™ competent cells (Gibco-BRL).
11. SOC medium: 20 g of bacto-tryptone, 5 g of bacto-yeast extract, 0.5 g of NaCl, and distilled water to 1 L; autoclave, and add 20 mL of 1 M glucose and 5 mL of 2 M MgCl$_2$.
12. LB agar plates: 10 g of bacto-tryptone, 5 g of bacto-yeast extract, 10 g of NaCl, distilled water to 1 L, and 15 g bacto-agar; autoclave, cool to 50°C, and add antibiotics containing 100 μg/mL of ampicillin (Sigma) and 50 μg/mL of Xgal (Sigma).

2.10. Second-Stage IVTT and Dideoxy Sequencing

1. LB medium: 10 g of bacto-tryptone, 5 g of bacto-yeast extract, 10 g of NaCl, and distilled water to 1 L; autoclave, cool to 50°C, and add antibiotics containing 50 μg/mL of ampicillin (Sigma).
2. TENS solution: 1 mL of 50X TE, 2.5 mL of 10% SDS, 1 mL of 5 M NaOH, sterile distilled water to 50 mL.
3. 3 M NaOAc, pH 5.2: 408.1 g of sodium acetate, 800 mL of distilled water, adjust pH to 5.2 using glacial acetic acid, make up volume to 1 L with distilled water, and autoclave.
4. Absolute ethanol.
5. TNT T7 coupled reticulocyte lysate system, RNasin (40 U/μL), EXPRE^{35}S^{35}S Translabel (*see* **Subheading 2.6.**).
6. (Optional) Sequenase™ Version 2.0 DNA sequencing kit (US Biochemical).

3. Methods

3.1. Specimens

Five to ten microliters of whole blood in EDTA or a minimum of 1 mL of aspirated bone marrow cells in a heparinized container is required. The use of preservative-free heparin is preferable. Specimens should be shipped at room temperature overnight, and cell separation ideally should be performed as soon as possible following receipt of the specimen. Frozen blood or bone marrow samples may also be used for RNA preparation; vials should contain at least 1×10^7 mononuclear cells and be thawed rapidly at 37°C to prevent degradation by RNases.

3.2. Mononuclear Cell Separation

1. Add an equal volume of culture medium to whole peripheral blood in a conical polypropylene tube. Dilute 1 vol of bone marrow with 3 vol of medium.
2. Carefully layer diluted whole blood or bone marrow onto an equal volume of Histopaque-1077 in a conical polypropylene tube, to avoid disturbing the interface.
3. Centrifuge at 2000g for 20 min at room temperature.
4. Using a Pasteur pipet, carefully aspirate the opaque interface ("buffy coat") into a clean 15-mL conical tube. Add medium to 10 mL. Centrifuge at 1000g for 7 min.
5. Aspirate off the supernatant and resuspend the cell pellet in 1 mL of medium. Count the cells. Cells not intended for immediate use should be frozen in an appropriate medium and stored in liquid nitrogen.

3.3. Preparation of RNA

RNA is prepared using TRIzol reagent according to the manufacturer's instructions, with minor modifications.

1. After counting, pellet the cells by centrifugation. Aspirate off the supernatant.
2. Add 1 mLof TRIzol reagent per 1×10^7 cells in a polypropylene tube. Using a syringe and a 25-gauge needle, aspirate the cells and TRIzol repeatedly in order to lyse the cells (seven or eight times is usually sufficient). At this point, the sample may be transferred to a 1.5-mL microcentrifuge tube if the required volume of TRIzol is 1 mL or less.
3. Incubate the lysed cells in TRIzol for 5 min at room temperature (15–30°C).
4. Add 0.2 mL of chloroform/mL of TRIzol and shake the tubes in order to mix the contents thoroughly. Incubate at room temperature for 2 to 3 min. Centrifuge at 4000g for 30 min at 4°C.
5. Aspirate off the upper aqueous phase and transfer to a clean tube. Avoid disturbing the interface, because this may result in contamination of the RNA preparation by DNA.
6. Add isopropanol to the aqueous phase (use 0.5 mL of isopropanol/mL of TRIzol used in **step 2**). Mix and incubate at room temperature for 10 min. Centrifuge at 4000g for 30 min at 4°C. The precipitated RNA should form a clear pellet at the bottom of the tube.
7. Aspirate off the supernatant and wash with 75% ethanol (use 1 mL of ethanol/mL of TRIzol used in **step 2**). Briefly vortex to expose the pellet to ethanol, and centrifuge at 4000g for 10 min.
8. Remove the supernatant and air-dry the RNA pellet for 10 min to allow any remaining ethanol to evaporate. Dissolve the pellet in an appropriate volume of RNase-free water; incubating the solution in a 55°C water bath for 10 min will facilitate this.

NF1 *Mutational Analysis by IVTT* 165

9. Determine the concentration of RNA in solution using a spectrophotometer at A_{260}. One A_{260} unit of single-stranded RNA corresponds to a concentration of 40 µg/mL. Pure RNA preparations should have an $A_{260}:A_{280}$ ratio of 2.0. RNA should be stored at $-70°C$ to prevent degradation.

3.4. First-Strand cDNA Synthesis

1. Add 1 µL of random hexamers (1 mg/mL of $pd(N)_6$) to an RNase-free 500-µL microcentrifuge tube, together with a volume of RNA constituting between 3 and 5 µg (to a maximum volume of 11.5 µL). Add RNase-free water to bring the total volume to 12.5 µL (*see* **Note 1**).
2. Incubate at 70°C for 10 min. Quench the reaction on ice for 2 min. Briefly spin and set back on ice.
3. To each tube, add 5 µL of first-strand buffer, 2 µL of 0.1 M DTT, 1 µL of 25 mM dNTPs, 0.5 µL of RNasin (40 U/µL), 1 µL of single-strand DNA-binding protein (0.5 mg/mL), and 1.5 µL of RNase-free water.
4. Add 1.5 µL of SuperScript II RNase H-Reverse Transcriptase (200 U/µL) to each tube and incubate at 37°C for 1 h. The total reaction volume should equal 25 µL.
5. Inactivate enzymes by heating to 65°C for 10 min.
6. Store synthesized cDNA at $-20°C$.

3.5. Polymerase Chain Reaction

1. Aliquot the following into a sterile 200-µL tube for each PCR reaction (total volume of 40 µL): 2 µL of first-strand cDNA template, 4 µL of 10X PCR buffer II, 3.2 µL of 25 mM $MgCl_2$, 1 µL of 10 mM dNTPs, 3 µL of forward primer (10 pmol/µL), 3 µL of reverse primer (10 pmol/µL), and 23.8 µL of sterile distilled water. A master mix using $n + 1$ (in which n is the number of samples to be analyzed) volumes of these reagents (excluding template) may be made.
2. Add one AmpliWax PCR Gem 100 to each tube, apply the caps, and incubate at 80°C for 5 min. Cool to 25°C for 10 min. **Step 2** should be performed in a thermocycling machine such as the Perkin-Elmer 9600 model.
3. Make up the top mix for the hot start PCR. For each reaction use (volume of 10 µL): 1 µL of 10X PCR buffer II, 0.8 µL of 25 mM $MgCl_2$, 0.5 µL of single-strand DNA-binding protein (0.5 mg/mL), 0.5 µL of AmpliTaq DNA polymerase (5 U/µL), and 7.2 µL of sterile distilled water. Again, a master mix using $n + 1$ (in which n is the number of samples to be analyzed) volumes of these reagents may be made.
4. Pipet 10 µL of the top mix onto the cooled AmpliWax gem taking care not to puncture the layer. Cap the tube.
5. Perform PCR amplification in a Perkin-Elmer 9600 thermocycling machine using the following conditions: initial denaturation step at 95°C for 1 min, followed by 40 cycles of PCR at 95°C for 30 s, 62.5°C for 30 s and 72°C for 90 s with a single final elongation step of 72°C for 10 min. Cool to 15°C.
6. Visualize the amplified PCR product in all the reactions by agarose gel electrophoresis. Use a 1% agarose gel and 1X TAE running buffer. Load 5 µL of PCR product plus 1 µL of 10X gel-loading dye and include a lane containing a λ*Hin*dIII

166   Side

marker in order to assess the size of the product. Run at 90 V until the dark blue dye front is approximately two-thirds down the gel.

7. Stain the gel with ethidium bromide. Visualize the DNA on an ultraviolet (UV) transilluminator and photograph the gel.

3.6. IVTT Reaction

1. Add 2 μL of PCR product to a sterile 500-μL microcentrifuge tube.
2. For each IVTT reaction use 4 μL of rabbit reticulocyte lysate, 0.33 μL of TNT buffer, 0.16 μL of amino acid mix minus methionine, 0.16 μL of RNasin, 1.14 μL of ^{35}S *trans*-labeled methionine (equivalent to 10 μCi/reaction), and 0.25 μL of T7 RNA polymerase. Make up a master mix using $n + 1$ volumes of these reagents, in which n is the number of samples to be analyzed.
3. Add 6 μL of the master mix to the 2-μL aliquot of PCR product in the microcentrifuge tube. Pipet to mix taking care not to introduce bubbles into the reaction.
4. Incubate in a 30°C water bath for 1 h. Reactions may be stored at 4°C for up to 24 h prior to electrophoresis.

3.7. Sodium Dodecyl Sulfate Polyacrylamide Gel Electrophoresis of IVTT Products

1. Make an SDS polyacrylamide (12.5%) gel for protein electrophoresis using 20×20 cm glass plates with 0.75-mm spacers. Set the apparatus vertically.
2. For the resolving gel, mix 9.375 mL of 40% acrylamide:bisacrylamide (37.5:1), 3.75 mL of resolving gel buffer (3 M Tris, pH 8.8), 0.3 mL of 10% SDS, 1.5 mL of 1.5% ammonium persulfate, and 15 mL of dH$_2$O. Add 0.015 mL of TEMED, swirl briefly, and pour. Layer with 0.2 mL of isobutanol. Allow the gel to polymerize (20–30 min). Rinse off the isobutanol using distilled water.
3. Mix reagents for the stacking gel (1.875 mL of 40% acrylamide:bisacrylamide [37.5:1], 5 mL of stacking gel buffer [0.5 M Tris, pH 6.8], 0.2 mL of 10% SDS, 1 mL of 1.5% ammonium persulfate, and 11.9 mL of dH2O). Add 0.015 mL of TEMED, swirl, and pour. Insert the comb. Allow at least 20 min to polymerize.
4. Make up 1X running buffer from 10X stock (Tris:glycine:SDS as per **Subheading 2.7.**). Remove the combs from the stacking gel and construct a vertical gel apparatus. Pour 1X buffer into the upper and lower reservoirs. Flush the wells of the stacking gel thoroughly with 1X running buffer taking care not to disrupt them.
5. Aliquot 25 μL of reducing sample buffer into sterile 500-μL microfuge tubes. Add 3 μL of the IVTT reaction product to each tube. Heat to 95°C for 5 min and then quench on ice. Spin briefly to collect the liquid at the bottom of the tubes and replace on ice. Load samples onto a 12.5% sodium dodecyl sulfate polyacrylamide gel electrophoresis (SDS-PAGE) gel immediately. A prestained protein marker should also be denatured and run on each gel in order to determine the size of any truncated protein product detected.
6. Run each gel at 30 mA of constant current until the dye front is close to the bottom of the gel. This should take approx 3.5–4 h.

NF1 *Mutational Analysis by IVTT* 167

3.8. Fixation and Development of SDS-PAGE Gels

1. Immerse the gel in a solution of 30% methanol, and 10% acetic acid for 30 min, preferably while gently agitating on a shaking table. Repeat.
2. (Optional). Enhance signal using an intensifying solution (Entensify, DuPont). Soak the gel in Entensify solution A, for 30 min, while shaking. Transfer the gel to Entensify solution B for 30 min, continuing to shake for the duration.
3. Affix the gel to filter paper and cover with cling film. Dry using a vacuum gel dryer at 65°C for 2 h.
4. Expose the gel to film overnight in a sealed cassette (less exposure time may be required if the signal has been enhanced). An in vitro synthesized truncated protein, if present, will appear as an additional smaller band compared to that of the full-length polypeptide (*see* **Note 2**).

3.9. Cloning into Plasmid Vector

1. Reverse transcriptase-PCR product (from **Subheading 3.5.**), which gives rise to a truncated peptide by IVTT should be purified from an agarose preparative gel prior to cloning into a plasmid vector. A 1% low melting point agarose gel run in 1X TAE buffer is suitable. Run the remaining PCR product (approx 45 μL) plus 5 μL of 10X gel-loading dye and include a lane containing a λ*Hind*III marker. Stain the gel with ethidium bromide, visualize the DNA on a UV transilluminator, and excise the correctly sized band from the gel.
2. Purify the PCR product from the agarose prep gel using a suitable method. We use the GENECLEAN kit according to the manufacturer's instructions. Check the DNA yield on a 1% agarose gel.
3. Clone purified DNA into a suitable plasmid vector. We use the pAMP1 vector using the CloneAmp kit according to the manufacturer's instructions, with minor modifications. However, if this method is to be used, PCR primers will need to be designed accordingly (*see* **Table 1**). To 100–200 ng of DNA add 1 μL of pAMP1 vector DNA, 1 μLof uracil DNA glycosylase, 0.75 μL of 10X annealing buffer, and sterile distilled water to a total volume of 10 μL. Incubate at 37°C for up to 2 h.
4. Use 5 μL of annealing reaction mix to transform competent cells according to the manufacturer's instructions. We find that DH5α subcloning efficiency competent cells provide a satisfactory transformation efficiency.

3.10. Second-Stage IVTT/Dideoxy Sequencing (see Note 3)

1. Culture individual colonies overnight in 2 mL of selective medium (LB containing 50 μg/mL of ampicillin). Harvest the cells by centrifugation and prepare plasmid miniprep DNA as in **step 2** or by a suitable alternative method.
2. Resuspend the cell pellet in 50 μL of supernatant. Add 300 μL of TENS and vortex. Add 150 μL of 3 *M* NaOAc, pH 5.2, vortex and spin in a microcentrifuge at 12,000–15,000 rpm for 2 min. Transfer the supernatant to a clean tube, add 900 μL of ice-cold 100% ethanol, vortex, and spin at 12,000–15,000 rpm for 3 min. Pour

off the supernatant, wash the pellet in 1 mL of 70% ethanol, air-dry, and resuspend in 30 µL of water.

3. Use 2 µL of plasmid DNA from **step 2** as template for a second IVTT reaction. Follow the protocol from **Subheadings 3.5.–3.8.** inclusive.

4. Plasmid-derived IVTT products should be separated by gel electrophoresis (*see* **Subheading 3.7.**) and the gel examined to determine whether the resulting polypeptides comigrate with either the normal full-length or abnormal truncated protein. Only plasmid DNA giving rise to a truncated protein need be sequenced.

5. Perform dideoxy sequencing reactions using the Sequenase Version 2.0 DNA sequencing kit according to the manufacturer's instructions, or an alternative automated method. The size of the truncated polypeptide should first be estimated by comparison to a prestained protein standard. Oligonucleotide primers for sequencing may then be designed to anneal approx 100 nt upstream of the predicted mutation site and the exact nucleotide sequence of the mutation determined (*see* **Notes 4** and **5**).

4. Notes

1. Regarding cDNA synthesis from a large transcript such as *NF1*, the use of random hexamers, as opposed to a gene-specific antisense primer or an oligo-dT primed reaction, appears to increase the efficiency of the reverse transcription step (Michael Luce, personal communication, and our own experience). In particular, we have found that this provides better representation of the 5' end of the gene. If IVTT is to be adapted for mutation screening of other genes, the method used for cDNA synthesis may need to be modified for optimal results.

2. Two exons of *NF1*, exons 23a and 48a *(14)*, are known to be alternatively spliced. In some tissues or samples, greater representation of alternatively spliced isoforms is a potential source of confusion when interpreting SDS-PAGE gels for the presence of truncated proteins *(12)*.

3. Prior to embarking on second-stage IVTT and sequencing of RT-PCR products giving rise to a truncated protein, we have performed duplicate RT-PCR and primary IVTT reactions on the sample. This is done to reduce the possibility of sequence alterations generated by *Taq* polymerase error being misinterpreted as potential truncating mutations.

4. To minimize the possibility of error, we recommend confirming the presence of mutations found in cDNA sequence in patient genomic DNA. For *NF1* we used intron-based primers to amplify short sequences of genomic DNA for cloning and dideoxy sequencing *(14,24)*. PCR products using these primers included the flanking splice acceptor and donor sequences, and in a number of our patients with NF1, this was the site of the mutation *(12,13)*.

5. Other groups *(25)* have documented the presence of abnormal RT-PCR products lacking part of the coding sequence and with breakpoints coincident with intron/exon boundaries. These products give rise to truncated peptides using IVTT, but the genomic DNA sequence from these patients is normal. They are thought to represent rare pre-mRNA species and should not be misinterpreted as mutations.

NF1 *Mutational Analysis by IVTT*

We have not encountered this problem with the conditions described above for RT-PCR of *NF1* sequence. However, we have found it to be a confounding factor with other candidate tumor suppressor genes that we have analyzed (L. Side, A. Banerjee, and K. M. Shannon, unpublished data). In this case, our approach has been to perform RT-PCR and IVTT on duplicate cDNA synthesis reactions from the same RNA sample. Since these aberrant pre-mRNA splicing products are rare, they are unlikely to give truncated proteins in duplicate reactions.

References

1. Riccardi, V. M. and Eichner, J. E. (1986) *Neurofibromatosis.* Johns Hopkins University Press, Baltimore, MD.
2. Passmore, S. J., Hann, I. M., Stiller, C. A., Ramani, P., Swansbury, G. J., Gibbons, B., Reeves, B., and Chessells, J. (1995) Pediatric myelodysplasia: a study of 68 children and a new prognostic scoring system. *Blood* **85,** 1743–1749.
3. Shannon, K. M., Watterson, J., Johnson, P., O'Connell, P., Lange, B., Shah, N., et al. (1992) Monosomy 7 myeloproliferative disease in children with neurofibromatosis, type 1: epidemiology and molecular analysis. *Blood* **79,** 1311–1318.
4. Stiller, C. A., Chessells, J. M., and Fitchett, M. (1994) Neurofibromatosis and childhood leukemia/lymphoma: A population-based UKCCSG study. *Br. J. Cancer* **70,** 969–972.
5. Haber, D. and Harlow, E. (1997) Tumour-suppressor genes: evolving definitions in the genomic age. *Nat. Genet.* **16,** 320–322.
6. Weinberg, R. A. (1991) Tumor suppressor genes. *Science* **254,** 1138–1146.
7. Knudson, A. G. (1993) All in the (cancer) family. *Nat. Genet.* **5,** 103,104.
8. Clurman, B. and Groudine, M. (1997) Killer in search of a motive? *Nature* **389,** 122,123.
9. Massague, J. and Weinberg, R. A. (1992) Negative regulators of growth. *Curr. Opin. Genet. Dev.* **2,** 28–32.
10. Knudson, A. G. (1971) Mutation and cancer: statistical study of retinoblastoma. *Proc. Natl. Acad. Sci. USA* **68,** 820–823.
11. White, R. L. (1998) Tumor suppressing pathways. *Cell* **92,** 591,592.
12. Side, L., Taylor, B., Cayouette, M., Connor, E., Thompson, P., Luce, M., and Shannon, K. M. (1997) Homozygous inactivation of *NF1* in the bone marrows of children with neurofibromatosis, type 1 and malignant myeloid disorders. *N. Engl. J. Med.* **336,** 1713–1720.
13. Side, L. E., Emanuel, P. D., Taylor, B., Franklin, J., Thompson, P., Castleberry, R. P., and Shannon, K. M. (1998) Mutations of the *NF1* gene in children with juvenile myelomonocytic leukemia without clinical evidence of neurofibromatosis, type 1. *Blood* **92,** 267–272.
14. Li, Y., O'Connell, P., Breidenbach, H. H., Cawthon, R., Stevens, J., Xu, G., et al. (1995) Genomic organisation of the neurofibromatosis 1 gene (*NF1*). *Genomics* **25,** 1–10.
15. Upadhyaya, M., Shaw, D., and Harper, P. (1994) Molecular basis of neurofibromatosis type 1 (NF1): mutation analysis and polymorphisms in the *NF1* gene. *Hum. Mut.* **4,** 83–101.

16. Heim, R., Silverman, L., Farber, R., Kam-Morgan, L., and Luce, M. (1994) Screening for truncated NF1 proteins. *Nat. Genet.* **8,** 218,219.

17. Heim, R., Kam-Morgan, L., Binnie, C., Corns, D., Cayouette, M., Farber, R., et al. (1995) Distribution of 13 truncating mutations in the neurofibromatosis 1 gene. *Hum. Mol. Genet.* **4,** 975–981.

18. Hahn, S., Schutte, M., Shamsul Hoque, A. T. M., Moskaluk, C. A., da Costa, L. T., Rozenblum, E., et al. (1996) *DPC4*, a candidate tumor-suppressor gene at human chromosome 18q21.1. *Science* **271,** 350–353.

19. Li, J., Yen, C., Liaw, D., Podsypanina, K., Bose, S., Wang, S. I., et al. (1997) *PTEN*, a Putative Protein Tyrosine Phosphatase Gene Mutated in Human Brain, Breast and Prostate Cancer. *Science* **275,** 1943–1946.

20. Roest, P. A. M., Roberts, R. G., Sugino, S., van Ommen, G.-J. B., and den Dunnen, J. T. (1993) Protein truncation test (PTT) for rapid detection of translation terminating mutations. *Hum. Mol. Genet.* **2,** 1719–1721.

21. Powell, S., Peterson, G., Krush, A., Booker, S., Jen, J., Giardiello, F., et al. (1993) Molecular diagnosis of familial adenomatous polyposis. *N. Engl. J. Med.* **329,** 1982–1986.

22. Muhlrad, D. and Parker, R. (1994) Premature translation termination triggers mRNA decapping. *Nature* **370,** 578–581.

23. Binnie, C. G., Kam-Morgan, L. N. W., Cayouette, M., Marra, G., Boland, C. R., and Luce, M. C. (1997) Rapid identification of RT-PCR clones containing translation-termination mutations. *Mut. Res.* **388,** 21–26.

24. Purandare, S. M., Breidenbach, H., Li, Y., Zhu, X. L., Sawada, S., Neil, S. M., Brothman, A., et al. (1995) Identification of neurofibromatosis type 1 (*NF1*) homologous loci by direct sequencing, fluoresence in situ hybridization, and PCR amplification of somatic cell hybrids. *Genomics* **30,** 476–485.

25. Fitzgerald, M. G., Bean, J. M., Hegde, S. R., Unsal, H., MacDonald, D. J., Harkin, D. P., et al. (1997) Heterozygous *ATM* mutations do not contribute to early onset of breast cancer. *Nat. Genet.* **15,** 307–309.

13

Mutation Analysis of Cancer Using Automated Sequencing

Amanda Strickson and Carrie Fidler

1. Introduction

There are a variety of methods for the detection and definition of mutations in disease states including cancer. For the detection of unknown mutations, several screening techniques are available including single-strand conformation polymorphism (SSCP) *(1)*, protein truncation test (PTT) *(2)*, heteroduplex analysis (HDA) *(3)*, temperature gradient gel electrophoresis (TGGE) *(4)*, denaturing gradient gel electrophoresis (DGGE) *(5)*, and more recently, denaturing high-performance liquid chromatography (DHPLC) *(6)*. Once detected, mutations are defined by DNA sequencing, and, thus, this is the "gold standard" method for mutation analysis. DNA sequencing, since its development in the late 1970s *(7,8)*, has become one of the most important and widely used tools in the molecular biology laboratory. Automated DNA sequencing was developed in the late 1980s and has the major advantages of a fluorescence-based detection system using a laser rather than radioactive detection, and automatic base-calling rather than manual base calling from a sequencing gel autoradiograph.

A number of sequencing protocols are available to the researcher, which utilize different sequencing enzymes and different labeling options. The protocol of choice is dependent on the sequencing application. Cycle sequencing is a reproducible method for the direct sequencing of polymerase chain reaction (PCR) products *(9)*. Direct sequencing is preferential for mutation analysis because it eliminates time-consuming subcloning procedures and avoids errors owing to the lower fidelity of thermostable polymerases that may show up in cloning of PCR products *(10)*. Until recently, cycle sequencing of PCR products was not ideal because uneven signals were generated when using *Taq* or

From: *Methods in Molecular Medicine, vol. 68: Molecular Analysis of Cancer*
Edited by: J. Boultwood and C. Fidler © Humana Press Inc., Totowa, NJ

similar thermostable enzymes. These uneven peaks were caused by uneven incorporation of nucleotides and made it difficult to search for heterozygous point mutations. However, new types of thermostable enzymes such as Thermo Sequenase are now available that give much more even incorporation of the nucleotides and have much improved the signal quality.

Several groups have successfully identified mutations in cancers and leukemias using cycle sequencing. *p53* is the most commonly mutated gene in human cancers with approx 90% localized to exons 5–8 *(9)*. *p53* gene mutations have been identified by cycle sequencing in breast and ovarian tumors *(11)*, as well as in the peripheral blood and spleens of patients with hairy cell leukemia *(12)*. Cycle sequencing has also been used successfully in the study of other gene mutations including ras and neurofibromatosis 1 (*NF1*) genes *(13)*. Luria et al. *(14)* identified an *NF1* germline mutation in exon 31 of a child who developed juvenile chronic myelogenous leukemia, and Garrett et al. *(15)* used cycle sequencing on papillary serous carcinoma of the peritoneum (PSCP) for *K-ras* mutations. Moreover, the multiple endocrine neoplasia 1 (*MEN1*) tumor suppressor gene was shown to harbour deleterious germline mutations by dideoxy fingerprinting and cycle sequencing *(16)*.

This chapter gives an example of a cycle sequencing protocol that uses the Thermo Sequenase™ Cy™5 Dye Terminator Kit (Amersham Pharmacia Biotech, Uppsala, Sweden) for use on the Alf*express* automated sequencer (Amersham Pharmacia Biotech).

2. Materials

2.1. Preparation and Purification of Template (see Note 1)

1. PCR kit (if DNA is the starting material) (e.g., Perkin-Elmer, Foster City,CA), or one-step reverse-transcriptase (RT)-PCR kit (if RNA is the starting material) (e.g., AbGene, Surrey, UK).
2. 10X Bromophenol blue loading dye: 0.25% bromophenol blue, 15% Ficoll (type 400; Amersham Pharmacia Biotech).
3. 1X TAE buffer: 45 mM Tris, 45 mM acetic acid, 0.5 mM EDTA, pH 8.0. Make as a 50X stock solution.
4. Low-melting-temperature agarose.
5. HyperLadder IV (100-bp ladder) (Bioline UK, London, UK).
6. Ethidium bromide: 10 mg/mL stock solution in distilled water.
7. Wizard PCR preps (Promega, Madison, WI).
8. Leuk syringes (2 mL) (Becton Dickinson UK, Oxford, UK).
9. 1X TAE buffer: 45 mM Tris, 45 mM acetic acid, 0.5 mM EDTA. Make as a 50X stock solution.
10. 1% Low EEO agarose in 1X TAE buffer.
11. Ethidium bromide: 10 mg/mL stock solution in distilled water.

Automated Sequencing for Analysis of Cancer 173

2.2. Preparation of dNTP/Cy5 ddNTP Mixes

1. Thermo Sequenase Cy5 Dye Terminator Kit (Amersham Pharmacia Biotech).

2.3. Sequencing Reactions

1. Thin-walled PCR tubes.
2. Primers (*see* **Note 2**).
3. Thermo Sequenase Cy5 Dye Terminator Kit.
4. Mineral oil.
5. Thermal cycler.

2.4. Precipitation of Samples

1. 7.5 *M* Ammonium acetate.
2. Glycogen (included in sequencing kit).
3. Absolute ethanol.
4. Lint- and dye-free tissues (e.g., Kimwipes; Merck, Leicester, UK).

2.5. Preparation of Polyacrylamide Gel and Loading of Samples

1. Distilled water.
2. Absolute ethanol.
3. Lint- and dye-free tissues (e.g., Kimwipes; Merck,).
4. Bind-Silane (2 mL of absolute ethanol, 7.5 µL of Bind-Silane, 0.5 mL of 10% acetic acid [v/v]).
5. ReproGel™ High Resolution gel mix (solution A and solution B).
6. 0.5X TBE buffer: 50 m*M* "ALF" Grade Tris, 41.5 m*M* "ALF" Grade boric acid, 0.5 m*M* "ALF" Grade EDTA. Make as a 10X stock solution.

3. Methods

3.1. Preparation and Purification of Template

1. Amplify target sequence from DNA or RNA using PCR or RT-PCR respectively (*see* **Note 3**).
2. Add 4 µL of 10X bromophenol blue loading dye to each reaction.
3. Load 50 µL of each reaction onto the 1% low-melting-temperature agarose gel in 1X TAE buffer/0.5 µg/mL of ethidium bromide. Load 2 µL of HyperLadder IV DNA marker. Run the gel at 40 V for approx 2 h.
4. Visualize the DNA on an ultraviolet (UV) transilluminator, and excise the band and purify using purification columns according to the manufacturer's instructions.
5. To a 0.5-mL microcentrifuge tube, add 1 µL of purified template, 1 µL of bromophenol blue loading dye, and 3 µL of distilled water to a final volume of 5 µL. Pipet up and down to mix.
6. Run all 5 µL on a 1% low EEO agarose gel in 1X TAE buffer at 100 V for approx 40 min. The purified product should be seen as a high-quality, single band.

3.2. Preparation of dNTP/Cy5 ddNTP Mixes (see Note 4)

1. Label four tubes "A Mix," "C Mix," "G Mix," and "T Mix," respectively for preparation of the dye terminator mixes.
2. To each tube, add 4 μL of 1.1 mM dNTP, 2 μL of the appropriate Cy5 ddNTP, and 16 μL of distilled water to a final volume of 22 μL. This volume is sufficient for 10 sequencing reactions.
3. Vortex the mixes and centrifuge briefly to collect the contents at the bottom of each tube.
4. Store the dNTP/Cy5 ddNTP mixes on ice in the dark until needed.

3.3. Sequencing Reactions (see Note 5)

1. For each template (1–10), label four 0.5-mL thin-walled PCR tubes "A," "C," "G," and "T," respectively. Alternatively, prepare a PCR microtiter plate.
2. Dispense 2 μL of the A Mix, C Mix, G Mix, and T Mix (prepared in **Subheading 3.2.**), respectively, into corresponding tubes.
3. For each template (set of four reactions: A, C, G, and T), prepare a master mix by combining the following in a 0.5-mL microcentrifuge tube: 1.0–20.5 μL of template DNA (*see* **Note 6**), 2 μL of primer (4 pmol) (*see* **Note 7**), 3.5 μL of reaction buffer, 1 μL of Thermo Sequenase DNA polymerase (10 U/μL), and distilled water to a final volume of 27 μL.
4. Vortex each tube gently, and then centrifuge briefly. Aliquot 6 μL of each template master mix into each of its A, C, G, and T mixes. Pipet up and down to mix. Overlay the reactions with mineral oil if required.
5. Perform 30 cycles of 95°C for 30 s; 60°C for 30 s (*see* **Note 8**); 72°C for 1 min, 20 s; and 4°C hold (*see* **Note 9**).

3.4. Precipitation of Samples (see Note 10)

1. If using a nonheated lid thermal cycler, transfer each reaction from underneath the mineral oil to a new 0.5-mL microcentrifuge tube.
2. Add 2 μL of 7.5 M ammonium acetate directly to each reaction.
3. Add 2 μL of glycogen solution to each tube.
4. Add 30 μL of ice-cold absolute ethanol to each tube.
5. Vortex each sample and incubate on ice for 20 min. Alternatively, incubate at –20°C overnight.
6. Centrifuge at full speed (10,000–16,000g) in a microcentrifuge for 15 min to pellet the DNA (*see* **Note 11**).
7. Remove the supernatant taking care not to touch the pellet, and add 200 μL of ice-cold 70% ethanol to each pellet.
8. Centrifuge at full speed for 5 min.
9. Carefully remove the supernatant, first with a 20- to 200-μL pipet tip, then with a 0.5- to 10-μL pipet tip. Any ethanol remaining in the tube should be removed with a clean, lint- and dye-free tissue taking care not to disturb the pellet (*see* **Note 12**).
10. Resuspend the pellet in 8 μL of stop solution by pipetting slowly up and down.

Automated Sequencing for Analysis of Cancer 175

3.5. Preparation of Polyacylamide Gel and Loading of Samples

1. Clean the gel plates twice with distilled water (*see* **Note 13**).
2. Clean the gel plates twice with absolute ethanol.
3. Wipe the top inch of both plates with Bind-Silane.
4. Clean the gel plates with absolute ethanol.
5. Clean 0.5-mm spacers with absolute ethanol and place securely on the bottom plate. Secure the plates with clips.
6. Clean the 0.5-mm comb with absolute ethanol and place between the plates.
7. Add ReproGel High Resolution gel mix Solution B to Solution A. Mix by inverting. Load the mix directly onto the gel plates.
8. Place the plates under the ReproSet™ and leave to polymerize for 10 min under UV light.
9. Heat the samples at 72°C for 3 min, and then immediately place the samples on ice (*see* **Note 14**).
10. Load the entire volume of each reaction (8 µL) into the appropriate well of the sequencing gel, and electrophorese under the appropriate conditions.

3.6. Processing Sequence Data on the ALFexpress Automated Sequencer

1. Process each clone (1–10) using the Extended Shift Function available in ALFwin™ Sequence Analyser 2.10 software. This process overcomes the effect known as "smiling" that is produced when samples in the first and last lanes move more slowly than those in the middle lanes (*see* **Note 15**).

4. Notes

1. This protocol describes the preparation and purification of PCR products. Plasmid DNA and cosmids may also be prepared for use as template.
2. Primers should be approx 50% GC and at least 19 bases in length. Additionally, the primer should contain either a G or C residue as the last 3'-base, and not have any regions that can self-anneal or form hairpin loops. Using the same primer in cycle sequencing as used to amplify the PCR product may produce good results, however, a nested sequencing primer is generally better because it adds specificity to the annealing and sequencing reactions. The increase in specificity results from the nested primer not annealing to any primer dimers or primer oligomers created in the PCR reaction. Dilute the primers in distilled water to a final concentration of 2 pmol/µL.
3. Use PCR/RT-PCR kits according to the manufacturer's instructions. Optimization of cycling conditions may be neccessary.
4. Prepare all reactions on ice.
5. Prepare all reactions on ice.
6. For amplified DNA, use 0.2–0.5 µg/kb of purified PCR product. We used between 1 and 4 µL of the purified template when a clear band was seen on the gel. We used up to 10 µL when the band was faint. Anything over 10 µL is not recom-

mended because the quality does not seem to be efficient. For templates up to 8 kb long, use at least 1 to 2 µg of plasmid DNA. For larger templates (>8 kb), such as cosmids, use at least 2–4 µg of template.

7. For purified PCR products and plasmid DNA, at least 2–5 pmol of primer should be used, and for cosmids, at least 4–10 pmol.

8. This annealing temperature is suggested as a start point. The annealing temperature is a critical parameter and must be determined for each new primer/template combination.

9. The optimal thermocycling conditions should be determined experimentally and depend on the primer(s) used; the amount and quality of PCR product; the degree of amplification required; and the length, GC content, and configuration of the PCR product.

10. Prepare all reactions on ice.

11. Centrifugation can be performed at room temperature; however, we found that centrifugation at 4°C helped prevent the pellet from dislodging.

12. Do not leave the pellets to dry for longer than 10 min, because overdrying will make the pellets difficult to resuspend. In addition, the pellet will turn from being bright white to transparent if left to dry for too long, making it less visible.

13. Use Kimwipe tissues at all times for cleaning the gel plates. Kimwipe tissues are used because they contain no dye and, therefore, prevent contaminating fluorescence.

14. Heating the samples at 95°C will degrade the signal from larger dye-terminated fragments.

15. Always process the data after the run has completed. Do not let the software process the data as a postrun action.

References

1. Beier, D. R. (1993) Single-strand conformation polymorphism (SSCP) analysis as a tool for genetic mapping. *Mammal. Genome* **11,** 627–631.

2. Roest, P. A., Roberts, R. G., Sugino, S., van Ommen, G. J., and den Dunnen, J. T. (1993) Protein truncation test (PTT) for rapid detection of translation-terminating mutations. *Hum. Mol. Genet.* **10,** 1719–1721.

3. Glavac, D. and Dean, M. (1995) Applications of heteroduplex analysis for mutation detection in disease genes. *Hum. Mutat.* **4,** 281–287.

4. Wartell, R. M., Hosseini, S. H., and Moran, C. P., Jr. (1990) Detecting base pair substitutions in DNA fragments by temperature-gradient gel electrophoresis. *Nucleic Acids Res.* **9,** 2699–2705.

5. Fodde, R. and Losekoot, M. (1994) Mutation detection by denaturing gradient gel electrophoresis (DGGE). *Hum. Mutat.* **2,** 83–94.

6. Liu, W., Smith, D. I., Rechtzigel, K. J., Thibodeau, S. N., and James, C. D. (1998) Denaturing high performance liquid chromatography (DHPLC) used in the detection of germline and somatic mutations. *Nucleic Acids Res.* **6,** 1396–1400.

7. Maxam, A. M. and Gilbert, W. (1977) A new method of sequencing DNA. *Proc. Natl. Acad. Sci. USA* **74,** 560–564.

8. Sanger, F., Nicklen, S., and Coulson, A. R. (1977) DNA sequencing with chain terminating inhibitors. *Proc. Natl. Acad. Sci. USA* **74,** 5463–5467.
9. Kretz K., Callen, W., and Hedden, V. (1994) Cycle sequencing. *PCR Methods Appl.* **5,** 107–112.
10. Gross, E., Arnold, N., Goette, J., Schwarz-Boeger, U., and Kiechle, M. (1999) A comparison of BRCA1 mutation analysis by direct sequencing, SSCP and DHPLC. *Hum. Genet.* **105,** 72–78.
11. Bharaj, B. S., Angelopoulou, K., and Diamandis, E. P. (1998) Rapid sequencing of the p53 gene with a new automated sequencer. *Clin. Chem.* **7,** 1397–1403.
12. Konig, E. A., Kusser, W. C., Day, C., Porzsolt, F., Glickman, B. W., Messer, G., et al. (2000) p53 mutations in hairy cell leukaemia. *Leukemia* **4,** 706–711.
13. Mok, S. C., Lo, K. W., and Tsao, S. W. (1993) Direct cycle sequencing of mutated alleles detected by PCR single-strand conformation polymorphism analysis. *Biotechniques* **5,** 790–794.
14. Luria, D., Avigad, S., Cohen, I. J., Stark, B., Weitz, R., and Zaizov, R. (1997) p53 mutation as the second event in juvenile chronic myelogenous leukemia in a patient with neurofibromatosis type 1. *Cancer* **10,** 2013–2018.
15. Garrett, A. P., Ng, S. W., Muto, M. G., Welch, W. R., Bell, D. A., Berkowitz, R. S., and Mok, S. C. (2000) ras gene activation and infrequent mutation in papillary serous carcinoma of the peritoneum. *Gynecol. Oncol.* **1,** 105–111.
16. Guru, S. C., Manickam, P., Crabtree, J. S., Olufemi, S. E., Agarwal, S. K., and Debelenko, L. V. (1998) Identification and characterization of the multiple endocrine neoplasia type 1 (MEN1) gene. *J. Intern. Med.* **6,** 433–439.

14

Detection of Differentially Expressed Genes in Cancer Using Differential Display

Yineng Fu

1. Introduction

It is estimated that the human genome contains 25,000–35,000 genes; however, only about 15% of these are expressed in any given cell and different cells and tissues express different gene subsets. Gene expression is tightly regulated under normal physiologic conditions but is often disrupted during malignant transformation and tumor progression. Analysis of differential gene expression in such events as cancer is essential to better understand these complicated processes so that new diagnoses and forms of treatment can be developed. RNA differential display technology offers a straightforward and efficient way to detect differential gene expression in a variety of physiologic and pathologic circumstances including cancer *(1,2)*. By comparing messenger RNA expression patterns between tumor cells and their normal counterparts on the same gel, altered gene expression in tumor cells can be easily detected. This technique has been widely and successfully applied not only in cancer research but also in many other areas of biologic research and has resulted in thousands of publications in the few years since it was developed *(3–5)*.

Differential display has several advantages over other technologies that have been developed to study differential gene expression such as subtractive or differential hybridization *(6,7)* and DNA microarray *(8)*. First, it requires no specialized equipment beyond that normally found in a standardly equipped laboratory. The experimental steps involved, including RNA extraction, reverse-transcription polymerase chain reaction (RT-PCR), gel electrophoresis, Northern hybridization, and cDNA cloning and sequencing, have all become routine. Second, gene sequence information is not required for performing differential display, whereas such information is essential for perform-

From: *Methods in Molecular Medicine, vol. 68: Molecular Analysis of Cancer*
Edited by: J. Boultwood and C. Fidler © Humana Press Inc., Totowa, NJ

ing DNA microarray. In fact, a distinguishing feature of differential display is that it enables the investigator to isolate and clone unknown genes that are differentially expressed. Another important feature of differential display is that multiple samples can be compared simultaneously on the same gel side by side, which not only increases flexibility (allows analysis of gene expression at various time points) but also helps to decrease the number of false positives.

Differential display also has certain limitations and drawbacks. The one that usually heads the list is false positives. According to some early reports, the false positive rate can be very high (*9,10*). Many factors can cause false positives. One of the most important of these is heterogeneity of the starting material, especially when crude tissue samples are used. However, with some modifications of technique and strict quality control at each step, false positive rates can be reduced to ~5% (*11*). Further details as to how to decrease experimental artifacts and minimize false positives are discussed below. Another potential disadvantage is that differential display is best suited to detect large differences in gene expression, those that can be identified on the gel with the naked eye; as a result, minor differences between samples are usually not detected or are ignored. As a result, rare RNA transcripts may not be efficiently amplified, and, therefore, they may be underrepresented. Finally, differential display is labor-intensive and time-consuming. Despite these drawbacks and limitations, with careful planning and precise execution, differential display can be and has been a valuable method for investigating differential gene expression in cancer.

Differential display was adapted and used successfully in my laboratory to study cancer gene expression as well as tumor-induced host cell gene expression (*3,12*). In this chapter, I present my experience with this technique and provide a detailed, step-by-step protocol.

2. Materials

2.1. Preparation of RNA

1. Diethylpyrocarbonate (DEPC) (Sigma, St. Louis, MO) (*see* **Note 1**).
2. TRIzol reagent (Gibco-BRL, Gaithersburg, MD).
3. RQ1 DNAse (Promega, Madison, WI).
4. RNasin RNase inhibitor 10 U/µL (Promega, Madison, WI).
5. Buffer-saturated phenol/chloroform/isoamyl alcohol, phenol/chloroform and chloroform (Sigma).
6. 3 M Sodium acetate: Dissolve 246.0 g of CH_3COONa in 800 mL of DEPC-treated distilled H_2O (DEPC-H_2O), adjust pH to 4.8 with glacial acetic acid, and bring to 1000 mL with DEPC-H_2O.
7. Glycogen (Sigma): 10 mg/mL in DEPC-H_2O. Store at –20°C.
8. 80% and absolute ethanol.
9. Polytron homogenizer (Brinkmann, Westbury, NY).

Differential Display in Cancer

2.2. RT-PCR and Differential Display

1. RNAimage kit (GenHunter, Nashville, TN) (*see* **Note 2**). This kit contains 5X reverse transcription buffer (200 µL), moloney murine leukemia virus (MMLV) reverse transcriptase (100 U/µL, 40 µL), dNTPs (250 µM, 200 µL), H-T$_{11}$G anchor primer (2 µM, 300 µL), H-T$_{11}$A anchor primer (2 µM, 300 µL), H-T$_{11}$C anchor primer (2 µM, 300 µL), 10X PCR buffer (500 µL), dNTPs (25 µM, 500 µL), H-AP1-8 arbitrary primers (2 µM, 150 µL each), control RNA (1 µg/µL), glycogen (10 mg/mL, 200 µL), dH$_2$O (1.2 mL), and loading dye (500 µL).
2. Ampli-Taq DNA polymerase (5 U/µL) (Perkin-Elmer, Foster City, CA).
3. α-[^{35}S]-dATP (1200 Ci/mmol) (Dupont/NEN, Boston, MA).
4. 6% Acryl-a-mix (acrylamide/urea gel mix) (Promega, Madison, WI).
5. 10% Ammonium persulfate: Dissolve 100 mg of ammonium persulfate in 1 mL of distilled H$_2$O; make fresh solution for each experiment.
6. TEMED (Sigma,).
7. 100 mM Dithiothreitol (DTT): Dissolve 309 mg of DTT in 20 mL of 0.01 M sodium acetate (pH 5.2), filter to sterilize, aliquot and store at –20°C.
8. Mineral oil (Sigma).
9. 10X Tris-borate EDTA buffer: Dissolve 108 g of Tris base and 55 g of boric acid in 800 mL of dH$_2$O, add 40 mL of 0.5 M EDTA, adjust to pH 8.0, and bring up to 1000 mL with dH$_2$O.
10. Kodak XAR-5 film (Kodak, Rochester, NY).
11. Sequencing gel apparatus.
12. Gel dryer.
13. Whatman 3MM filter paper.
14. Automated thermal cycler (Perkin-Elmer).

2.3. Differential Display Band Selection, Expression Confirmation, and Sequence Analysis

1. AmpliTaq DNA polymerase (5 U/µL) and 10X PCR buffer (Perkin-Elmer).
2. dATP, dCTP, dGTP, and dTTP (10 mM each) (Gibco-BRL).
3. TaqStart antibody (Clontech, Palo Alto, CA).
4. γ-[^{32}P]-dCTP (3000 or 6000 Ci/mol) (Dupont/NEN).
5. Quick-spin column for DNA (Boehringer Mannheim, Mannheim, Germany).
6. GeneScreen plus hybridization transfer membranes (DuPont/NEN).
7. Wizard DNA cleanup system (Promega).
8. TA cloning system (Promega).
9. Sequenase DNA sequencing kit (US Biomedical).
10. 20X Saline sodium citrate: Dissolve 175.3 g of NaCl and 88.2 g of trisodium citrate dihydrate in 800 mL of dH$_2$O. Adjust pH to 7.0 with 1 N HCl. Bring the final volume up to 1000 mL with dH$_2$O and autoclave.
11. 10% Sodium dodecyl sulfate (SDS): Dissolve 100 g of electrophoresis-grade SDS in 900 mL of sterile distilled water, and bring the volume up to 1000 mL. Do not autoclave.

12. 0.5 *M* EDTA: Add 186.1 g of disodium EDTA dihydrate to 800 mL of distilled water. Adjust pH to 8.0 with NaOH tablets. Add water to a final volume of 1000 mL and autoclave.
13. Salmon sperm DNA denatured and fragmented (Sigma).
14. Ultraviolet-crosslinker (Strategene, La Jolla, CA).
15. Computer equipment with Internet Web access.

3. Methods

3.1. Preparation of RNA (see Note 3)

The quality of the starting tissue or cells is the most important factor in the success of differential display experiments. Both cell lines and fresh tissue samples have been used with success. If cell lines are to be compared, culture conditions should be identical (same culture medium, incubator, type of culture dish/flask, and stage of growth phase) except for the true variables being compared. In vitro cultures are useful when studying cellular responses to exogenous treatments such as drugs or chemicals. Of course, cultured cells may not always accurately represent the actual in vivo state; for example, gene expression in cultured tumor cells may be very different from that of tumors growing in vivo. For this reason, freshly obtained tissue samples may be preferred because changes detected in such samples will more closely represent events that are occurring in vivo. However, fresh tissue samples are much harder to deal with than established cell lines, because they are made up of mixed populations of both parenchymal and stromal cells and also include connective tissue stroma. The complexity and heterogeneity of fresh tissues have been a major obstacle to the application of differential display even though successes have been reported *(4,5)*. Separation of tumor cells from host cells and stroma in solid tumors to obtain a pure cellular population is difficult in practice. Enzyme digestion and gradient centrifugation may enrich the cellular component, but one usually is still left with a heterogeneous mixture of cell types. At present, tissue microdissection appears to be the best way to isolate the desired cell fraction from solid tumors, and it has been used to obtain starting material for differential display experiments *(13,14)*. The recently developed laser assisted microdissection technique *(15,16)* has greatly increased the efficiency and accuracy of microdissection and is at present the approach of choice when dealing with solid tumors.

Total RNA is preferred over mRNA for differential display, since total RNA is much easier to purify and gives lower background on a differential display gel, although both can be used *(2,9)*. RNA samples should be treated with DNase to destroy possible contaminating DNA before reverse transcription. It should be obvious, but nonetheless deserves emphasis, that for proper comparison RNA samples should be prepared with the same method and at the same time.

Differential Display in Cancer 183

3.1.1. Total RNA Extraction (see **Note 4**)

1. Place 100 mg of tissue, or 10×10^6 cultured cells in a 17×100 mm round-bottomed Falcon plastic tube.
2. Add 1.0 mL of TRIzol reagent (*see* **Note 5**).
3. Immediately homogenize samples with a power homogenizer (Polytron) with a setting at medium to high speed for 45 s (for tissue samples) or 15–20 s (for cell lines).
4. Incubate homogenized samples at room temperature (25°C) for 5 min.
5. Add 0.2 mL of buffer-saturated chloroform/mL of TRIzol used. Cap securely, shake the tubes vigorously for 15 s, and let the tubes stand at room temperature for 3 min.
6. Transfer each of the mixtures to a 1.5-mL centrifuge tube.
7. Centrifuge at 12,000g for 15 min at 2–8°C.
8. Transfer the upper colorless aqueous phase to a fresh 1.5-mL centrifuge tube.
9. Add 0.5 mL of isopropyl alcohol, and incubate samples at room temperature for another 10 min.
10. Centrifuge at 12,000g for 10 min at 2–8°C to precipitate RNA.
11. Remove the supernatant carefully; wash the RNA pellet with 1.0 mL of 80% ethanol twice.
12. After the last wash, remove supernatant and leave the tubes on the bench with the caps open for 5–15 min to air-dry the RNA. Dissolve the RNA in 50 μL of DEPC-H_2O.
13. Dilute 1 μL of RNA in 500 μL of DEPC-H_2O and quantitate with a spectrophotometer at $A260/280$.
14. Determine RNA integrity by running 1.0 μg of RNA on a 1% agarose/formaldehyde gel.
15. Store the RNA samples at −80°C.

3.1.2. Removal of Contaminating DNA

A clean RNA sample without DNA contamination is critical if false positives are to be minimized.

1. Add to a 1.5-mL sterile centrifuge tube 5.0 μL of RNA (10–20 μg), 6.0 μL of 5X reverse transcription buffer, 1.0 μL of RNase inhibitor, 3.0 μL of RQ-1 DNase, and 15 μL of DEPC-H_2O.
2. Mix and incubate at 37°C in a water bath for 30 min.
3. Add 30 μL of buffer-saturated phenol/chloroform/isoamyl alcohol, vortex for 30 s and centrifuge for 2 min at top speed in a minicentrifuge (~13,000 rpm).
4. Transfer the upper aqueous phase to a fresh 1.5-mL centrifuge tube, and extract with chloroform/isoamyl alcohol once.
5. Transfer the upper aqueous phase to a fresh centrifuge tube, and add 3.0 μL of 3 M sodium acetate, 1 μL of 10 mg/mL glycogen, and 100 μL of cold 100% ethanol. Incubate at −80°C for 3 h. The RNA samples can be stored in this form until the next reverse transcription step, or they can be precipitated and dissolved in DEPC-H_2O and be kept at −80°C.
6. The RNA concentration should be measured again as above before starting reverse transcription.

3.2. Reverse Transcription

1. For each RNA sample, label three 0.5-mL thin-walled PCR tubes designated for the three 3'-anchor primers (H-T11A, H-T11C, and H-T11G) set up on ice (*see* **Note 6**).
2. Prepare a reaction core mix volume sufficient for the number of reactions planned to run. Generally, about 20% more reaction mix than calculated should be prepared (e.g., for 10 reactions, make reagents mix enough for 12 reactions). The reagents used for each individual reaction are as follows: 0.5 µL of RNasin, 4.0 µL of 5X RT buffer, 2.0 µL of 100 mM DTT, 1.6 µL of 250 µM dNTPs, and 1.0 µL of 200 U/µL MMLV reverse transcriptase. Prepare this reaction mix immediately before use and store on ice.
3. Add to each tube 8.9 µL of RNA (0.5–1 µg) and 2.0 µL of H-T11 3'-anchor primer. Mix and spin briefly to bring down all the solution. Incubate at 65°C for 10 min. Leave the reaction tubes at room temperature (25°C) for 2 min.
4. Add to each tube 9.1 mL of the reaction mix prepared at **step 2**, mix, and spin briefly. Incubate at 37°C for 1 h, and then transfer the tubes to a 75°C water bath and incubate for 5 min.
5. Store on ice and proceed to the next step, differential display PCR. Alternatively, the reaction tubes can be stored at –20°C for up to 2 wk.

3.3. Differential Display PCR

1. Thaw [α-^{35}S] dATP at room temperature.
2. For each RNA sample and primer set, label one thin-walled PCR tube (*see* **Note 7**).
3. Similar to reverse transcription, to minimize artificially induced difference among samples owing to pipetting error, a reaction core mix of all reagents except cDNA (reverse transcription product) and the 5'-AP arbitrary primer should be prepared. Prepare reagent core mix for each 3'-HT anchor primer. A typical reaction contains 7.4 µL of dH$_2$O, 2.0 µL of 10X PCR buffer, 1.6 µL of 25 µM of each of the dNTPs, 2.0 µL of 3'-HT primer, 0.8 µL of [α-^{35}S] dATP, and 0.2 µL of 5.0 U/µL AmpliTaq DNA polymerase (*see* **Note 8**). Prepare the reagent mix immediately before use.
4. Add to each PCR tube 2.0 µL of 5'-AP arbitrary primer, 2.0 µL of cDNA (reverse transcription products), and 16 µL of the reagent core mix.
5. Vortex to mix and centrifuge briefly to bring down all solution. Seal with a drop (50–100 µL) of mineral oil.
6. Set up and run PCR reactions as follows: 95°C for 5 min, for 1 cycle; 94°C for 1 min; 40°C for 2 min, 72°C for 1 min, for 40 cycles; 72°C for 10 min; and then soak at 4°C.

3.4. Gel Electrophoresis (see Note 9)

Electrophoresis can be carried out with a standard sequencing gel apparatus with a square-toothed comb.

1. Prepare a 6% denaturing acrylamide/urea gel the night before.
2. Remove the comb and rinse the wells with tap water. Set up the gel apparatus and rinse the wells again with running buffer immediately before loading the samples.

Differential Display in Cancer 185

3. To a fresh 0.5-mL centrifuge tube, add 3.5 μL of PCR product, and 2.0 μL of gel-loading dye, and incubate at 95°C for 2 min. Centrifuge the tubes briefly to bring down all the solution.

4. Load the samples onto the gel and run it in 1X TBE buffer at a constant power of 60 W until xylene cyanol dye reaches within 2 cm of the bottom of the gel.

5. Carefully remove one glass plate without disturbing the gel on the other plate. Place an appropriately sized Whatman 3MM filter paper firmly on top of the gel. Carefully remove any air bubbles in between the gel and filter paper.

6. Take the filter with the attached gel and place onto a vacuum gel dryer with the gel face up. Then cover the gel with Saran Wrap and dry for about an hour at 80°C.

7. Remove the Saran Wrap and replace with a new one, and make three triangular marks on the gel with either radioactive ink or by another method before exposing to X-ray film. Expose the gel to X-ray film overnight at −80°C.

3.5. Recovery of Differentially Expressed Gene Fragments

1. Examine exposed film carefully to identify differentially expressed genes.

2. Align the gel with the film precisely with the help of the marking points.

3. Cut the bands of interest out of the gel through the film with a razor blade (*see* **Note 10**).

4. Place the gel slice in a 1.5-mL centrifuge tube containing 100 μL of dH$_2$O. Incubate at room temperature for 10–15 min.

5. Boil the tube for 15 min, and then centrifuge at top speed in a minicentrifuge (~13,000 rpm) for 2 min at 4°C.

6. Transfer the supernatant (~100 μL) to a fresh 1.5-mL centrifuge tube, and add 10 μL of 3 *M* sodium acetate, 5.0 μL of 10 mg/mL glycogen, and 400 μL of cold 100% ethanol. Incubate the tube at −80°C for at least 1 h (it can be left at −80°C overnight or even longer).

7. Centrifuge at top speed in a minicentrifuge for 10 min at 4°C.

8. A white DNA plus glycogen pellet will be seen at the bottom of the tube. Carefully remove the supernatant with a pipet without disturbing the pellet, and add 1.0 mL of 80% ethanol to wash the pellet once. Vacuum-dry the DNA samples and dissolve in 10 μL of dH$_2$O. They can be stored at 4°C (on ice) for immediate use or at −20°C for later use.

3.6. Analysis of Differentially Expressed Gene Fragments

Differentially expressed bands identified on a differential display gel may not represent the actual in vivo expression pattern owing to variations in in vitro culture conditions, heterogeneity of the tissue samples, as well as artifacts introduced during experiments such as pipetting error. Therefore, it is essential to confirm the differential expression pattern by other methodologies such as Northern hybridization. For this purpose, isolated DNA fragments from the differential display are labeled radioisotopically and hybridized to RNA blots prepared from the samples being compared. Sequence information can also be obtained either before or after Northern confirmation, depending on the approach one chooses. Whenever sequence information is available, databases such as GeneBank can be searched to find homology to known genes. With the rapid progress of the Human Genome Project, increasing amounts of information will be readily obtainable by a simple search. Different approaches have been used to analyze the differential display bands to achieve those goals. In the original differential display protocol described by Liang and Pardee (*see* **refs. *1*, *2*,** and ***9***), these selected fragments from differential display were first PCR reamplified and cloned into a TA cloning vector, and the cloned inserts were labeled with radioisotope and used as probes for Northern confirmation. DNA sequences were obtained only after differential expression was confirmed by Northern hybridization. We have successfully adapted this strategy in our laboratory for the differential display experiments *(3,12)*. This strategy works well when the expected false positive rate is low, such as when pure cellular materials (cultured cell lines) are compared. However, when solid tumors or other crude cell mixtures are studied, the false positive rate can be high. In such cases, many of the cloned fragments are likely to turn out to be false positives after Northern confirmation, and much of the work in cloning becomes a wasted effort.

Several other approaches have been developed and utilized successfully. These include direct sequencing *(17)* and reverse Northern assay *(18,19)*. Although direct sequencing provides rapid sequence information, not all differential display bands can be easily sequenced directly. Also, given the fact that each individual differential display band may contain more than one species of DNA fragments *(20)*, it is possible that the sequence obtained from direct sequencing may actually have come from a contaminating fragment. Reverse Northern is an excellent approach to eliminate false positives before sequencing. The differential display bands still need to be cloned before reverse Northern confirmation.

In our later differential display experiments, we adapted another approach that we feel is more time-efficient and can be applied in situations when high false positives are expected. Briefly, differential display bands were PCR-amplified and labeled with ^{32}P to probe Northern blots without initial cloning. Probes that showed differential expression on Northern blots were recovered directly from the Northern blot by cutting out the membrane and reamplified by PCR *(10)*. This PCR product can then be cloned and sequenced. In this approach, Northern hybridization serves as both expression confirmation and specific DNA probe capturing. Avoiding cloning before Northern confirmation can save enormous amounts of time and effort. This approach is described in detail in the following section. It is my belief that all the approaches already mentioned may work well under appropriate circumstances. The choice of

Differential Display in Cancer

approach depends on the goals of the project, and on particulars of the experiments such as the nature of the starting material. Also, choice of methodology may simply be a matter of a researcher's personal preference. Readers are referred to **refs.** *1*, *17–19*, and *21* for details of approaches that are not described here.

3.6.1. Reamplification of Differential Display Bands with PCR

Differential display bands are reamplified by PCR using the same sets of 3'-anchor and 5'-arbitrary primers used for the original differential display PCR.

1. Set on ice properly labeled thin-walled PCR tubes.
2. Prepare the reagent core mix containing all reagents except DNA and both primers. For each reaction add 20.5 μL of dH$_2$O, 4.0 μL of 10X PCR buffer, 3.2 μL of 250 μM dNTPs, 0.3 μL of *Taq* DNA polymerase. Prepare 20% more reagents than calculated.
3. Add to each PCR tube sequentially 4.0 μL of 3'-anchor primer, 4.0 μL of 5'-arbitrary primer, 28 μL of reaction mix, and 4.0 μL of DNA recovered from the differential display gel.
4. Set up and run the PCR as follows: 95°C for 5 min, one cycle; 94°C for 30 s, 40°C for 1 min, 72°C for 45 s, for 40 cycles; 72°C for 10 min; then soak at 4°C.
5. Purify the PCR products using a Quick-spin column according to the manufacturer's instructions (*see* **Note 11**).

3.6.2. Probe Preparation by Single-Primer PCR (see **Note 12**)

It is important to generate probes that are of the same length as the identified differential display fragments to ensure subsequent successful recovery from the Northern membrane and PCR reamplification. The single-primer PCR method is adapted and modified for this purpose (*22*).

1. Set up PCR tubes on ice.
2. To each tube add 30 μL of dH$_2$O; 5.0 μL of 10X PCR buffer; 1.0 μL of each 10 mM dATP, dGTP, dTTP; 0.2 μL of 10 mM dCTP; 1.8 μL of *Taq* polymerase and TaqStart antibody mix (0.4 μL of *Taq* plus 1.4 μL of antibody); 1.0 μL of 6000 Ci/mol [^{32}P] dCTP; 4.0 μL of 3'-anchor primer specific to the differential display band under analysis; and 5.0 μL of DNA from (*see* **Subheading 3.6.1., step 5**) differential display reamplification (*see* **Note 13**).
3. Run the PCR using the same program used in the differential display reamplification.
4. Purify the probes by running through a Quick-spin column.
5. Measure the radioactivity of the probe by mixing 1.0 μL of column-purified probe with 3.0 mL of scintillation fluid. Then count in a β-counter under the program used for ^{32}P.
6. Use the probes immediately or store at –20°C for up to 1 wk (*see* **Note 14**).

3.6.3. Northern Blot Confirmation and Probe Recovering

1. Run 10–20 μg of total RNA samples on a 1.0% agarose/formaldehyde gel and transfer onto GeneScreen plus nylon membrane. Carry out Northern hybridization according to a standard protocol (*23*).

188   *Fu*

2. For each hybridization, use probes at a concentration of 10^6 cpm/mL.
3. Expose the hybridized membrane to X-ray film at –80°C overnight. Make three (triangular) reference marks on the membrane with radioactive ink before exposing to ensure precise matchup between the film and membrane after exposure.
4. Identify the Northern confirmed band on the film, and align the film with the Northern membrane using the reference marks.
5. Cut out the membrane strip corresponding to the band on the film.
6. Put the membrane strip into a 1.5-mL centrifuge tube containing 100 μL of dH_2O.
7. Boil the tube for 10 min, centrifuge briefly, and transfer the supernatant to a fresh 1.5-mL tube.
8. Add 10 μL of 3 M NaOAc (10%), 5 μL of 10 mg/mL glycogen (5.0 μg/mL), and 450 μL of 100% cold ethanol. Store at –80°C overnight.
9. Centrifuge the tubes at 10,000g for 10 min at 4°C.
10. Remove the supernatant and wash the pellet with 85% ethanol once. Dry the pellet under vacuum.
11. Dissolve the pellet in 10 μL of dH_2O (*see* **Note 15**).

3.6.4. PCR Amplification, Cloning, and Sequencing (see **Note 16**)

1. Set up labeled PCR tubes on ice.
2. Prepare the PCR reaction as follows: 18 μL of dH_2O, 4.0 μL of 10X PCR buffer, 3.2 μL of 25 μM dNTPs, 1.8 μL of *Taq* and TaqStart antibody mix, 4.0 μL of 3'-anchor primer, 4.0 μL of 5'-arbitrary primer (*see* **Note 17**), 5.0 μL of DNA (probes recovered from **Subheading 3.6.3.**). As described earlier, it is helpful to prepare a core mix of all reagents except DNA and both primers to minimize pipetting error.
3. Run the PCR reaction as described in differential display reamplification (*see* **Subheading 3.6.1.**).
4. Run the PCR products on 1.2% low-melting point agarose gel (*see* **Note 18**).
5. Cut out the gel band and purify by using Promega's DNA cleanup system (*see* **Note 19**).
6. Using Promega's TA-cloning system, clone the fragments into pGEM-T vector according to the manufacturer's instructions.
7. Amplify five colonies from each ligation, and digest with appropriate restriction enzymes to confirm the presence and size of the inserts. Use one clone for sequencing.
8. Sequence the clones using either a sequenase DNA sequencing kit or an automated DNA sequencer.

3.6.5. Sequence Analysis

Sequences of the cloned fragments are searched for in available databases. The goals are to identify fragments that are part of known genes or have homologies that suggest functional relationships. The best website on the Internet for this task is the National Center for Biotechnology Information Website: (http://www.ncbi.nlm.nih.gov/BLAST/). With the BLAST program, one can perform similarity searches through the entire human genomes and

Differential Display in Cancer

genomes of other species. Expression sequence tags can also be searched through this site. With the rapid progress of the Human Genome Project, valuable information such as chromosomal location of a new gene can be obtained easily through the search. Depending on the goals of the project, one can use the isolated differential display fragments as probes to screen an appropriate library to clone the full-length cDNA, or one can obtain gene expression profiles for certain types of tumors to generate expression patterns that have diagnostic or prognostic importance.

4. Notes

1. DEPC-treated distilled water should be used in all reagents that are prepared in the laboratory.
2. GenHunter's RNAimage kits contain all the necessary reagents except for RNA samples, *Taq* DNA polymerase, and [^{35}S]-dATP to carry out RT-PCR and differential display. Each kit has eight arbitrary 5' primers. Additional arbitrary primers up to a total of 80 can be ordered separately. It is a good idea to start with one RNAimage kit (eight arbitrary primers), work out the conditions through the entire differential display process, then expand the experiment to the desired number of primer sets. Although 80 arbitrary primers are estimated to cover >90% of genes, by decreasing the arbitrary primer number to 40, which reduces the workload by half, one may still be able to detect about 80% of genes. The user can also design and make his or her own primers in the laboratory, especially when gene-specific primers are needed, as when doing targeted differential display *(24)*. These self-designed arbitrary primers should have a GC content of about 50% and a G or C at the 3' terminus. The length of the primer should also be considered since longer primers may increase specificity but decrease the number of genes covered.
3. It is mandatory that gloves be worn at all steps during differential display experiments.
4. Since the size of tissue fragments and cell numbers can be variable, adjust TRIzol reagent volume accordingly. Many methods used for RNA extraction can be used for differential display. We found no major differences between the TRIzol method and the standard guanidinium isothiocyanate/CsCl method. However, the TRIzol reagent offers several advantages over the CsCl method. It is simple to perform, permits simultaneous processing of multiple specimens, and is especially suitable when dealing with small amounts of starting material. There are many commercially available RNA extraction kits that offer simple, fast, and reliable RNA extraction with high quality. The key, however, is to use the same method to extract RNA for all the samples to be compared.
5. Use protective equipment such as glasses or face shields when working with TRIzol reagents and homogenizer.
6. Random primers can also be used at the reverse transcription step especially if gene-specific primers are used in subsequent differential display PCR. Such primers are commercially available from many sources.

7. Duplicate reactions for the same RNA samples or same tumor types displayed on the same gel can significantly decrease false positives especially when dealing with tissue samples *(21)*. However, this will significantly increase the workload.

8. Factors such as the source of *Taq* DNA polymerase can greatly affect the differential display banding pattern *(25)*. The quality and consistency of differential display banding can be improved by using approaches that improve the PCR reaction, such as hot-start PCR or TaqStart antibodies.

9. Although most people use denaturing gels, nondenaturing gels may also be used. Some feel that nondenaturing gels can decrease the frequency of double binding for the same cDNA fragment, a phenomenon that occurs in denaturing gels especially for small DNA fragments (<200 bases) *(2)*.

10. Narrow gel bands should be cut out instead of wide ones in order to minimize contamination by nearby irrelevant DNA fragments. Some users reexpose the gel to another X-ray film after removal of the bands to ensure that the appropriate bands were excised *(26)*. We found this approach to be of potential value in trouble-shooting when there is consistent difficulty in getting products in the next PCR reamplification step, but to be cumbersome and time-consuming if used routinely.

11. PCR products can also be purified through standard gel electrophoresis, allowing confirmation of the presence and size of PCR products. This approach is preferable if only a small number of samples need to be processed.

12. Single-primer PCR labeling should be used to generate a full-length probe for later recovery from Northern membranes and subsequent PCR amplification. Make sure that the 3'-anchor primer is used instead of the 5'-arbitrary primer. Double-primer PCR labeling can also be used but usually leads to increased background. Random primer labeling is not appropriate for subsequent probe recovery and PCR amplification and should be avoided.

13. To minimize pipetting error, it is helpful to prepare a reagent core mix including all reagents except DNA and the specific 3'-anchor primer. The use of TaqStart antibody can greatly improve the quality of the PCR reaction. Premixed *Taq* enzyme and antibody are also commercially available.

14. Although probes stored in the freezer at –20°C for a few days can be used, it is better to prepare fresh probes for consistent results. A good probe should have an activity approaching 100,000 cpm in 1 μL. Lower radioactivity may be usable but can result in higher backgrounds and lower specific signals on Northern blots.

15. The recovered probes should be PCR amplified as soon as possible without prolonged storage since the concentration of DNA is usually very low.

16. The recovered probes either can be sequenced directly *(17)* or can be cloned into a vector first and then sequenced by conventional methods. Direct sequencing is fast but the results are not always consistent, depending on the sequence of the fragment and the nature of the primers. Since there will not be many false positives at this stage, I prefer the "clone first and then sequence" approach.

17. Both 3'-anchors and 5'-arbitrary primers are the same pairs used in the original differential display PCR specific for the band recovered.

Differential Display in Cancer

18. If PCR fails to amplify the fragment, the following steps should be taken. First, reexpose the Northern blot after the bands were excised to ensure that the removed membrane slice contains the target. Second, use 10 µL of recovered probe instead of 5 µL. Third, run two or more positive samples to capture maximum amounts of probes. In our experience, if a positive band can be seen on Northern blot after overnight exposure, there will be no problem on PCR reamplification.

19. Many other conventional methods and commercially available kits can be used to purify DNA from agarose gels.

Acknowledgments

I gratefully acknowledge Dr. Harold F. Dvorak for his support of the work and critical reading the manuscript as well as invaluable suggestions. I also thank Drs. Olivier Kocher and Tina Haliotis for critical reading the manuscript and helpful discussions.

References

1. Liang, P. and Pardee, A. B. (1992) Differential display of eukaryotic messenger RNA by means of the polymerase chain reaction. *Science* **257,** 967–971.
2. Liang, P., Bauer, D., Averboukh, L., Warthoe, P., Rohrwild, M., Muller, H., et al. (1995) Analysis of altered gene expression by differential display. *Meth. Enzymol.* **254,** 304–321.
3. Fu, Y., Comella, N., Tognazzi, K., Brown, L. F., Dvorak, H. F., and Kocher, O. (1999) Cloning of DLM-1, a novel gene that is up-regulated in activated macrophages, using RNA differential display. *Gene* **240,** 157–163.
4. Guan, R. J., Ford, H. L., Fu, Y., Li, Y., Shaw, L. M., and Pardee, A. B. (2000) Drg-1 as a differentiation-related, putative metastatic suppressor gene in human colon cancer. *Cancer Res.* **60,** 749–755.
5. Silva, I. D., Salicioni, A. M., Russo, I. H., Higgy, N. A., Gebrim, L. H., and Russo, J. (1997) Tamoxifen down-regulates CD36 messenger RNA levels in normal and neoplastic human breast tissues. *Cancer Res.* **57,** 378–381.
6. St. John, T. P. and Davis, R. W. (1979) Isolation of galactose-inducible DNA sequences from Saccharomyces cerevisiae by differential plaque filter hybridization. *Cell* **16,** 443–452.
7. Zimmermann, C. R., Orr, W. C., Leclerc, R. F., Barnard, E. C., and Timberlake, W. E. (1980) Molecular cloning and selection of genes regulated in Aspergillus development. *Cell* **21,** 709–715.
8. Schena, M., Shalon, D., Davis, R. W., and Brown, P. O. (1995) Quantitative monitoring of gene expression patterns with a complementary DNA microarray. *Science* **270,** 467–470.
9. Liang, P., Averboukh, L., and Pardee, A. B. (1993) Distribution and cloning of eukaryotic mRNAs by means of differential display: refinements and optimization. *Nucleic Acids Res.* **21,** 3269–3275.

10. Li, F., Barnathan, E. S., and Kariko, K. (1994) Rapid method for screening and cloning cDNAs generated in differential mRNA display: application of northern blot for affinity capturing of cDNAs. *Nucleic Acids Res.* **22,** 1764,1765.
11. Martin, K. J., Kwan, C. P., O'Hare, M. J., Pardee, A. B., and Sager, R. (1998) Identification and verification of differential display cDNAs using gene-specific primers and hybridization arrays. *Biotechniques* **6,** 1018–1026.
12. Kocher, O., Cheresh, P., Brown, L. F., and Lee, S. W. (1995) Identification of a novel gene, selectively up-regulated in human carcinomas, using the differential display technique. *Clin. Cancer Res.* **1,** 1209–1215.
13. Chuaqui, R. F., Englert, C. R., Strup, S. E., Vocke, C. D., Zhuang, Z., Duray, P. H., et al. (1997) Identification of a novel transcript up-regulated in a clinically aggressive prostate carcinoma. *Urology* **50,** 302–307.
14. Chakravarty, G., Roy, D., Gonzales, M., Gay, J., Contreras, A., and Rosen, J. M. (2000) P190-B, a Rho-GTPase-activating protein, is differentially expressed in terminal end buds and breast cancer. *Cell Growth Differ.* **11,** 343–354.
15. Schutze, K., Posl, H., and Lahr, G. (1998) Laser micromanipulation systems as universal tools in cellular and molecular biology and in medicine. *Cell Mol. Biol.* **44,** 735–746.
16. Suarez-Quian, C. A., Goldstein, S. R., Pohida, T., Smith, P. D., Peterson, J. I., Wellner, E., et al. (1999) Laser capture microdissection of single cells from complex tissues. *Biotechniques* **26,** 328–335.
17. Wang, X. and Feuerstein, G. Z. (1995) Direct sequencing of DNA isolated from mRNA differential display. *Biotechniques* **18,** 448–453.
18. Mou, L., Miller, H., Li, J., Wang, E., and Chalifour, L. (1994) Improvements to the differential display method for gene analysis. *Biochem. Biophys. Res. Commun.* **199,** 564–569.
19. Zhang, H., Zhang, R., and Liang, P. (1997) Differential screening of differential display cDNA products by reverse northern. *Meth. Mol. Biol.* **85,** 87–93.
20. Callard, D., Lescure, B., and Mazzolini, L. (1994) A method for the elimination of false positives generated by the mRNA differential display technique. *Biotechniques* **16,** 1096–1103.
21. Martin, K. J. and Pardee, A. B. (1999) Principles of differential display. *Meth. Enzymol.* **303,** 234–258.
22. Kalman, M., Kalman, E. T., and Cashel, M. (1990) Polymerase chain reaction (PCR) amplification with a single specific primer. *Biochem. Biophys. Res. Commun.* **167,** 504–506.
23. Sambrook, J., Fritsch, E. F., and Maniatis, T. (1989) Extraction, purification, and analysis of messenger RNA from eukaryotic cells, in *Molecular Cloning, A Laboratory Manual,* 2nd ed., Cold Spring Harbor Laboratory Press, Plainview, NY, pp. 7.2–7.87.
24. Donohue, P. J., Alberts, G. F., Guo, Y., and Winkles, J. A. (1995) Identification by targeted differential display of an immediate early gene encoding a putative serine/threonine kinase. *J. Biol. Chem.* **270,** 10,351–10,357.

Differential Display in Cancer

25. Haag, E. and Raman, V. (1994) Effects of primer choice and source of Taq DNA polymerase on the banding patterns of differential display RT-PCR. *BioTechniques* **17,** 226–228.

26. Zimmermann, J. W. and Schultz, R. M. (1994) Analysis of gene expression in the preimplantation mouse embryo: use of mRNA differential display. *Proc. Natl. Acad. Sci. USA* **91,** 5456–5460.

15

Genomewide Gene Expression Analysis Using cDNA Microarrays

Chuang Fong Kong and David Bowtell

1. Introduction

Understanding when and where the constellation of genes in a genome are expressed provides important information about the state of a tissue. Changes in gene expression are a driving force in cell differentiation, proliferation, and death. Abnormal gene expression as a direct consequence of genomic amplification or deletion, or indirectly, owing to mutation in regulatory proteins, underlies many diseases. Cancer is the exemplar of this concept (*see* CGAP: http://www.ncbi.nlm.nih.gov/ncicgap/). RNA expression analysis can be broadly divided into two approaches: the monitoring of expression of an individual gene and parallel analysis of many genes. This distinction is not simply a matter of degree. Detailed expression analysis of an individual gene, usually cloned by some functional criteria, is performed as part of a systematic characterization of the gene. When many genes are analyzed in parallel, the aim is often to concentrate on differences in gene expression between two samples, such as tumor vs normal, which may contribute to phenotypic differences. Such studies can be a powerful means of systematically searching for new prognostic markers or for genes that are central to disease initiation or progression *(1–6)*. Comprehensive profiling of RNA expression patterns can provide a "global" report on the state of a cell or tissue, e.g., the direction of metabolic processes in a cell *(7)* or its response to stress or other stimuli *(8)*.

There are several ways that differences in RNA expression patterns can be analyzed between two samples, including differential display *(9)*, representational difference analysis (RDA) *(10,11)*, serial analysis of gene expression *(12)*, and mass sequencing of cDNA *(13)*. Recently an additional technique for RNA expression analysis has been introduced that employs hybridization of

From: *Methods in Molecular Medicine, vol. 68: Molecular Analysis of Cancer*
Edited by: J. Boultwood and C. Fidler © Humana Press Inc., Totowa, NJ

probes generated from RNA to high-density arrays of immobilized DNA. cDNA arrays have a high throughput and high degree of quantitative precision compared with differential display or RDA, which involve more lengthy procedures and may suffer from polymerase chain reaction (PCR)-based distortion and bias. DNA array analysis is limited, however, to the genes that are arrayed, whereas the other techniques can isolate novel genes. As the identification of all genes within major genomes of interest is achieved, this limitation of cDNA arrays becomes less significant.

High-density cDNA arrays on membrane filters were first used to demonstrate that immobilized DNA targets could be used to quantitatively measure differences in RNA expression over a wide dynamic range *(14)*. Recently, such filters have become available commercially. Major advances have also been made recently in producing other types of high-density DNA arrays. Affymetrix perfected the synthesis *in situ* of very high-density oligonucleotide arrays (GeneChips) using photolithographic methods *(15,16)*. GeneChip arrays are a powerful and sophisticated approach to RNA expression analysis, but the high costs of these arrays and the fact that their composition is determined by the supplier are major impediments to their current widespread use. A competing technology of spotting purified cDNA samples onto glass slides has been developed *(8)*. Separate DNA samples, encoding thousands of individual genes, are arrayed at high density on glass slides with an XYZ robot or arrayer. The slides are hybridized with fluorescently labeled probes generated from RNA, and after washing, they are read with a scanning confocal microscope or reader. Gene expression profiles from different tissue samples, such as tumor vs normal, are compared by hybridization with probes labeled with different fluorophores, usually Cy3 and Cy5 *(17)*. Under optimal conditions, glass slide arrays can detect twofold or greater differences in gene expression for genes expressed at as little as five copies per cell *(8)*. High-density glass slide arrays can be produced in an academic laboratory setting and are relatively cheap to manufacture and use once major pieces of hardware are in place. These features, plus the high degree of compositional flexibility, make them a powerful and versatile tool for a wide range of biological studies. While establishing a microarray laboratory is a substantial undertaking, the recent introduction of purpose-built equipment for producing and reading glass slide arrays has greatly facilitated the process. Issues related to the assembly of a complete array system have been reviewed recently *(18)*. This chapter describes some of the protocols for producing and using glass slide arrays for RNA expression analysis.

2. Materials
1. 96-Well PCR plates.
2. Thermocycler with 96-well platform.

cDNA Microarrays in Gene Expression Analysis

3. 10X PCR buffer: 100 mM Tris-HCl, pH 8.4, 500 mM KCl, 1% Triton X-100.
4. 25 mM MgCl2.
5. dNTP cocktail for PCR: 250 μM each of dATP, dCTP, dTTP, and dGTP.
6. Forward primer (for UniGene clone set purchased from Research Genetics): 5'-GTG AGC GGA TAA CAA TTT CAC ACA GGA AAC AGC-3' (100 pmol/μL).
7. Reverse primer (for UniGene clone set purchased from Research Genetics: 5'-GTG CAA GGC GAT TAA GTT GGG TAA C-3' (100 pmol/μL).
8. 3 M Sodium acetate, pH 6.0 (for precipitation of PCR products).
9. 100% EtOH.
10. *Taq* DNA polymerase (2 U/μL).
11. dH$_2$O.
12. EtOH/acetate precipitation mix: 5 μL of 3 M NaOAc, pH 6.0 and 100 μL of EtOH.
13. Slide-cleaning solution: 400 g of NaOH in 400 mL of dH$_2$O then add 600 mL of 95% EtOH.
14. Poly-L-lysine solution: 70 mL of 0.1% (w/v) poly-L-lysine, 70 mL of tissue culture phosphate-buffered saline (PBS)–Mg–Ca, 560 mL of dH$_2$O.
15. 3X Saline sodium citrate (SSC): dilute from 20X SSC.
16. TAE: 40 mM Tris acetate, 1 mM EDTA.
17. Polyacrylamide.
18. Ultraviolet (UV) Stratalinker (Stratagene).
19. Slide-blocking solution: 70 mM succinic anhydride in *n*-methylpyrrollinode.
20. Diethylpyrocaronate (DEPC)-treated dH$_2$O.
21. GITC solution (50 mL final volume): 85 mg of sodium acetate and 23.64 g of guanidine isothiocyanate. Dissolve in 27.5 mL of DEPC-treated dH$_2$O, add 2.5 mL of 10% sarkosyl, adjust the pH to 5.5 with acetic acid, and add 0.77 mg of dithiothreitol (DTT) just before use.
22. CsCl solution: 95.97 g of CsCl (5.7 M), 0.83 mL of 3 M sodium acetate, pH 6.0, and 100 μL of DEPC. Dissolve in 100 mL of dH$_2$O.
23. SuperScript II Rnase H$^-$ reverse transcriptase: 200 U/μL (Gibco-BRL, Gaithersburg MD).
24. Oligo (dT)$_{20}$ (0.5 mg/mL).
25. 50X lowT dNTP mix: 25 mM each of dATP, dCTP, dGTP; 10 mM dTTP.
26. 5X Reverse transcriptase (RT) buffer (comes with SSII RT enzyme).
27. 0.1 M DTT (comes with SSII RT enzyme).
28. [α^{33}P] dCTP: >2500 Ci/mmol.
29. 0.5 M EDTA.
30. 1 M NaOH.
31. 1 M Tris-HCl.
32. Biospin-6 chromatography column (Bio-Rad, Hercules, CA).
33. Microcon 30 filtration unit (Millipore).
34. TE: 10 mM Tris-HCl, pH 7.4, 1 mM EDTA.
35. Scintillation counter.
36. Incomplete hybridization buffer: 50% formamide, 2X SSC, 10% dextran sulfate.
37. Poly d(A)$_{12-16}$ (8 mg/mL).

38. *Escherichia coli* tRNA (4 mg/mL).
39. Cot-1 DNA (10 mg/mL).
40. Wash buffer 1: 0.5X SSC, 0.01% sodium dodecyl sulfate (SDS).
41. Wash buffer 2: 0.06X SSC.
42. Molecular Dynamics Storm or Bio-Rad FX fluorescence scanner.
43. Molecular Dynamics Storm or Bio-Rad FX phosphorimager.
44. 50X Denhardt's: 5 g of Ficoll, 5 g of polyvinyl pyrrolidone, 5 g of bovine serum albumin in 500 mL of dH_2O.
45. 20X SSC: 350.6 g of NaCl, 176.5 g of sodium citrate in 2 L of dH2O.

3. Methods

3.1. Amplification and Purification of cDNAs for Microarray Manufacture

1. Label a PCR plate to match the template plate label.
2. Add 99 µL of PCR mix containing 10 µL of 10X PCR buffer, 1 µL of forward primer, 1 µL of reverse primer, 2 µL of dNTP cocktail, 10 µL of 25 mM $MgCl_2$, 1 µL of *Taq* polymerase, and 74 µL of dH_2O.
3. Add 1 µL of template into each well.
4. Seal the PCR plate with PCR plate sealer and place in a PCR machine.
5. Denature at 95°C for 3 min and amplify the cDNA using 30 rounds of PCR (94°C, 30 s; 55°C, 30 s; 72°C, 60 s) with a further 5 min extension at 72°C at the end of 30 cycles.
6. Run 2 µL of PCR products from each well on a 2% TAE agarose gel to assess amount and purity of cDNA present.
7. Transfer 50 µL of PCR product to a 96-well plate labeled to match the PCR plate label and add 105 µL of EtOH/acetate precipitation mix to each well. Precipitate at −80°C for 1 h to overnight. Centrifuge the plates in a benchtop centrifuge equipped with 96-well plate carriers at 2500 rpm for 45 min.
8. After centrifugation, remove the ethanol/water supernatant and wash the pellet with 70% ethanol, decant, and dry the plates overnight in a drawer covered with a clean paper towel.
9. Add 20 µL of 3X SSC to each well, seal the plates with plate sealer, and allow the PCR product to dissolve into solution by shaking on a plate shaker for 2 h. Store the plates at −20°C.

3.2. Preparation of Poly-L-Lysine Coated Slides (see Note 1)

1. Place the slides in a slide holder and submerge the slide holder in the cleaning solution (*see* **Note 2**).
2. Shake for 2 h.
3. Rinse five times for 5 min with dH_2O.
4. Submerge the slides in poly-L-lysine solution and shake for 1 h.
5. Rinse once for 1 min with dH_2O.
6. Spin-dry the slides in a benchtop centrifuge equipped with 96-well plate carriers at 800 rpm for 3 min.

cDNA Microarrays in Gene Expression Analysis

7. Transfer the slides to a clean plastic slide box (*see* **Note 3**).
8. Allow slides to age for 2 wk before printing (*see* **Note 4**).

3.3. Microarray Printing and Processing

1. Print the cDNA resuspended in 3X SSC (*see* **Note 5**) prepared as previously described using an arrayer according to the manufacturer's instructions.
2. Allow the printed microarrays to dry overnight and leave to age for 1 wk in a slide box in a drawer (*see* **Note 6**).
3. Bake the slides in an oven for 30 min at 80°C.
4. Hydrate the slides by holding over a 37°C water bath for 5 s (array side down), heat snap on top of a 100°C hot plate for 3 s (array side up), and cool to room temperature. Hydrate the slides again as above, and UV-crosslink at 450×100 μJ with a UV Stratalinker.
5. Block the slides with slide-blocking solution at room temperature with agitation for 25 min (*see* **Note 7**).
6. Denature the slides by immersing directly into a 95°C dH_2O bath for 2 min and then into cold 95% EtOH for 1 min.
7. Spin-dry the slides in a benchtop centrifuge equipped with 96-well plate carriers at 800 rpm for 3 min.

3.4. Preparation of Total RNA: CsCl Method (see Note 8)

1. For cells, pellet 1×10^6 to 1×10^8 cells at 300 rpm for 5 min. For tissue, quick-freeze 0.5 g of tissue in liquid nitrogen and grind to a fine powder; take care to keep the tissue frozen at all times.
2. Add 5 mL of cold GITC to cells or ground tissues and lyse the cells (*see* **Note 9**).
3. Into SW41 tubes, dispense 4 mL of CsCl and remove any air bubbles.
4. Carefully layer the GITC-lysed sample on top.
5. Fill and balance the tubes with GITC.
6. Spin for 16–24 h in SW41 rotor at 32,000 rpm at 20°C.
7. Carefully remove rotor from the centrifuge.
8. Carefully remove the GITC and CsCl from the top carefully with a wide-bore plastic Pasteur pipet. The RNA is the clear, gelatinous pellet at the bottom of the tubes.
9. Cut off the tubes about 10 mm from the base.
10. Wash the pellet twice with 500 μL of 70% EtOH at room temperature.
11. Dissolve the pellet in 400 μL of DEPC-treated dH_2O, and leave to dissolve on ice for several hours.
12. Transfer to a microcentrifuge tube, and add 40 μL of 3 M sodium acetate and 1 mL of EtOH to precipitate overnight at –70°C.
13. Spin at 4°C for 30 min at 13,000 rpm in a microcentrifige.
14. Dissolve the pellet in 50 μL of DEPC-treated dH_2O (*see* **Note 10**).

3.5. Preparation of Fluorescently Labeled Probes from Total RNA

1. In a 0.2-mL PCR tube, mix 17 μL of total RNA (100 μg) and 2 μL of oligo $(dT)_{20}$. Denature at 65°C for 10 min in a PCR machine.

2. Return to ice and add to the tube 1 µL of RNAsin, 8 µL of 5X RT buffer, 4 µL of lowT dNTP mix, 4 µL of 0.1 M DTT, and 3 µL of Cy3-dUTP or Cy5-dUTP to respective primer-annealed RNAs.
3. Vortex and quick-spin to remove air bubbles.
4. Return to the PCR machine and bring the temperature to 42°C.
5. After 2 min at 42°C, add 2 µL of SSII and mix the enzyme well into the reaction mix. Incubate at 42°C for 25 min.
6. Add an additional 2 µL of SSII and mix the enzyme well into the reaction mix. Incubate at 42°C for 35 min.
7. Add 5 µL of 0.5 M EDTA to stop the reaction.
8. Add 10 µL of 1M NaOH and incubate at 65°C for 60 min to hydrolyze the residual RNA (*see* **Note 11**).
9. Cool to room temperature.
10. Add 25 µL of 1 M Tris-HCl and 18 µL of dH$_2$O.
11. Place 500 µL of TE into each of two Microcon 30 filtration units. Add labeling reaction to each and centrifuge at 10,000 rpm in a microcentrifuge to concentrate to a 10- to 20-µL volume.
12. Wash once with 300 µL of TE and concentrate to 10- to 20-mL volume.
13. Invert the Microcon 30 into a fresh tube and centrifuge at 3000 rpm for 3 min in a microcentrifuge to harvest the labeled probes.
14. Run 2 µL of cy5-labeled probes on a 2% TAE agarose gel with minimal dye added in the loading buffer.
15. Scan the gel on a Molecular Dynamics Storm or Bio-Rad FX fluorescence scanner. Successful labeling produces a dense smear of probe from 400 to >1000 bp, with little pileup of low molecular weight transcripts.

3.6. cDNA Microarray Hybridization and Washing: Fluorescently Labeled Probes

1. The volume required for hybridization is dependent on the size of the array used. Use 15–20 µL for half slide and 30 µL for a full slide.
2. Combine Cy3- and Cy5-labeled probes and add to that 1 µL of poly d(A)$_{12-16}$, 1 µL of tRNA, 1 µL of Cot-1 DNA, 1 µL of 50X Denhardt's, and 4.5 µL of 20X SSC to give a total volume of 30 µL.
3. Heat at 95°C for 3 min.
4. Cool on ice for 2 min and add 0.1 vol of 10% SDS.
5. Centrifuge for 10 min at 13,000 rpm at 4°C in a microcentrifuge.
6. Apply to the array avoiding any particulate matter at the bottom of the tube.
7. Apply a cover slip.
8. Hybridize at 65°C for 16–24 h in a sealed, humidified chamber (*see* **Note 12**).
9. Remove the residual unbound probe from the slides by washing twice for 3 min each at room temperature in wash buffer 1 and once for 3 min in wash buffer 2.
10. Spin-dry the slide in a slide holder at 800 rpm for 3 min on a benchtop centrifuge equipped with 96-well plate carriers.

cDNA Microarrays in Gene Expression Analysis

3.7. Data Acquisition and Analysis with Microarrays: Fluorescently Labeled Probes

1. Scan the microarray with a microarray scanner to collect fluorescence emission (*see* **Note 13**).
2. Quantitate the fluorescence emission at each position within the microarray.
3. Assign gene expression values by comparing the experimental data to the appropriate controls (*see* **Note 14**).

3.8. Preparation of ^{33}P-Labeled Probes from Total RNA

1. In a 0.2-mL PCR tube, mix 13.5 µL of total RNA (10 µg) and 2 µL of oligo (dT)$_{20}$ and denature at 65°C for 10 min in a PCR machine.
2. Return to ice and add to the tube 1 µL of RNAsin, 8 µL of 5X RT buffer, 4 µL of lowT dNTP mix, 4 µL of 0.1 *M* DTT, and 5 µL of [α^{33}P] dCTP (*see* **Note 15**).
3. Vortex and quick-spin to remove air bubbles.
4. Return to the PCR machine and bring the temperature to 42°C.
5. Add 2 µL of SSII and mix the enzyme well into the reaction mix. Incubate at 42°C for 25 min.
6. Add an additional 2 µL of SSII and mix the enzyme well into the reaction mix. Incubate at 42°C for 35 min.
7. Add 5 µL of 0.5 *M* EDTA to stop the reaction.
8. Add 10 µL of 1 *M* NaOH and incubate at 65°C for 60 min to hydrolyze the residual RNA.
9. Cool to room temperature.
10. Add 25 µL of 1 *M* Tris-HCl and 18 µL of dH$_2$O. Purify the labeling reaction mixture in a Biospin-6 chromatography column.
11. Add 11 µL of 3 *M* NaOAc and 300 µL of EtOH to the 100-µL purified probe and incubate at –20°C for 1 h.
12. Spin in a microcentrifuge for 15 min at 13,000 rpm at 4°C.
13. Remove the supernatant and wash with 70% EtOH. Spin again at 13,000 rpm for 10 min.
14. Air-dry the pellet and dissolve it in 20 µL of incomplete hybridization buffer.
15. Count 1 µL of probe in a scintillation counter (we routinely obtain ~5 × 10^6 to 1 × 10^7 total counts from 10 µg of total RNA).

3.9. cDNA Microarray Hybridization and Washing: ^{33}P-Labeled Probes

1. The volume required for hybridization is dependent on the size of array used: Use 15–20 µL for a half slide and 30 µL for a full slide.
2. Add 40 µg of poly d(A), 20 µg of tRNA, and 50 µg of Cot-1 DNA to incomplete hybridization buffer to make 50 µL of complete hybridization buffer.
3. Add 5 × 10^6 to 1 × 10^7 count of probe to complete hybridization buffer.
4. Heat at 95°C for 5 min.
5. Spin for 2 min at 13,000 rpm at room temperature in a microcentrifuge tube.

6. Apply to the array avoiding any particulate matter at the bottom of the tube.
7. Apply a coverslip.
8. Hybridize at 42°C for 16–24 h in a sealed, humidified chamber.
9. Remove the residual unbound probe from the slides by washing three times for 5 min each at 55°C in wash buffer 1 and once for 5 min wash in wash buffer 2.
10. Air-dry the slides in a slide holder with the array sides down.

3.10. Data Acquisition and Analysis with Microarrays: ^{33}P-Labeled Probes

1. Tape the dried hybridized slides onto 3MM paper uncovered.
2. Place this in a bleached Phosphorimager cassette.
3. Expose overnight and scan in a Molecular Dynamics Storm or Bio-Rad FX Phosphorimager at 50-μ resolution.
4. Quantitate radioactivity at each position within the microarray.

4. Notes

1. Precoated poly-L-lysine slides can be purchased from Sigma (St. Louis, MO) or BDH.
2. It is important to wear powder-free gloves when handling slides. Make sure gloves are clean and grease free.
3. It is important to use a plastic slide box with no cork.
4. Aged slides become hydrophobic, that is, water drops leave no trail when moving across the slide surface.
5. The optimal concentration of cDNA for printing is 0.2–0.5 mg/mL.
6. Aging slides after printing seems to help cDNA binding to the slides and results in better hybridization.
7. It is crucial to block the slides with blocking solution to reduce background and increase signal/noise.
8. Alternative RNA preparation methods: Qiagen RNeasy or Ambion RNAqueous work well in our hands to produce quality RNA for labeling.
9. We routinely homogenize tissues after adding GITC to ensure good lysis.
10. If RNA looks dirty or 260/280 is <1.9, extract once with phenol/CHCl3 and EtOH precipitate.
11. Alternatively, RNase H can be used to degrade RNA.
12. A humid chamber can be purchased from Telechem or you can make your own by placing wet 3MM paper in a plastic box with a tight lid.
13. Several scanners are available commercially—Axon, Genetic MicroSystems, GSI Luminors, and Virtex—or you can build your own following instructions available from http://cmgm.stanford.edu/pbrown/index.html.
14. Various commercial software packages are available for image analysis. Free software can be downloaded from http://rana.stanford.edu.au or http://chroma.mbt.washington.edu/mod_www/tools/index.html.
15. Based on specific activity of $[\alpha^{33}P]$ dCTP >2500 Ci/mmol.

cDNA Microarrays in Gene Expression Analysis

References

1. Ramsay, G. (1998) DNA chips: state-of-the art. *Nat. Biotechnol.* **16,** 40–44.
2. Zhou, W., Sokoll, L. J., Bruzek, D. J., Zhang, L., Velculescu, V. E., Goldin, S. B., et al. (1998) Identifying markers for pancreatic cancer by gene expression analysis. *Cancer Epidemiol. Biomarkers Prev.* **7,** 109–112.
3. Gress, T. M., Muller-Pillasch, F., Geng, M., Zimmerhackl, F., Zehetner, G., Friess, H., et al. (1996) A pancreatic cancer-specific expression profile. *Oncogene* **13,** 1819–1830.
4. Schena, M., Shalon, D., Davis, R. W., and Brown, P. O. (1995) Quantitative monitoring of gene expression patterns with a complementary DNA microarray. *Science* **270,** 467–470.
5. Derisi, J., Penland, L., Brown, P. O., Bittner, M. L., Meltzer, P. S., Ray, M., et al. (1996) Use of a cDNA microarray to analyse gene expression patterns in human cancer. *Nat. Genet.* **14,** 457–460.
6. DeRisi, J., Penland, L., Brown, P. O., Bittner, M. L., Meltzer, P. S., Ray, M., et al. (1996) Use of a cDNA microarray to analyse gene expression patterns in human cancer. *Nat. Genet.* **14,** 457–460.
7. DeRisi, J. L., Iyer, V. R., and Brown, P. O. 1997. Exploring the metabolic and genetic control of gene expression on a genomic scale. *Science* **278,** 680–686.
8. Schena, M., Shalon, D., Heller, R., Chai, A., Brown, P. O., and Davis, R. W. (1996) Parallel human genome analysis: microarray-based expression monitoring of 1000 genes. *Proc. Natl. Acad. Sci. USA* **93,** 10,614–10,619.
9. Liang, P. and Pardee, A. B. (1992) Differential display of eukaryotic messenger RNA by means of the polymerase chain reaction. *Science* **257,** 967–971.
10. Lisitsyn, N. and Wigler, M. (1993) Cloning the differences between two complex genomes. *Science* **259,** 946–951.
11. Hubank, M. and Schatz, D. G. (1994) Identifying differences in mRNA expression by representational difference analysis of cDNA. *Nucleic Acids Res.* **22,** 5640–5648.
12. Velculescu, V. E., Zhang, L., Vogelstein, B., and Kinzler, K. W. (1995) Serial analysis of gene expression. *Science* **270,** 484–487.
13. Lennon, G., Auffray, C., Polymeropoulos, M., and Soares, M. B. (1996) The I.M.A.G.E. Consortium: an integrated molecular analysis of genomes and their expression. *Genomics* **33,** 151–152.
14. Gress, T. M., Hoheisel, J. D., Lennon, G. G., Zehetner, G., and Lehrach, H. (1992) Hybridization fingerprinting of high-density cDNA-library arrays with cDNA pools derived from whole tissues. *Mamm. Genome* **3,** 609–619.
15. Pease, A. C., Solas, D., Sullivan, E. J., Cronin, M. T., Holmes, C. P., and Fodor, S. P. (1994) Light-generated oligonucleotide arrays for rapid DNA sequence analysis. *Proc. Natl. Acad. Sci. USA* **91,** 5022–5026.
16. Fodor, S. P., Read, J. L., Pirrung, M. C., Stryer, L., Lu, A. T., and Solas, D. (1991) Light-directed, spatially addressable parallel chemical synthesis. *Science* **251,** 767–773.

17. Shalon, D., Smith, S. J., and Brown, P. O. (1996) A DNA microarray system for analyzing complex DNA samples using two-color fluorescent probe hybridization. *Genome Res.* **6,** 639–645.
18. Bowtell, D. L. (1999) Options available—from start to finish—for obtaining expression data by microarray. *Nat. Genet.* **21,** 25–32.

16

Gene Expression Profiling in Cancer Using cDNA Microarrays

Javed Khan, Lao H. Saal, Michael L. Bittner, Yuan Jiang, Gerald C. Gooden, Arthur A. Glatfelter, and Paul S. Meltzer

1. Introduction

The principle of cDNA microarray hybridization takes advantage of the property of DNA to form duplex structures between two complementary strands. In this technique (**Fig. 1**), the cDNA probes, which are arrayed onto a glass slide and represent the sequence of known genes or expressed sequence tags (ESTs), interrogate fluorescently labeled cDNA targets synthesized from extracted mRNA. In two-color microarray experiments, the differentially labeled cDNA targets (e.g., from tumor and normal tissue) hybridize to their respective cDNA probe sequences tethered to the slide. After imaging the microarray slide for signal intensities in each color channel, the relative expression ratio for each arrayed gene can be determined. In contrast to traditional gene-by-gene expression monitoring (such as Northerns), the cDNA microarray technique is limited only by the number of genes printed on the slide and, therefore; allows the analysis of gene expression on a truly genomewide scale (*see* **Note 1**).

In 1994, Drmanac et al. *(1,2)*, who used radioactive targets hybridized onto filter-immobilized polymerase chain reaction (PCR)-amplified cDNA probes, described gene expression monitoring using microarrays. In 1995, Schena et al. *(3)* first described the hybridization of two-color fluorescently labeled targets to cDNA microarrays printed on glass. The two-color detection scheme has the advantage over radioactively labeled targets by allowing rapid and simultaneous differential expression analysis of two biologic samples, with one color used as a reference for normalization purposes. The reference allows for compensation of target-to-target and slide-to-slide variations in intensity

From: *Methods in Molecular Medicine, vol. 68: Molecular Analysis of Cancer*
Edited by: J. Boultwood and C. Fidler © Humana Press Inc., Totowa, NJ

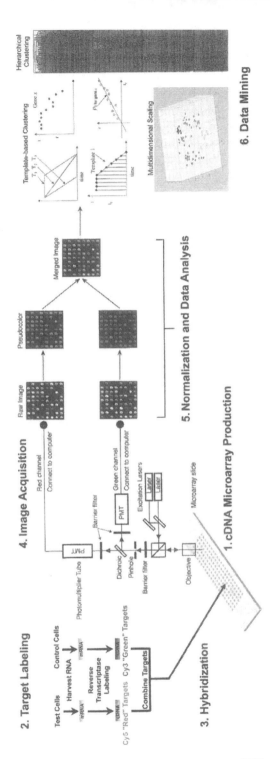

Fig. 1. The entire microarray process is summarized. (1) Plasmid DNA is extracted from the bacterial clones, and the cDNA insert PCR amplified using vector primers. The products are purified and printed onto immobilized slides using robots. Expression arrays containing up to 30,000 genes can be printed onto a microscope glass slide. (2) Total RNA extracted from test and reference cells is fluorescently labeled using oligo dT-primed reverse transcription by utilizing nucleotides tagged with either Cy3 or Cy5, respectively. (3) The probe mixture is hybridized to the microarray on the glass slides. (4) Fluorescence intensities at the immobilized targets are measured using laser confocal microscopes with the appropriate excitation lasers and emission filters. Each of the images is arbitrarily assigned a pseudo-color (i.e., Cy5 = red and Cy3 = green). A normalization process is performed to compensate for differential efficiencies of labeling and detection of Cy3 and Cy5. The two fluorescent images thus constitute the raw data from which differential gene expression ratio values are calculated. (5) Data mining tools are being developed depending on the experimental design. For instance, template-based clustering can identify genes sequentially expressed in time. Multidimensional scaling allows visualization of the similarity of expression profiles between experiments where the distance between the experiments correspond as closely as possible to 1 minus the Pearson correlation coefficient of the gene expression. Similarly, the relationships between genes and experiments can also be visualized by hierarchical clustering.

Microarrays in Gene Expression Profiling

owing to DNA concentrations and hybridization efficiencies, and thereby permits comparisons among multiple biologic samples across many experiments.

With more than 2,800,000 human EST sequences available (http://www.ncbi.nlm.nih.gov/dbEST/dbEST_summary.html) at the latest UniGene build 137, representing 50–90% of all human genes, it is now possible to uncover the gene expression profiles of human cancers, querying the expression of thousands of genes in a single experiment. Global gene expression of different types of cancer may allow the development of expression profiles unique for a cancer *(4–7)* and may lead to the development of rapid diagnostic assays. It may also identify secreted and membrane proteins *(8)* that can be used for early diagnosis and for monitoring therapy. Gene expression profiles can also be correlated with clinical data to help predict biologic behavior *(9)* and may allow us to direct therapy. In addition, this information may be useful in dissecting out the pathways involved in therapy failure *(10)*, or malignant transformation with oncogenic transcription factors *(11)*, and may ultimately provide novel therapeutic targets. Interest in microarray technology has risen in the pharmaceutical industry for new cancer drug discovery and for monitoring the effects of novel therapeutic agents *(12)*. The list of potential uses of this technique is endless and is not limited to cancer research *(13,14)*.

The steps involved in microarray analysis are summarized in **Fig. 1**. In brief, it involves cDNA microarray production, making fluorescent targets, hybridization, image acquisition, normalization and data analysis, and data mining.

The following protocols are meant to be a general guide to setting up a microarray facility; other kits, reagents, and protocols may be substituted where necessary.

2. Materials

All materials may be stored at room temperature unless otherwise noted.

2.1. cDNA Microarray Production

2.1.1. Clone Production

1. Luria-Bertani (LB) broth (cat. no. 359-000; Biofluids Division, BSI, Rockville, MD).
2. Superbroth (cat. no. 371-000; Biofluids Division).
3. 96-Well round-bottomed plates (cat. no. 3799; Corning, Corning, NY).
4. ThinSeal Plate Sealers (cat. no. STR-THIN-PLT; Excel Scientific, Wrightwood, CA).
5. 96-Well Culture Blocks (cat. no. 4050066; Edge BioSystems, Gaithersburg, MD).
6. Airpore Tape Sheets (cat. no. 19571; Qiagen, Valencia, CA).
7. Carbenicillin.
8. Ampicillin.
9. 96-Pin inoculation stamp.
10. 100% Ethanol.

2.1.2. Isolation of Plasmid DNA

1. 96-well Alkaline Lysis Miniprep Kit (cat. no. 91528; Edge BioSystems). Store all buffers at 4°C.
2. 1 *M* Tris-HCl, pH 8.0 (cat. no. 5568UA; Gibco-BRL, Rockville, MD).
3. 0.5 *M* EDTA, pH 8.0 (cat. no. 750009; Research Genetics, Huntsville, AL).
4. 100% Ethanol.

2.1.3. PCR Amplification of Clones

1. Cycleplate thin-walled PCR plate (cat. no. 1038-00-0; Robbins Scientific, Sunnyvale, CA).
2. Cycleseal PCR Plate Sealer (cat. no. 1038-00-0; Robbins Scientific).
3. MJ Research (DNA Engine Tetrad) PTC-225 Peltier Thermal Cyclers.
4. 10X PCR Buffer (cat. no. N808-0189; Perkin-Elmer, Wellesley, MA) (4°C).
5. Ampli Taq Polymerase (cat. no. N808-4015; Perkin-Elmer) (–20°C).
6. dNTPs (100 m*M* stocks) (cat. no. 27-2035-02; Amersham Pharmacia, Piscataway, NJ) (–20°C).
7. Diethylpyrocarbonate (DEPC)-treated H_2O (cat. no. 750024; Research Genetics).
8. AEK M13 forward (F) and reverse (R) primers, a custom oligo (Midland Certified, Midland, TX) (–20°C):
   a. AEK M13F: 5'-GTTGTAAAACGACGGCCAGTG-3' (stock concentration of 1 m*M*).
   b. AEK M13R: 5'-CACACAGGAAACAGCTATG-3' (stock concentration of 1 m*M*).

2.1.4. Quantification of PCR Product

1. FluoReporter Blue Fluorometric dsDNA Kit (cat. no. F-2962; Molecular Probes, Eugene, OR) (4°C).
2. Microfluor 2 White 96-well U-bottomed plates (cat. no. 7105; Dynex, Chantilly, VA).
3. Lambda *Hind*III fragments (cat. no. 15612-013; Gibco-BRL) (–20°C).
4. Perkin-Elmer Luminescence Spectrometer LS50B.

2.1.5. Purification of PCR Product

1. 96-Well V-bottom plates (cat. no. 3894; Corning).
2. Cyclefoil plate sealers (cat. o. 1044-39-3; Robbins Scientific).
3. Super T21 Centrifuge (Sorvall, Newtown, CT).
4. 1575 ImmunoWash (Bio-Rad, Hercules, CA).
5. 100% Ethanol and 70% ethanol.
6. 3 *M* Sodium acetate buffered to pH 6.0.
7. 3X Saline sodium citrate (SSC): 20X SSC stock: 3 *M* NaCl, 0.3 *M* sodium citrate. Dilute accordingly.
8. Quart-size heat-sealable bags and (cat. no. 404; Kapak, Minneapolis, MN).
9. Electric sealer.

2.1.6. Poly-L-Lysine Pretreatment of Glass Slides

1. Gold Seal slides: These slides have consistently low intrinsic fluorescence (cat. no. 3011; Becton Dickinson, Franklin Lakes, NJ).

Microarrays in Gene Expression Profiling

2. 50-Slide stainless steel slide racks and glass tanks (cat. no. 900400; Wheaton, Millville, NJ).
3. Sodium hydroxide (pellets).
4. 100% Ethanol: The source alcohol should be examined in a fluorometer to ensure that it has very low levels of contaminating fluorescent organic compounds.
5. 0.1% (w/v) Poly-L-lysine (cat. no. P8920; Sigma, St. Louis, MO).
6. Tissue culture phosphate-buffered saline (PBS): 8 g/L of sodium chloride, 0.2 g/L of potassium chloride, 1.44 g/L of sodium phosphate dibasic anhydrous, 0.24 g/L of potassium phosphate monobasic (sterilized and filtered).
7. 25-Slide plastic slide racks and plastic tanks with lids (cat. no. 195 and no. 196; Shandon Lipshaw, Pittsburgh, PA).

2.1.7. Blocking Slides After Printing with Succinic Anhydride

1. 1-Methyl-2-pyrrolidinone (cat. no. 32,863-4; Aldrich, Milwaukee, WI).
2. Succinic anhydride (cat. no. 23,969-0; Aldrich).
3. 1 M Sodium borate, pH 8.0. Adjust pH of boric acid with sodium hydroxide.
4. Stratagene UV Stratalinker 2400.
5. 30-Slide stainless steel slide rack (cat. no. 900234; Wheaton).
6. 30-Slide glass submersion tanks (cat. no. 900303; Wheaton).
7. 100% Ethanol.
8. Glass beakers (500-mL) and stir bars.
9. Large glass dish (14-in. casserole).
10. Large round Pyrex dishes (8-in. diameter).
11. Plastic slide box.

2.2. RNA Extraction and Target Production

2.2.1. RNA Extraction

1. Virsonic 100 with microprobe (conical titanium probe, 1.8-mm-diameter tip) (cat. no. 346411; Virtis, Gardiner, NY).
2. RNeasy Midi Kit (cat. no. 75142; Qiagen).
3. TRIzol (cat. no. 15596-018; Gibco-BRL) (4°C).
4. Microcon-30 (cat. no. 142410; Millipore, Bedford, MA).
5. β-Mercaptoethanol (cat. no. 806445; ICN Biomedicals, Aurora, OH).
6. DEPC H_2O (cat. no. 750024; Research Genetics).
7. Chloroform.
8. Isopropanol.
9. 50 mM Sodium hydroxide.
10. 70% Ethanol.

2.2.2. Direct Labeling of cDNA with Fluorescent Dyes

1. 10X Low T dNTPs nucleotide mix (–20°C): 25 μL each of dGTP, dATP, and dCTP for a 0.5 mM final (1/10) concentration; 10 μL of dTTP for a 0.2 mM (1/10) concentration; and 415 μL of DEPC H_2O for a total volume of 500 μL (100 mM dNTPs from Amersham Pharmacia; cat. no. 27-2035-02).

210 Khan et al.

2. FluoroLink Cy3-dUTP 1 mM (cat. no. PA53022; Amersham Pharmacia) (photosensitive) (–20°C).
3. FluoroLink Cy5-dUTP 1 mM (cat. no. PA55022; Amersham Pharmacia) (photosensitive) (–20°C). Cye dyes are also available from NEN Life Sciences, Boston, MA.
4. SuperScript II reverse transcriptase (RT) enzyme, 5X First Strand Buffer, 0.1 M dithiothreitol (DTT) (cat. no. 18064-014; Gibco-BRL) (–20°C).
5. Anchored oligo-dT (d-20T-d[AGC]) (1 µg/µL) primer (–20°C).
6. Rnase Inhibitor RNAsin (cat. no. N211A; Promega, Madison, WI) (–20°C).
7. DEPC H$_2$O (cat. no. 750024; Research Genetics).

2.2.3. Target Purification

1. 0.5 M EDTA, pH 8.0 (cat. no. 750009; Research Genetics).
2. 1 M Tris-HCl, pH 7.5 (cat. no. 351-006-100; Quality Biological, Gaithersburg, MD).
3. 1 M Sodium hydroxide.

2.3. Microarray Assembly

1. Poly dA (10 mg/mL) (cat. no. P9403; Sigma) (–20°C).
2. Yeast tRNA (4 mg/mL) (cat. no. 15401-011; Gibco-BRL) (–20°C).
3. Human Cot-1 DNA (concentrated to 10 mg/mL) (cat. no. 15279-011; Gibco-BRL) (–20°C).
4. 50X Denhardt's (cat. no. 750018; Research Genetics) (–20°C).
5. 10% Sodium dodecyl sulfate (SDS) (cat. no. 750008; Research Genetics).
6. Slide hybridization chamber (cat. no. AHC-1; TeleChem, Sunnyvale, CA).
7. 20X SSC: 3 M NaCl, 0.3 M sodium citrate.

2.4. Posthybridization Slide Washes

1. Glass Coplin staining jars (cat. no. 900470; Wheaton).
2. 25-Slide plastic slide racks (cat. no. 195; Shandon Lipshaw).
3. Wash Solution #1: 0.1% SDS + 0.5X SSC in ddH$_2$O (filtered).
4. Wash Solution #2: 0.01% SDS + 0.5X SSC in ddH$_2$O (filtered).
5. Wash Solution #3: 0.06X SSC in ddH$_2$O (filtered).

3. Methods

3.1. cDNA Microarray Production

The choice of which genes or ESTs to print are user specified. For human cancer profiling, we are currently using the "22K" human gene set comprising 22,320 human UniGene clones available from the IMAGE consortium and distributed by Research Genetics. Within the set are approx 4000 clones corresponding to known genes; the rest are unknown genes or ESTs. Currently, arrays of up to 15,000 probes are printed. The probe DNA is made from the IMAGE clones, which are arrayed in 96-well format and are used as template for PCR amplification.

Microarrays in Gene Expression Profiling 211

Currently, prefabricated high-density microarrays can be purchased from a number of sources such as TeleChem (http://www.arrayit.com). Companies such as Incyte (http://www.incyte.com/) offer microarray hybridization and analysis services to investigators who provide the RNA. The Affymetrix GeneChips (http://www.affymetrix.com) are high-density arrays of oligonucleotide probes synthesized simultaneously on a large glass wafer by photolithography. Protocols for RNA preparation and microarray hybridization for these commercial solutions vary considerably.

3.1.1. Clone Production

3.1.1.1. PREGROWTH OF CLONES TO ENSURE MAXIMUM PLASMID PRODUCTION (*SEE* NOTE 2)

1. In sterile 96-well round-bottomed plates, add 100 µL of LB broth/well with 100 µg/mL of carbenicillin.
2. Thaw frozen 96-well library plates containing source bacterial cultures and spin briefly for 2 min at 200 rcf to remove condensation and droplets from the sealer.
3. Sterilize the 96-pin inoculation stamp between samples using 100% ethanol, and flame the pins using appropriate safety precautions.
4. After briefly allowing the inoculation block to cool, dip the pins in the library plate, and then inoculate the equivalent LB plate ensuring correct orientation. Sterilize the inoculation pins as in **step 3**.
5. Reseal the library plates with plate sealers (ThinSeal). Store the library plates at −70°C.
6. Incubate the growth plates in a humidified oven overnight at 37°C.

3.1.1.2. INOCULATION OF DEEP-WELL CULTURE BLOCKS

1. Add 1 mL of Superbroth, containing 100 µg/mL of carbenicillin, to each well of the 96-well culture blocks using an eight-channel pipettor.
2. Using the 96-pin inoculation stamp, inoculate the 96-well culture blocks.
3. Cover (Airpore sheets) and place the blocks in a 37°C shaker incubator (200 rpm) for 24 h.

3.1.2. Isolation of Plasmid DNA

1. Isolate plasmid DNA from the cultures using the miniprep kit according to the manufacturer's protocol.
2. Resuspend the plasmid DNA in 200 µL of T. low E. (10 mM Tris-HCl, 0.1 mM EDTA).
3. Store the DNA at −20°C and use as template for PCR amplification (*see* **Subheading 3.1.3.**).

3.1.3. PCR Amplification of Clones

The isolated DNA is used as a template for PCR amplification with vector primers (AEK-M13) using a 96-well format, typically 12 plates at a time.

1. Make a PCR reaction mix by combining the components in **Table 1** (*see* **Note 3**).
2. Using a multichannel pipet, transfer 99 μL of the master mix to each well of the PCR plates (Cycleplates).
3. Using a multichannel pipet, transfer 1 μL of appropriate template DNA in each well taking care to retain the plates orientation and order (*see* **Note 4**).
4. Cover the plates with sealers (Cycleseal) and place in a thermocycling device.
5. Amplify the templates using the following cycle conditions:
   a. Step 1. 96°C for 30 s.
   b. Step 2. 94°C for 30 s.
   c. Step 3. 55°C for 30 s.
   d. Step 4. 72°C for 150 s.
   e. Step 5. Repeat **steps 2–4**, 24 times.
   f. Step 6. 72°C for 5 min.

3.1.4. Quantification of PCR Product

1. Analyze 2 μL of each PCR product by electrophoresis on a 2% TAE agarose gel containing 0.5 μg/mL of ethidium bromide. We obtain a digital image of the gel under UV illumination and analyze the electrophoresis products to ensure that a single band of distinct size is produced for each sample. The intensity of the band gives an estimate of the relative amount of product.
2. Quantify the PCR products using fluorometric quantitation (*see* **Note 5**). Expected yield is ~100 μg/mL.

3.1.5. Purification of PCR Product Purification

1. Prepare an ethanol/acetate precipitation mix (150 m*M* sodium acetate, pH 6.0, in ethanol). Add 200 mL of the precipitation mix to each well of a V-bottomed 96-well plate.
2. Using a multichannel pipettor, transfer the remaining (approx 97 mL) PCR products to their corresponding wells containing the precipitation mix (*see* **Note 6**).
3. Place the plates in the –80°C for 1 h, or overnight at –20°C, to precipitate the DNA.
4. Allow the plates to thaw (to reduce brittleness and melt any ice), and spin in a high-speed swinging-holder centrifuge (Sorvall Super T21). We typically spin stacks of three plates at 1600 rcf for 1 h (*see* **Note 7**).
5. After centrifugation, remove the supernatant from plates, and dispense a 70% ethanol wash, 150 mL/well, using a plate-processing station such as the Bio-Rad 1575 ImmunoWash.
6. Centrifuge the plates as in **step 4** at 1600 rcf for 1 h, and remove the supernatant. In a dust-free area, allow the plates to dry overnight without lids and covered with clean paper towels.
7. Resuspend the PCR products in 40 μL of 3X SSC. Seal the plates with foil sealer making sure that all wells are tightly sealed. Place the plates in an airtight heat-sealed bag with a moistened paper towel, and place in a 65°C oven for 2 h (*see* **Note 8**).
8. Remove the cooled plates and store at –20°C.

Microarrays in Gene Expression Profiling

Table 1
Components for PCR Reaction Mix

Reagent	Stock	Final	Volume per 1000 reactions (mL)
PCR buffer	10 X	1 X	10
dATP	100 mM	0.2 mM	0.2
dTTP	100 mM	0.2 mM	0.2
dGTP	100 mM	0.2 mM	0.2
dCTP	100 mM	0.2 mM	0.2
AEK M13F	1000 µM	0.5 µM	0.05
AEK M13R	1000 µM	0.5 µM	0.05
Ampli Taq Polymerase	5 U/µL	0.05 U/µL	1
DEPC H$_2$O			87.1

3.1.6. Poly-L-Lysine Pretreatment of Glass Slides

Treatment of slides with a coat of poly-L-lysine allows the target DNA to adhere to the surface and minimize loss during hybridization (*see* **Note 9**).

1. Place new Gold Seal microscope slides into a stainless steel 50-slide rack.
2. Prepare cleaning solution in a large glass beaker (500 mL is required per 50-slide glass tank): 400 mL of ddH$_2$O, 100 g of NaOH, of 600 mL of 95% ethanol. Dissolve NaOH in water, and then add ethanol. Stir until the solution is clear. If the solution does not clear, add H$_2$O until it does.
3. Dispense the cleaning solution into 50-slide glass tanks. Submerge the rack in the cleaning solution and shake for 2 h on an orbital shaker.
4. Remove the slides and rinse with fresh ddH$_2$O for 2–5 min. Repeat the wash four times, each time using fresh ddH$_2$O (*see* **Note 10**).
5. Move the clean slides to 25-slide plastic racks.
6. Prepare the poly-L-lysine solution as follows (for two boxes of 25 slides each): 35 mL of poly-L-lysine (0.1% [w/v]), 35 mL of tissue culture PBS, 280 mL of ddH$_2$O.
7. Dispense the poly-L-lysine solution into plastic 25-slide containers. Submerge the rack in poly-L-lysine solution, cover with a lid, and shake for 1 h.
8. Rinse once in ddH$_2$O for 1 min.
9. Centrifuge the rack in a low-speed swinging-holder centrifuge to remove free liquid.
10. Immediately transfer to a clean slide box.
11. Allow the slides to age for 2 wk before printing (*see* **Note 11**).

3.1.7. Microarray Slide Printing

The next stage is printing of DNA probes on the coated glass slides. The printing process refers to the robot-driven sequential transfer of individual purified PCR-amplified fragments from a 96-well microtiter tray to exact, predefined locations on glass slides. Several arrayers are available from commercial companies: Affymetrix 417 Arrayer (http://www.affymetrix.com/products/spotted.html), Cartesian Technologies (http://www.cartesiantech.com/), Beecher Instruments (http://www.beecherinstruments.com/), Genomic Solutions (http://www.genomicsolutions.com/), BioRobotics (http://www.biorobotics.co.uk/). It is also possible to build you own arrayer for approx US $25,000 (http://cmgm.stanford.edu/pbrown/), and arrayers have been built in several academic settings *(15)*.

The Cancer Genetics Branch custom-built arrayers, using "quill"-type pens, print sequentially up to 16 spots at once on each of 48 or 96 slides, wash and dry the print pens before picking up the next set of cDNAs, and repeat until a complete 96-well plate of probe DNA has been printed *(13)*. At this time, 96-well plates must be manually changed; however, an autoloading mechanism is in development. Each pen collects approx 200–500 nL and deposits between 2 and 3 nL (0.2–0.5 ng) of PCR product.

After printing is complete, identifying marks are etched along the top of each slide (print number and slide number) with a diamond scriber and the slides are placed in plastic slide box (use simple plastic slide boxes with no paper or cork to shed particles) (*see* **Note 12**).

3.1.8. Blocking Slides After Printing with Succinic Anhydride

To reduce nonspecific binding of strongly negatively charged target on microarray slides, the positively charged amine groups on poly-L-lysine-coated slides are passivated by reaction with succinic anhydride. We routinely process 48 slides at a time (*see* **Note 13**).

1. Age the slides for 1 wk at room temperature after printing (*see* **Note 14**).
2. Place the slides in a glass casserole dish and cover with plastic wrap. UV-crosslink printed cDNA with a dose of 450 mJ of UV energy (Strategene Stratalinker).
3. Place the slides in stainless steel 30-slide racks, and place the racks in clean glass tanks. Prepare the passivation reaction (for one tank) in a dedicated, dry 500-mL beaker: 6 g of succinic anhydride, 325 mL of 1-methyl-2-pyrrolidinone, 25 mL of 1 M sodium borate, pH 6.0. When succinic anhydride has completely dissolved, add 25 mL of 1 M sodium borate buffer while mixing, and quickly pour onto the slides (*see* **Note 15**).
4. Shake the slides for 20–30 min on an orbital shaker—some precipitation will occur. While blocking, boil ddH$_2$O in a clean Pyrex dish using a hot plate, so that it will be ready after the reaction (*see* **Note 16**).
5. Remove the slide holder from the passivation reaction, and dunk immediately in boiling ddH$_2$O to denature the DNA. Turn off the heat source and let stand for 2 min in the nearly boiling ddH$_2$O bath. Remove the slide holder, and dunk in a fresh glass tank with 100% ethanol to dehydrate the slides.

Microarrays in Gene Expression Profiling

6. After 3–5 min in ethanol, remove the slides and centrifuge dry in a low-speed swinging-holder centrifuge.
7. Place the dry slides in a clean slide box.

3.2. RNA Extraction and Target Production

RNAs isolated from the cells or tissue one wishes to analyze are used as the template for synthesis of fluorescently labeled cDNA targets. For cell lines, RNA first extracted using a Qiagen RNeasy kit followed by a further round of purification using TRIzol yields excellent results (two rounds of TRIzol extraction is recommended for tissues). The amount of total RNA in each channel required for a microarray experiment varies from 50 to 200 µg, with the precise amount varying with the size of the array and fluorescent nucleotide used (*see* **Note 17**).

Considerable thought should be given to what reference cell line or tissue to use for your microarray experiments. The reference should be abundant and offer at least a minimal intensity for all genes printed on your array (if a gene has no intensity in the reference channel, then ratios and other statistical calculations cannot be computed because the denominator cannot be zero).

3.2.1. RNA Extraction

1. For the RNeasy kit, follow the manufacturer's guidelines. At the final elution stage, elute with two successive aliquots of 150 µL of RNase-free water (*see* **Note 18**).
2. Determine the concentration of your RNA in 50 mM NaOH. At this time it may be convenient to aliquot out appropriate quantities (55–220 µg) of your RNA before beginning the second round of purification (*see* **Note 19**).
3. Extract the eluted RNA a second time by adding 1 mL of TRIzol/0.3 mL of eluent, vortexing, and following manufacturer guidelines for RNA extraction. You may leave the precipitated RNA in isopropanol at –80°C for later use.
4. If the RNA is to be used immediately, wash the RNA pellet twice with 70% ethanol, remove the ethanol, and dry the pellet (air-dry or Speedvac) (*see* **Note 20**).
5. Resuspend the dried RNA pellet (50–200 µg) in 400 µL of RNase-free H$_2$O. Take 1 µL for final RNA concentration measurement, and make sure the total amount of RNA for labeling with Cy3 is 80–100 µg, and 150–200 µg for Cy5.
6. Transfer the RNA to a Microcon-30 and centrifuge at 14,000 rcf for 7–12 min to concentrate the RNA. Concentrate the RNA to <14 µL (*see* **Note 21**).
7. Elute the RNA and bring to a final volume of 14 µL with DEPC H$_2$O.

3.2.2. Direct Labeling of cDNA Using Fluorescent Dyes

The labeling of complex probes is accomplished by direct incorporation of fluorescent nucleotides during an RT reaction. Currently, the factors of labeling efficiency, fluorescent yield, spectral separation, and nonspecific binding make the Cy3/Cy5 pair the most useful for our detection system. Although a number of conjugated fluorophores are available (dCTP, dUTP, amino-allyl dUTP RT coupled to monofunctional dyes), we have found that Amersham Pharmacia dUTP-conjugated Cy3/Cy5 yields consistent results. Other labeling systems are being tested.

1. Preanneal RNA with anchored oligo-dT (d-20T-d[AGC]) (1 μg/μL) primer: 14 μL of RNA, 3 μL of anchored oligo-dT primer. Incubate in a thermocycler at 70°C for 5 min and cool to 42°C.
2. Mix the RT labeling reaction: 4 μL of Cy3 *or* Cy5-dUTP (1 m*M*), 8 μL of 5X First-Strand Buffer, 4 μL of 10X low T dNTP mix, 4 μL of 0.1 *M* DTT, 1 μL of Rnase Inhibitor RNAsin, 2 μL of SSII RT.
3. Add RT labeling mix to the preannealed RNA.
4. Incubate at 42°C for 30–60 min.
5. Add 2 μL of SII RT enzyme, incubate at 42°C for another 30–60 min, and cool to room temperature.

3.2.3. Target Purification

The labeled target reaction must be purified to remove unincorporated nucleotides.

1. To stop the labeling reaction, add 5 μL of 0.5 *M* EDTA, pH 8.0, and mix well.
2. To hydrolyze the RNA, add 10 μL of 1 *M* sodium hydroxide and mix well. Incubate at 65°C for 20–30 min, then cool to room temperature.
3. Add 25 μL of 1 *M* Tris-HCl, pH 7.5, to neutralize the NaOH.
4. Purify each labeled color individually for the first purification. In Microcon-30 spin columns, add labeled target and bring up to a total volume of 400 μL with DEPC H$_2$O. Spin the column at 16,000 rcf for about 8 to 9 min to a volume of approx 50 μL (*see* **Note 22**).
5. Recover each target. For the second purification, pool the Cy3- and Cy5-labeled targets for an experiment in a new Microcon-30 column, and bring up to a total volume of 400 μL of H$_2$O.
6. Concentrate the combined targets to a 25-μL final volume for hybridization.

3.3. Hybridization

Hybridization volumes may vary depending on array size. The following is based on a 20 × 40 mm array. Adjust volumes proportionally and use appropriate sized cover slips for smaller/larger arrays.

3.3.1. Microarray Assembly

1. Make the hybridization mixture containing competitor DNA (to reduce nonspecific binding and background): 25 μL of pooled Cy5/Cy3 labeled targets, 1.5 μL of poly dA (10 mg/mL), 1.5 μL of yeast tRNA (4 mg/mL), 1.5 μL of human Cot-1 DNA (10 mg/mL), 1.5 μL of 50X Denhardts, 5 μL of 20X SSC (*see* **Note 23**).
2. Denature at 98°C for 2 min and cool on wet ice for 10 s.
3. Add 0.8 μL of 10% SDS.

Microarrays in Gene Expression Profiling

4. Pipet hybridization targets up and down several times until well mixed, and place the mixture on a microarray under a 24 × 50 mm glass coverslip (*see* **Note 24**).
5. Place the microarray slide in a hybridization chamber with 15–20 μL of 3X SSC to maintain humidity within the chamber.
6. Incubate the microarray hybridization chamber in a 65°C water bath for 12–18 h.

3.3.2. Posthybridization Slide Washes

After hybridization, the hybridization solution and any unbound target must be removed from the surface of the slide to reduce background.

1. Remove the microarray hybridization chamber from the water bath (*see* **Note 25**).
2. Dispense wash solutions into Coplin staining jars. Open the hybridization chamber and immediately place the slide in Wash #1 until the coverslip slips off. Once the coverslip comes off, agitate gently for 2 min (*see* **Note 26**).
3. Transfer the slide to Wash #2 and agitate gently for 2 min.
4. Transfer the slide to Wash #3 and agitate gently for 2 min.
5. Place the slide in a plastic 25-slide rack and spin in a centrifuge equipped with a swinging carrier (horizontal) that can hold the slide holder. Spin immediately (900 rcf for 2 min at room temperature).
6. Scan the slide as soon as possible.

3.4. Image Acquisition

Target fluorescence intensities at the immobilized probes can be measured using a variety of commercially available scanners (*16*). The following is a brief list scanners and contact information:

1. Affymetrix: 418 Array Scanner—Scanning laser digital imaging epifluorescence microscope; 5320 nm (350 mW) and 6350 nm (350 mW) lasers with 3-min scan time per slide. Cost: US $50,000 (http://www.affymetrix.com/).
2. Agilent: Under development (http://www.agilent.com/).
3. Axon: GenePix 4000—532-nm (20-mW) and 635-nm (15-mW) lasers with 10-μm pixel resolution and 5-min scan time per slide. Cost: US $50,000 (http://www.axon.com/).
4. Beecher Instruments: Scanner—laser confocal, two simultaneous photomultiplier tube channels, three lasers: 488 nm at 75 mW, 532 nm at 100 mW, 633 nm at 35 mW with 10- to 100-μm pixel resolution (http://www.beecherinstruments.com/).
5. Genomic Solutions: GeneTAC LS IV and GeneTAC 2000—Charge-coupled device camera with high-energy xenon light source; can scan up to four fluors per slide. Cost: US $60,000 (http://www.genomicsolutions.com/).
6. GSI Lumonics: ScanArray LITE, ScanArray 4000, ScanArray 5000—Scanning confocal laser GHeNe 543 nm (Cy3) and RHeNe 632 nm (Cy5) (http://www.genscan.com/).
7. Molecular Dynamics: Array Scanner—Confocal optics, nine-element lens; HeNe and NdYag lasers; scanning time per slide: 5 min for single color, 11 min for two color. Cost: US $110,000 (http://www.moleculardynamics.com/).

218   Khan et al.

8. Packard Instruments: BioChip Imager—Epifluorescence confocal scanning laser system. 543 nm (Cy3) and 633 nm (Cy5) HeNe lasers with 50-, 20-, or 10-μm pixel resolution (http://packardinst.com/).

The scanners used by our laboratory are Beecher Instruments or Agilent custom-built dual-laser confocal microscopes that generate two-color simultaneous digital scans saved to an IBM PC. Intensity data are integrated in 10- to 15-μm square pixels and recorded at 16 bits.

3.5. Image Analysis and Normalization

The two image files generated by the scanner are analyzed using software tools (Array Suite) developed by Chen et al. *(17)* for the ScanAlytics IPLab image-processing package. These software tools can be used with any image file format to extract raw target intensity information as well as to compute background-corrected intensities and expression ratios, confidence intervals (CI), and to allow for data integration of all clone information. As each probe is roboticly printed to a predefined position, the scanned images are overlaid with a grid that divides the images into segments, each containing a target spot. All clone information, including gene name, clone identification number, chromosome and radiation hybrid–mapped location, and source microplate position, is attached to each segment by this process. Each of the images is assigned a pseudo-color (e.g., Cy5 = red and Cy3 = green). The probe spot is identified within each segment, and the target fluorescent intensity is calculated for each color by averaging the intensities of every pixel inside the detected spot region. The local background intensity around each spot in each color is also measured within each segment. For every spot in each color channel, the final target intensity values are derived by subtracting the local background intensity from the average fluorescent intensity.

Next, a normalization constant is determined to compensate for differential efficiencies of labeling and detection of Cy3 and Cy5. The process involves calculating the average intensity, in both color channels, for a set of internal controls consisting of 88 housekeeping genes. These genes are preselected and have been verified on numerous hybridizations as being stable for most experiments (red:green ratio = 1.0). The normalization constant is then derived and used to calculate a calibrated red:green ratio for each cDNA spot within the image. In addition the ratio variance of the 88 control genes is used to calculate 99% CIs in which the ratios are statistically no different from 1. The output of the analysis is in the form of a pseudo-colored image of the entire array. Individual spots can be highlighted using the mouse cursor, and information including gene name, clone identity, intensity values, intensity ratios, normalization constant, and user-defined CIs can be obtained. A spreadsheet of expression ratio data for each spot is generated. For more information about

Microarrays in Gene Expression Profiling

this process and to download free software and tools, *see* our website (http://www.nhgri.nih.gov/DIR/LCG/15K/HTML/).

3.5.1. Sensitivity and Specificity

It is estimated that that the sensitivity of this method allows the detection of mRNA species comprising 1:10,000 of the mass of poly (A)+. Comparisons among the microarray experiments with Northern hybridizations have confirmed this technique to be reliable *(11,13,14,18)*. Our experience to date has indicated the high consistency of microarray data for determining ratio changes; however, there is some variation in the exact value of the ratios obtained by these two methods. In some instances, the ratio obtained by microarray analysis underestimates that obtained by Northern analysis. Possible causes for this underestimation include reaching a probe intensity saturation limit at the highest intensities under our current detection system. Additionally, the largest ratio changes frequently have one of the measurements near the lower limit of detection, and at these levels the effects of background and nonspecific binding are more apparent, causing variance at the higher ratio measurements. Other causes of discrepancy may be owing to nonlinear binding characteristics of target to probe. Currently, we can detect up to 300-fold ratio changes with accuracy.

3.6. Data Mining and Statistical Analysis

All data from each experiment can be downloaded into a relational database such as FileMaker Pro (Claris) and further parsed for comparing data across experiments as well as for extracting data from individual array hybridizations. It is obvious that large-scale, high-throughput experimental methods require information processing coupled to a variety of analysis tools. Software tools such as ArrayDB *(19)* can also be used to integrate information from many Internet sources, such as NCBI Entrez, UniGene, and KEGG databases, with experimental gene expression data. Hierarchical clustering of biologic samples and genes *(14,20,21)* is a commonly applied mathematical strategy to organize gene expression data. Algorithms such as multidimensional scaling are proving to be an informative way to visualize expression profiles *(14)*. More complex data analysis systems *(22–25)* are currently being devised for complex clustering of data; however, a description of this is beyond the scope of this chapter.

4. Notes

1. There currently exists in the literature a confusing interchangeable nomenclature system for referring to hybridization partners termed probes and targets. For the purpose of this chapter we refer to the tethered DNA (of known iden-

tity) on the microarray slide as the probe, and the fluorescently labeled cDNA (synthesized from unknown mRNA messages) as the hybridization targets.

2. Use extreme care to avoid cross-contamination. Cross-contamination will be evident when PCR products are gel electrophoresed and present multiple bands. Contaminated clones will require restreaking and sequencing.

3. It is recommended that a slight excess of PCR reaction mix than what is actually required be made.

4. Take care to remove air bubbles and ensure proper mixing of the reaction mix.

5. We use the FluoReporter Blue Fluorometric dsDNA kit, Dynex Microfluor plates, lambda *Hin*dIII fragments for standards, and a Perkin-Elmer Luminescence Spectrometer LS50B.

6. Ensure proper mixing of the PCR solution with the precipitation mix. Failure to do so will decrease the concentration of DNA yield.

7. Use rubber pads between the stacked plates to prevent cracking and breakage.

8. Heat and cool the plates slowly to prevent condensation on the sealer and upper rim of the well.

9. It is important to wear powder-free gloves at all times and avoid contact with detergents or other compounds that may cause background fluorescence.

10. It is important to remove all traces of cleaning solution. Failure to do so will hinder poly-L-lysine coating the reaction and will adversely affect microarray results (low-intensity spots, high background).

11. Aged slides will be very hydrophobic (water drops leave no trail when they move across the surface).

12. A new slide should be marked for use as a template to line up the coverslip when putting together the microarray experiment, because the printed spots will not be visible after the slide-blocking procedure.

13. The reaction solution must be prepared in completely dry containers. All glassware, stir bars, and graduated cylinders should be dedicated to slide blocking and should not be cleaned with detergents, which can adversely affect this reaction.

14. A number of groups have found that rapid or slow hydration of the DNA on the slide after printing followed by a quick-drying step improves DNA distribution or signal strength. This has not been observed for materials prepared by our procedure, so it is routinely omitted.

15. When water is added, the anhydride will begin to rapidly decompose, so add the mix to the slides very quickly. It is helpful to dispense the sodium borate buffer from a prealiquoted 50-mL conical tube.

16. Cover the dish with aluminum foil to reduce evaporation and simultaneously boil ddH_2O in a microwave to replenish evaporative loss.

17. High-quality RNA is crucial to the success of a microarray experiment. It is also possible to use $2-4$ µg of poly(A)-purified mRNA in the target synthesis reaction. Smaller quantities of RNA may be used in conjunction with RNA amplification techniques, which are currently under development.

18. Cell lines should be harvested under consistent conditions and lysed rapidly. It is recommended that you sonicate the very viscous lysate with several 5-s bursts to

Microarrays in Gene Expression Profiling

disrupt the genomic DNA before applying to the RNeasy column. We use the microprobe (conical titanium probe 1.8-mm-diameter tip) at a setting of 5, dissipated power approx 5–10 W. When extracting RNA from tissue add the frozen sample directly to the TRIzol without thawing with immediate homogenization.

19. Factor in an approx 10% loss of RNA from each TRIzol purification round.
20. Overdrying may make resuspension of RNA difficult and may adversely affect results.
21. Do not concentrate to dryness, because the sample may be lost or difficult to recover. Proper volume is when the filter is partially dry on visual inspection.
22. The flowthrough may be saved at this step for high-performance liquid chromotography recovery of unincorporated fluorophores.
23. Appropriate competitor DNA should be used for microarrays of clones from other organisms, such as mouse.
24. For the best results, apply pooled targets to the center of the coverslip, and then, using the template slide as a guide (*see* **Subheading 3.1.7.**), place the inverted microarray slide from above.
25. Use paper towels and vacuum suction to completely dry the outer surface of the chamber.
26. Take care that the coverslip does not scratch the microarray surface.

References

1. Drmanac, S. and Drmanac, R. (1994) Processing of cDNA and genomic kilobase-size clones for massive screening, mapping and sequencing by hybridization. *Biotechniques* **17**, 328,329, 332–336.
2. Drmanac, S., Stavropoulos, N. A., Labat, I., Vonau, J., Hauser, B., Soares, M. B., and Drmanac, R. (1996) Gene-representing cDNA clusters defined by hybridization of 57,419 clones from infant brain libraries with short oligonucleotide probes. *Genomics* **37**, 29–40.
3. Schena, M., Shalon, D., Davis, R. W., and Brown, P. O. (1995) Quantitative monitoring of gene expression patterns with a complementary DNA microarray. *Science* **270**, 467–470.
4. Khan, J., Simon, R., Bittner, M., Chen, Y., Leighton, S. B., Pohida, T., et al. (1998) Gene expression profiling of alveolar rhabdomyosarcoma with cDNA microarrays. *Cancer Res.* **58**, 5009–5013.
5. Perou, C. M., Jeffrey, S. S., van de Rijn, M., Rees, C. A., Eisen, M. B., Ross, D. T., et al. (1999) Distinctive gene expression patterns in human mammary epithelial cells and breast cancers. *Proc. Natl. Acad. Sci. USA* **96**, 9212–9217.
6. Golub, T. R., Slonim, D. K., Tamayo, P., Huard, C., Gaasenbeek, M., Mesirov, J. P., et al. (1999) Molecular classification of cancer: class discovery and class prediction by gene expression monitoring. *Science* **286**, 531–537.
7. Ross, D. T., Scherf, U., Eisen, M. B., Perou, C. M., Rees, C., Spellman, P., et al. (2000) Systematic variation in gene expression patterns in human cancer cell lines. *Nat. Genet.* **24**, 227–235.
8. Diehn, M., Eisen, M. B., Botstein, D., and Brown, P. O. (2000) Large-scale identification of secreted and membrane-associated gene products using DNA microarrays. *Nat. Genet.* **25**, 58–62.

9. Alizadeh, A. A., Eisen, M. B., Davis, R. E., Ma, C., Lossos, I. S., Rosenwald, A., et al. (2000) Distinct types of diffuse large B-cell lymphoma identified by gene expression profiling. *Nature* **403,** 503–511.

10. Bubendorf, L., Kolmer, M., Kononen, J., Koivisto, P., Mousses, S., Chen, Y., et al. (1999) Hormone therapy failure in human prostate cancer: analysis by complementary DNA and tissue microarrays. *J. Natl. Cancer Inst.* **91,** 1758–1764.

11. Khan, J., Bittner, M. L., Saal, L. H., Teichmann, U., Azorsa, D. O., Gooden, G. C., et al. (1999) cDNA microarrays detect activation of a myogenic transcription program by the PAX3-FKHR fusion oncogene. *Proc. Natl. Acad. Sci. USA* **96,** 13,264–13,269.

12. Scherf, U., Ross, D. T., Waltham, M., Smith, L. H., Lee, J. K., Tanabe, L., et al. (2000) A gene expression database for the molecular pharmacology of cancer. *Nat. Genet.* **24,** 236–244.

13. Khan, J., Saal, L. H., Bittner, M. L., Chen, Y., Trent, J. M., and Meltzer, P. S. (1999) Expression profiling in cancer using cDNA microarrays. *Electrophoresis* **20,** 223–229.

14. Khan, J., Bittner, M. L., Chen, Y., Meltzer, P. S., and Trent, J. M. (1999) DNA microarray technology: the anticipated impact on the study of human disease. *Biochim. Biophys. Acta* **1423,** M17–28.

15. Cheung, V. G., Morley, M., Aguilar, F., Massimi, A., Kucherlapati, R., and Childs, G. (1999) Making and reading microarrays. *Nat. Genet.* **21,** 15–19.

16. Bowtell, D. D. (1999) Options available—from start to finish—for obtaining expression data by microarray (published erratum appears in *Nat. Genet.* 1999 Feb;21[2]:241). *Nat. Genet.* **21,** 25–32.

17. Chen, Y., Dougherty, E. R., and Bittner, M. L. (1997) Ratio-based decisions and the quantitative analysis of cDNA microarray images. *Biomed. Optics.* **2,** 364–374.

18. DeRisi, J., Penland, L.,. Brown, P. O, Bittner, M. L., Meltzer, P. S., Ray, M., et al. (1996) Use of a cDNA microarray to analyse gene expression patterns in human cancer. *Nat. Genet.* **14,** 457–460.

19. Ermolaeva, O., Rastogi, M., Pruitt, K. D., Schuler, G. D., Bittner, M. L., Chen, Y., et al. (1998) Data management and analysis for gene expression arrays. *Nat. Genet.* **20,** 19–23.

20. Spellman, P. T., Sherlock, G., Zhang, M. Q., Iyer, V. R., Anders, K., Eisen, M. B., et al. (1998) Comprehensive identification of cell cycle-regulated genes of the yeast Saccharomyces cerevisiae by microarray hybridization. *Mol. Biol. Cell* **9,** 3273–3297.

21. Eisen, M. B., Spellman, P. T., Brown, P. O., and Botstein, D. (1998) Cluster analysis and display of genome-wide expression patterns. *Proc. Natl. Acad. Sci. USA* **95,** 14,863–14,868.

22. Toronen, P., Kolehmainen, M., Wong, G., and Castren, E. (1999) Analysis of gene expression data using self-organizing maps. *FEBS Lett.* **451,** 142–146.

23. Brown, M. P., Grundy, W. N., Lin, D., Cristianini, N., Sugnet, C. W., Furey,T. S., et al. (2000) Knowledge-based analysis of microarray gene expression data by using support vector machines. *Proc. Natl. Acad. Sci. USA* **97,** 262–267.

24. Gaasterland, T. and Bekiranov, S. (2000) Making the most of microarray data [news]. *Nat. Genet.* **24,** 204–206.

25. Aach, J., Rindone, W., and Church, G. M. (2000) Systematic management and analysis of yeast gene expression data. *Genome Res.* **10,** 431–445.

17

Wilms Tumor Gene *WT1* as a Tumor Marker for Leukemic Blast Cells and Its Role in Leukemogenesis

Haruo Sugiyama

1. Introduction

Patients with acute leukemia have a total of approx 10^{12} leukemic cells at the time of diagnosis, and still have as many as 10^{10} leukemic cells in complete remission. The most important problem in the treatment of leukemia patients is the uncertainty of whether leukemic cells have been totally eradicated when complete remission has been achieved. Through accurate assessment of a small number of leukemic cells (minimal residual disease [MRD]) that still remained in complete remission *(1)*, individual patients will be able to be treated with different protocols based on the extent of the MRD, resulting in improvement of cure rates.

In this chapter, I focus on the clinical usefulness of the WT1 assay (quantitation of expression levels of Wilms tumor gene *WT1*) not only for the detection of MRD of leukemia but also for the diagnosis of hematopoietic malignancies. Also, I discuss an oncogenic function of the *WT1* gene in leukemogenesis and tumorigeneis rather than a tumor suppressor gene function.

1.1. Wilms Tumor Gene WT1

The *WT1* gene is a candidate gene for Wilms tumor, a childhood renal tumor that is thought to arise as a result of inactivation of both alleles of the *WT1* gene located at chromosome 11p13 *(2–4)*. The *WT1* gene has been considered to be a tumor suppressor gene on the basis of the following data *(5–9)*: intragenic deletions or mutations in Wilms tumor, germline mutations in patients with leukemia predisposition syndromes, and WT1-mediated growth suppression of Wilms tumor cells expressing a WT1 splicing variant. The *WT1* gene

From: *Methods in Molecular Medicine, vol. 68: Molecular Analysis of Cancer*
Edited by: J. Boultwood and C. Fidler © Humana Press Inc., Totowa, NJ

encodes a zinc-finger transcription factor that represses transcription of growth factor [platelet-derived growth factor-A chain *[10]*, colony-stimulating factor-1 *[11]*, and insulin-like growth factor-2 *[12]*) and growth factor receptor [IGF-IR *[13]* and epidermal growth factor receptor *[14]*) genes, and the other genes (RARα *[15]*, c-myb *[16]*, c-myc *[17]*, and bcl-2 *[17]*).

Tumor suppressor genes such as *Rb* and *p53* are expressed ubiquitously. On the other hand, expression of the *WT1* gene is restricted to a limited set of tissues, including gonads, uterus, kidney, and mesothelial structures, but it is highest in the developing kidney, reflecting the significant role of WT1 in renal development *(18–20)*. WT1 knockout mice were shown to have defects in the urogenital system and to die at embryonic d 3.5, probably owing to heart failure *(21)*.

1.2. WT1 *Gene Expression in Leukemias*

Miwa et al. *(22)* examined the expression of the *WT1* gene in leukemias using Northern blot analysis. The *WT1* gene expression was detected in 15 of 22 acute myelogenous leukemias (AMLs), in 7 of 16 acute lymphoid leukemias (ALLs), and in 8 of 10 chronic myelogeneous leukemias (CMLs) in blastic crisis. Miyagi et al. *(23)* also detected the WT1 transcript in 4 of 10 AMLs, in 1 of 9 ALLs, and in 1 of 6 CMLs in accelerated-phase or blastic crisis. These two reports have shown that the *WT1* gene is expressed in some cases of myeloid or lymphoid leukemias.

Inoue et al. *(24)* provided a new development for the significance of the *WT1* gene expression in leukemias by the quantitation of the expression levels of the *WT1* gene using quantitative reverse transcriptase polymerase chain reaction (RT-PCR). Forty-five patients with AML, 22 with ALL, 6 with acute mixed lineage leukemia (AMLL), and 23 with CML (8 chronic phase, 5 accelerated phase, and 10 blast crisis) were quantitated for the expression levels of the *WT1* gene using quantitative RT-PCR. In all the leukemia samples examined, significant levels of *WT1* gene expression were found, and the levels were approx 1000 and 100,000 times higher than those in normal bone marrow or in normal peripheral blood, respectively. In CML, the levels increased as the disease progressed. A clear correlation between the WT1 expression levels (<0.6 vs ≥0.6) and the prognosis of acute leukemia was observed (WT1 expression level in K562 cells was defined as 1.0). Patients with levels of <0.6 had significantly higher rates of complete remission, and disease-free and overall survivals than those with levels of ≥0.6. All seven patients with levels of *WT1* gene expression of >1.0 did not achieve complete remission. Bergmann et al. *(25)* also reported the correlation between the WT1 expression levels and the prognosis. Brieger et al. *(26)* detected WT1 transcript in 41 of 52 (79%) AML patients, while most of the 14 patients studied in complete remission lost

Wilms Tumor Gene WT1 *in Leukemia*

their WT1 expression. In three of the four patients in complete remission, the reappearance of WT1 expression preceded their relapse. Menssen et al. *(27)* also found *WT1* gene expression in 53 of 57 (93%) AML patients, 12 of 14 (86%) pre-pre-B ALL patients, 33 of 41 (80%) cALL patients, and 23 of 31 (74%) T-ALL patients. They confirmed the *WT1* gene expression in leukemic blast cells by an immunofluorescence assay using WT1-specific antibodies *(28)*. Patmasiriwat et al. *(29)* quantitated WT1 expression levels in 62 AML samples and found that 82% strongly expressed WT1. Im et al. *(30)* studied WT1 expression in children with acute leukemia by means of RT- PCR *(30)*. WT1 was detectable in all 3 AML and 7 of 10 ALL patients, but not in 2 ALL patients in remission. The expression levels were higher for AML than for ALL. These reports demonstrated that the *WT1* gene expression is a novel tumor marker for leukemic blast cells in both children and adults and a new prognostic factor for acute leukemia.

1.3. Detection of MRD of Leukemia by Quantitation of Expression Levels of WT1 Gene

The average levels of the WT1 expression in leukemic cells were approx 3 logs higher than those in normal bone marrow cells and more than 5 logs higher than those in peripheral blood cells *(24)*. This striking difference in WT1 expression levels between leukemic and normal cells made it possible to detect MRD of leukemia by the quantitation of the expression levels of the *WT1* gene (WT1 assay). To determine the sensitivity of the WT1 assay, RNA from the leukemic cells (WT1 expression level = 0.58) of acute promyelocytic leukemia (APL) with the *PML/RARα* fused gene was serially diluted with RNA from normal bone marrow or peripheral blood cells, and then WT1 and PML/RARα mRNAs were quantitated by RT-PCR with the respective primers *(24)*. The WT1 mRNA was quantitated in parallel with the PML/RARα mRNA along with dilutions. This meant that the amount of the WT1 mRNA directly reflected that of APL blast cells, confirming that WT1 mRNA is a tumor marker for APL blast cells. The detection limit of leukemic cells by RT-PCR with the PML/RARa primer was 10^{-4} for both bone marrow and peripheral blood samples, whereas that by RT-PCR with the WT1 primer was 10^{-3} to 10^{-4} for bone marrow samples and 10^{-5} for peripheral blood samples. Therefore, the detection sensitivity of APL blast cells was superior in te RT-PCR method with the WT1 primer to the RT-PCR method with the PML/RARα primer. Tamaki et al. *(31)* found that WT1 expression levels increased at relapse and that the levels at relapse were significantly higher than those at diagnosis (mean: 0.73 ± 0.12 vs 0.38 ± 0.04; $p < 0.01$). In nine AML patients from whom paired samples were obtained at both diagnosis and relapse, the average WT1 expression level at relapse (1.05) was 4.5 times higher than that assayed at diagnosis (0.23) (maximal change: 27.7-fold increase from 0.013 to 0.360; minimal change: 1.9-fold increase from 0.44 to 0.85). Accordingly, these results should mean an increase in detection sensitivity of MRD by the WT1 assay as relapse nears.

A clean correlation existed between the MRD detected in the paired bone marrow and peripheral blood samples for various types of leukemia (AML, ALL, and CML), with MRD in peripheral blood samples being approx one-tenth of that in bone marrow samples *(30)*. Since background levels of WT1 expression in peripheral blood is less than one hundredth of those in bone marrow, peripheral blood samples should be, in practice, superior to bone marrow samples for the detection of MRD *(32)*.

1.4. Long-Term Follow-Up of MRD of Leukemia by WT1 Assay

Thirty-one patients (27 AML, 2 ALL, and 2 AMLL) treated with conventional chemotherapy (CHT) and 23 patients (13 AML, 5 ALL, and 5 CML) treated with allogeneic bone marrow transplantation (BMT) were monitored for WT1 expression levels in bone marrow and peripheral blood using RT-PCR over a long-term period (mean: 29 mo for CHT and 24 mo for BMT) *(32)*. Nineteen patients (16 CHT and 3 BMT) who achieved complete remission eventually relapsed. In 10 of these patients, WT1 expression that had returned to normal bone marrow background levels ($<10^{-3}$) at complete remission either gradually or rapidly increased again to abnormal levels 1–18 mo (mean 7 mo) before their clinical relapse. In nine patients, WT1 expression never returned to normal bone marrow background levels even during complete remission, and their subsequent relapse was accompanied by a rapid increase in WT1 expression to levels higher than 10^{-2}. On the other hand, the remaining 35 patients (15 CHT and 20 BMT) maintained their complete remission. In 29 (11 CHT and 18 BMT) of these, WT1 expression either gradually or rapidly decreased to normal bone marrow background levels, whereas in the other 6 patients (4 CHT and 2 BMT), low levels of WT1 mRNA (10^{-3}–10^{-2}) still remained detectable, but no clinical signs of relapse were evident. These results showed that clinical relapse is impending when there is a rapid or gradual increase in WT1 expression levels to or over 10^{-2} after an initial return to normal bone marrow background levels in complete remission, or when there is retention of the WT1 expression at levels near or over 10^{-2} in the bone marrow without a return to normal bone marrow background levels even during complete remission. The absolute levels of WT1 that predict with certainty that a patient will relapse are 10^{-2} levels in bone marrow and 10^{-3} levels in peripheral blood. Patients with these signs should be immediately and appropriately treated before clinical relapse becomes apparent. Bergmann et al. *(33)* also found that patients achieving complete remission after chemotherapy usually

Wilms Tumor Gene WT1 in Leukemia

lose detectable signals of WT1, and in relapse of the disease, recurrence of WT1 mRNA can be determined in almost all patients with initially detectable WT1 mRNA. Detectable levels of WT1 during follow-up in AML patients have been shown to be useful as a marker for MRD or even to predict relapse of AML *(33)*.

In a patient with AML who recieved allogeneic BMT, WT1 expression levels gradually increased to 5.9×10^{-3} in bone marrow (normal range: $<1.0 \times 10^{-3}$) and 2.4×10^{-3} in peripheral blood (normal range: $<1.0 \times 10^{-5}$) on d 367 post-BMT *(34)*. However, bone marrow aspiration showed no evidence of relapse (100% donor type chromosomes). Since the increase in WT1 expression levels over 10^{-2} in bone marrow or 10^{-3} in peripheral blood predicts that clinical relapse is impending, we diagnosed this patient as having molecular relapse on d 367 and performed donor leukocyte transfusion (DLT). Leukemic blast cells increased and reached a maximum (50%) 29 d after DLT, but thereafter rapidly decreased and became undetetable 39 d after DLT and complete remission was achieved. The patient showed no evidence of graft-vs-host disease or other complications. Note that the patient did not manifest marrow aplasia, which is a common complication of DLT. The WT1 expression levels rapidly decreased from 29 d post-DLT and returned to normal range 60 d post-DLT. The patient was in complete remission with a normal range of WT1 expression levels for more than 21 mo after DLT. This case clearly demonstrated that early application of DLT at molecular relapse is essential for the improvement of the efficacy of DLT for relapsed AML after BMT, confirming the availability of the WT1 assay for the monitoring of MRD of leukemia.

Taken together, the WT1 assay has made it possible to rapidly assess the effectiveness of treatment, to evaluate the degree of eradication of leukemic cells, and to diagnose molecular relapse in individual leukemia patients. Thus, treatment for leukemia patients can be individualized by the monitoring of MRD by the WT1 assay, resulting in the improvement of cure rates.

1.5. Continuous Assessment of Disease Progression of Myelodysplastic Syndromes by WT1 Assay

The WT1 expression levels were examined for 57 patients with myelodysplastic syndromes (MDS) (refractory anemia, 35; refractory anemia with excess of blasts [RAEB] 14; RAEB in transformation [RAEB-t]), 6; and MDS with fibrosis, 2) and 12 patients with AML evolved from MDS *(35)*. These levels significantly increased in proportion to the disease progression of MDS from refractory anemia to overt AML via RAEB and RAEB-t in both bone marrow and peripheral blood, demonstrating that the WT1 expression levels directly reflect the disease progression of MDS. WT1 expression levels in peripheral blood, but not in bone marrow, significantly correlated with the evolution of RAEB or RAEB-t to overt AML within 6 mo. An increase in WT1 expression levels to 10^{-2} in peripheral blood means that disease progression to overt AML is impending within 6 mo. Thus, the WT1 expression levels in peripheral blood are superior to those in bone marrow for early prediction of the evolution to AML by the means of the WT1 assay. Furthermore, WT1 expression in peripheral blood of overt AML patients was significantly decreased by effective chemotherapy or allogeneic stem cell transplantation and became undetectable in long-term survivors. Interestingly, the WT1 expression levels in bone marrow did not correlate with the percentages of morphologically leukemic blast cells in bone marrow in RAEB or RAEB-t patients, suggesting that the WT1 expression levels reflect the amount of not only morphologically leukemic blast cells but also of abnormal, transformed cells that are undetectable morphologically as blast cells. These results showed that WT1 expression levels are a tumor marker for both morphologically leukemic blast cells and abnormal cells that are undetectable morphologically as blast cells in MDS and thus reflect the disease progression of MDS. Monitoring of WT1 expression levels has made continuous assessment of the disease progression of MDS possible, as well as the prediction of the evolution of RAEB or RAEB-t to overt AML within 6 mo. The WT1 assay is also useful for diagnosis of MRD of MDS with high sensitivity, thus making it possible to evaluate the efficacy of treatment for MDS.

1.6. Differential Diagnosis Between Reactive and Leukemic Leukocytosis by WT1 Assay

Juvenile chronic myeloid leukemia (JCML) and infantile monosomy 7 syndrome (IMo7), which belong to childhood MDS, have common clinical features such as a male predominance, prominent hepatosplenomegaly, the presence of immature precursors in peripheral blood, an excessive proliferation of myeloid progenitor cells, and poor prognosis. The etiology and classification of both diseases, however, have been the subject of controversy. Two JCML and two IMo7 patients with characteristic clinical features were examined on the WT1 expression levels in bone marrow and peripheral blood by the WT1 assay *(36)*. The WT1 expression levels ($2.4-7.2 \times 10^{-2}$) in bone marrow of these four patients were significantly elevated in comparison with the levels ($<10^{-3}$) in normal bone marrow and equivalent to those in bone marrow of the patients with AML, ALL, or CML at blastic crisis. In two patients who were successfully treated with allogeneic peripheral blood stem cell transplantation, the WT1 expression returned to normal background levels in bone marrow and to undetectable levels in peripheral blood. Abnormally increased WT1 expression levels, which were equivalent to those in acute leukemias, in both JCML and IMo7 strongly indicated that both the diseases are defined as an etiologically similar entity and result from leukemic transformation of hematopoietic progenitor cells. The results that the WT1 expression levels in both JCML and IMo7 were approx 10 times higher than those in CML at chronic phase are compatible with clinical findings that the clinical course of JCML is much more aggressive than that of CML at chronic phase. The WT1 assay may become a clinical test indispensable for the discrimination between JCML and CML, and between myeloproliferative disorders and reactive leukocytosis in childhood such as congenital viral infection and persistent Epstein-Barr virus infection, both of which present a picture quite similar to JCML, because WT1 expression levels significantly increase in leukemic growth, but not in reactive states.

Acute eosinophilic leukemia (AEoL) is a rare form of AML that presents with a substantially increased series of left-shifted but maturing eosinophilic precursors and an increased number of blasts in bone marrow. By contrast, the idiopathic hypereosinophilic syndrome consists of a heterogeneous group of nonmalignant myeloproliferative disorders of unknown origin that is characterized by persistent overproduction of mature and sometimes immature eosinophilic cells, leukocytosis, and eosinophilic organ infiltrations. Reactive eosinophilia usually can be discriminated from AEoL. However, the distinction between AEoL and hyperoscinophilic syndrome is known to be difficult, because clinical and hematological features do not necessarily differ between the two diseases. Menssen et al. *(37)* analyzed WT1 expression levels in patients with AEoL, hyperoscinophilic syndrome, or reactive eosinophilia by means of RT-PCR. They found that the WT1 expression was restricted to AEoL patients and that isolated central nervous system–related leukemia could be diagnosed by detecting WT1 mRNA transcript in the cerebrospinal fluid in an AEoL patient. Thus, the WT1 assay is a powerful complementary diagnostic tool to distinguish AEoL from hyperoscinophilic syndrome.

1.7. WT1 Expression in Various Types of Solid Tumors

WT1 gene expression was examined in 34 solid tumor cell lines and four freshly isolated lung cancers and detected in 3 of the 4 gastric cancer cell lines, all of the 5 colon cancer cell lines, 12 of the 15 lung cancer cell lines, 2 of the 4 breast cancer cell lines, 1 germ tumor cell line, 2 ovarian cancer cell lines, 1 uterine cancer cell line, 1 thyroid cancer cell line, and 1 hepatocellular carcinoma cell line *(38)*. Therefore, of the 34 solid tumor cell lines examined, 28 (82%) expressed WT1. Furthermore, WT1 expression was examined in fresh lung cancer tissues *(38)*. Tissue masses resected from lung cancer patients were separated into two parts: normal-appearing tissues and cancer cell–rich tissues. WT1 expression levels in three paired normal-appearing and cancer cell–rich tissues obtained from three lung cancer patients were $<10^{-5}$, and 3.9×10^{-3},

4.1 × 10^{-4}, and 3.6 × 10^{-2}, and 1.4 × 10^{-4}, and 1.2 × 10^{-3}, respectively. The WT1 expression level of cancer cell–rich tissues from another lung cancer patient was 1.4 × 10^{-3}. These results demonstrated that WT1 expression is significantly higher in cancer cell–rich tissues than in normal-appearing tissues, suggesting abnormal expression of the *WT1* gene not only in the cultured cancer cell lines but also in fresh lung cancer cells.

1.8. WT1 Gene Exerts an Oncogenic Function in Leukemogenesis and Tumorigenesis

The *WT1* gene originally was defined as a tumor suppressor gene. However, Inoue et al. *(24,39)* have recently proposed that the *WT1* gene has basically two functional aspects—that of a tumor suppressor gene and that of an oncogene—but that in leukemias and various types of solid tumors mentioned earlier, it performs an oncogenic rather than a tumor suppressor gene function on the basis of the following data: high levels of expression of wild-type WT1 in leukemic blast cells and various types of solid tumor cells *(38)*; a clear inverse correlation between WT1 expression levels and the prognosis of leukemia *(24)*; increased WT1 expression at relapse *(31)*; growth inhibition not only of leukemic cells *(40)* but also of various types of solid tumor cells *(38)* by treatment with WT1 antisense oligomers; and blocking of differentiation but induction of proliferation in response to granulocyte colony-stimulating factor in both 32D cl3 myeloid progenitor cells *(41)* and normal myeloid progenitor cells *(42)*, both of which constitutively express WT1 as a result of transfection with the *WT1* gene. Furthermore, molecular analysis of dimethylbenz anthracene (DMBA)–induced rat leukemia by Osaka et al. *(43)* has supported our hypothesis. WT1 expression was detected in 15 (71%) of 21 DMBA-induced erythroblastic leukemias, and cells with high expression levels of WT1 tended to develop into leukemia. Differences in the interactions of the WT1 protein with other regulatory proteins might determine whether the *WT1* gene acts as a tumor suppressor gene or performs an oncogenic function, because the WT1 protein does interact with regulatory proteins such as P53 *(44)*, par-4 *(45)*, and Ciao 1 *(46)*.

Inoue et al. *(24)* examined whether the *WT1* gene overexpressing in leukemias has mutations or deletions. Samples from 12 acute leukemia patients were subjected to PCR single-strand conformation polymorphism (SSCP) analysis. However, no point mutations were found *(24)*. Algar et al. *(47)* also found no tumorigeneic point mutations or small deletions or insertions in the *WT1* gene when they examined 15 AML and 33 ALL patients. Concerning WT1 mutations in CML, Carapeti et al. *(48)* examined 39 patients with CML blast crisis, and they concluded that dominant-negative mutations of the zinc-finger region of the *WT1* gene are uncommon in CML blast crisis. On the other hand, King-Underwood et al. *(49)* found mutations in the *WT1* gene in 4 of 36 acute leukemias by SSCP analysis. The

Wilms Tumor Gene WT1 in Leukemia

mutations comprised small insertions or a nonsense mutation. Furthermore, they extended their study and found that WT1 mutations occur in 14% of AML and 20% of biphenotypic leukemias, but are rare in ALL *(50)*. In AML, the presence of a WT1 mutation is associated with failure to achieve complete remission and a lower survival rate. Miyagawa et al. *(51)* also found WT1 mutations in 6 of 46 (13%) AMLs, but they were rare in ALL. Concerning the biologic significance of *WT1* gene mutations in leukemias, note that the majority of leukemias expressing high levels of WT1 have no mutations in the *WT1* gene, indicating that wild-type *WT1* gene expression plays an important role in leukemogenesis.

1.9. WT1 Protein is a Tumor-Specific Antigen Capable of Eliciting Cytotoxic T-Lymphocyte Responses

The *WT1* gene is expressed at high levels not only in leukemias but also in various types of solid tumors and exerts an oncogenic function in these malignancies. To determine whether the WT1 protein can serve as a target antigen for tumor-specific immunity, 9-mer WT1 peptides, which contain major histocompatibility complex (MHC) class I binding motifs and have a comparatively higher binding affinity for MHC class I molecules, were tested for the induction of cytotoxic T-lymphocytes (CTLs) against these WT1 peptides. Immunization in vivo of C57BL/6 mice (MHC class I: H-2D^b) with WT1 peptide Db126 (RMFPNAPYL) elicited CTLs against the WT1 peptide *(52)*. The CTLs specifically lysed not only Db126-pulsed target cells but also WT1-expressing murine leukemic cells in an MHC class I (H-2D^b)–restricted fashion. The mice immunized with this WT1 peptide completely rejected the challenges by WT1-expressing leukemic cells and survived for a long time with no signs of organ damage by autoimmunity mediated by the CTLs. Also, in vitro stimulation of human peripheral blood mononuclear cells with the WT1 peptide Db126 elicited CTLs against the WT1 peptide *(53)*. The CTLs specifically killed WT1-expressing human leukemic cells as well as WT1 peptide-pulsed target cells in an human leukocyte antigen class I–restricted manner. Therefore, the WT1 protein was identified as a novel tumor antigen of leukemia and various types of solid tumors. Immunotherapy targeting the WT1 protein should find clinical application not only for leukemias but also for solid tumors.

2. Materials

2.1. Sample Preparation

1. Phosphate-buffered saline (PBS): Dissolve 0.2 g of KCl, 0.2 g of KH$_2$PO$_4$, and 8 g of NaCl in 800 mL water. Adjust the pH to 7.2, and make up to 1 L with water.
2. Ficol-Paque (Pharmacia, Uppsala, Sweden).
3. Solution D: 4 mol/L of guanidin thiocyanate, 25 mmol/L of sodium citrate, pH 7.0, 0.5% sarcosyl, 0.1 mol/L of 2-mercaptoethanol.

2.2. Reverse Transcriptase Polymerase Chain Reaction

1. Diethylpyrocarbonate (DEPC)-treated water.
2. RT buffer: 50 mM Tris-HCl, pH 8.3, 70 mM KCl, 3 mM MgCl$_2$, 10 mM dithiothreitol.
3. Moloney murine leukemia virus (MMLV) RT (Gibco-BRL, Gaithersburg, MD).
4. Deoxynucleotide triphosphates.
5. Oligo dT primers.
6. RNase inhibitor (Boehringer Mannheim).
7. Agarose.
8. Ethidium bromide (10 mg/mL).
9. Polaroid 664 film.

3. Methods

3.1. Sample Preparation

1. Mix heparinized bone marrow aspirates or peripheral blood cells with isovolumes of PBS and centrifuge on Ficol-Paque.
2. Gather mononuclear cells from the mononuclear cell layer and wash twice with PBS to remove platelets.
3. Dissolve cells (1×10^6 to 1×10^7) in 0.5 mL of solution D and store at $-80°$C until use.

3.2. Reverse-Transcriptase Polymerase Chain Reaction

RT-PCR was performed as described previously *(35)*.

1. Isolate total RNA with the acid-guanidine-phenol-chloroform method, dissolve in DEPC-treated water, and quantitate spectrometrically with absorbance at 260 nm.
2. Heat 2 µg of total RNA in 12.5 µL of DEPC-treated water at 65°C for 5 min.
3. Mix with 17.5 µL of RT buffer containing 600 U of MMLV RT, 500 µM of each deoxynucleotide triphosphate, 750 ng of oligo dT primers, and 40 U of RNase inhibitor.
4. Incubate the reaction mixture at 37°C for 90 min, heat at 100°C for 5 min, and then store at $-20°$C until use.
5. Perform PCR on a DNA thermal cycler under the following optimized conditions: denaturation at 94°C for 1 min, primer annealing at 64°C for 1 min, and then chain elongation at 72°C for 1.5 min.
6. Separate the PCR products on 1.3% agarose gels containing 0.05 µg/mL of ethidium bromide, and photograph with Polaroid 665 film.
7. Develop the negative film at 25°C for 5 min, and measure the band density (densitometric units) with a densitometer.

Optimal conditions for PCR to quantitate WT1 expression levels were determined as follows. PCR was performed for various cycles using WT1 primers (sense primer for exon 7: 5'-GGCATCTGAGACCAGTGAGAA-3'; antisense primer for exon 10, 5'-GAGAGTCAGACTTGAAAGCAGT-3') with serial dilutions of the cDNA prepared from total RNA of K562 human leuke-

Wilms Tumor Gene WT1 in Leukemia

mic cells, which highly express WT1. PCR amplification for 36, 33, 30, and 27 cycles was exponential from 4×10^{-4} to 4×10^{-2} ng of RNA (equivalent to 10^{-5}–10^{-3} levels when the WT1 expression level of K562 leukemic cells was defined as 1.0), from 8×10^{-3} to 4×10^{-1} ng of RNA (2×10^{-4}–10^{-2} levels), from 8×10^{-2} to 4×10^{0} ng of RNA (2×10^{-3}–10^{-1} levels), and 8×10^{-1} to 4×10^{1} ng of RNA (2×10^{-2}–10^{0} levels), respectively. Therefore, PCR was performed for 36, 33, 30, or 27 cycles according to WT1 expression levels in samples under exponential amplification conditions.

Similarly, to determine optimal conditions for PCR to quantitate β-actin expression levels, PCR was performed for various cycles using β-actin primers (sense primer, 5'-GTGGGGCGCCCCAGGCACCCA-3'; antisense primer, 5'-GTCCTTAATGTCACGCACGATTTC-3') with serial dilutions of the cDNA prepared from total RNA of K562 leukemic cells. Exponential amplification was observed for 19 cycles of PCR in the range from 8×10^{-1} to 4×10^{1} ng of RNA, in which β-actin expression levels in almost all samples were included. To normalize the differences in RNA degradation for individual samples and in RNA loading for RT-PCR, the value of *WT1* gene expression divided by that of β-actin gene expression was defined as the WT1 expression level in the samples. Calibration curves were shown in every experiment and the WT1 expression levels were quantitated according to the curves. The expression level of the *WT1* gene in K562 leukemic cells was defined as 1.0, and the WT1 expression level in the samples were relatively shown compared with that in K562 cells.

References

1. Campana, D. and Pui, C.-H. (1995) Detection of minimal residual disease in acute leukemia: Methodologic advances and clinical significance. *Blood* **85,** 1416–1434.
2. Call, K. M., Glaser, T., Ito, C. Y., Buckler, A. J., Pelletier, J., Haber, D. A., Rose, E. A., et al. (1990) Isolation and characterization of a zinc finger polypeptide gene at the human chromosome 11 Wilms' tumor locus. *Cell* **60,** 509–520.
3. Gessler, M., Poustka, A., Cavenee, W., Neve, R. L., Orkin, S. H., and Bruns, G. A. P. (1990) Homozygous deletion in Wilms tumours of a zinc-finger gene identified by chromosome jumping. *Nature* **343,** 774–778.
4. Menke, A. L., van der Eb, A. J., and Jochemsen, A. G. (1998) The Wilms' tumor gene: oncogene or tumor suppressor gene? *Intl. Rev. Cytol.* **181,** 151–212.
5. Coppes, M. J., Campbell, C. E., and Williams, B. R .G. (1993) The role of WT1 in Wilms tumorigenesis. *FASEB J.* **7,** 886–895.
6. Rauscher, F. J. III. (1993) The WT1 Wilms tumor gene product: a developmentally regulated transcription factor in the kidney that functions as a tumor suppressor. *FASEB J.* **7,** 896–903.
7. Haber, D. A., Park, S., Maheswaran, S., Englert, C., Re, G. G., Hazen-Martin, D. J., et al. (1993) WT1-mediated growth suppression of Wilms tumor cells expressing a WT1 splicing variant. *Science,* **262,** 2057–2059.

8. Algar, E. M., Kenney, M. T., Simms, L. A., Smith, S. I., Kida, Y., and Smith, P. J. (1995) Homozygous intragenic deletion in the WT1 gene in a sporadic Wilms' tumour associated with high levels of expression of a truncated transcript. *Hum. Mutat.* **5**, 221–227.
9. Little, M. and Wells, C. (1997) A clinical overview of WT1 gene mutations. *Hum. Mutat.* **9**, 209–225.
10. Gashler, A. L., Bonthron, D. T., Madden, S. L., Rauscher, F. J. III., Collins, T., and Sukhatme, V. P. (1992) Human platelet-derived growth factor A chain is transcriptionally repressed by the Wilms tumor suppressor WT1. *Proc. Natl. Acad. Sci. USA* **89**, 10,984–10,988.
11. Harrington, M. A., Konicek, B., Song, A., Xia, X.-L., Fredericks, W. J., and Rauscher, F. J. III. (1993) Inhibition of colony-stimulating factor-1 promoter activity by the product of the Wilms' tumor locus. *J. Biol. Chem.* **268**, 21,271–21,275.
12. Drummond, I. A., Madden, S. L., Rohwer-Nutter, P., Bell, G. I., Sukhatme, V. P., and Rauscher, F. J. III. (1992) Repression of the insulin-like growth factor II gene by the Wilms tumor suppressor WT1. *Science* **257**, 674–678.
13. Werner, H., Re, G. G., Drummond, I. A., Sukhatme, V. P., Rauscher, F. J. III., Sens, D. A., et al. (1993) Increased expression of the insulin-like growth factor I receptor gene, IGF1R, in Wilms tumor is correlated with modulation of IGF1R promoter activity by the WT1 Wilms tumor gene product. *Proc. Natl. Acad. Sci. USA* **9**, 5828–5832.
14. Englert, C., Hou, X., Maheswaran, S., Bennett, P., Ngwu, C., Re, G. G., et al. (1995) WT1 suppresses synthesis of the epidermal growth factor receptor and induces apoptosis. *EMBO J.* **14**, 4662–4675.
15. Godyer, P., Dehbi, M., Torban, E., Bruening, W., and Pelletier, J. (1995) Repression of the retinoic acid receptor-α gene by the Wilms tumor suppressor gene product, wt1. *Oncogene* **10**, 1125–1129.
16. McCann, S., Sullivan, J., Guerra, J., Arcinas, M., and Boxer, L. M. (1995) Repression of the c-myb gene by WT1 protein in T and B cell lines. *J. Biol. Chem.* **270**, 23,785–23,789.
17. Hewitt, S. M., Hamada, S., McDonnel, T. J., Rauscher, F. J. III., and Saunders, G. F. (1995) Regulation of the proto-oncogenes bcl-2 and c-myc by the Wilms' tumor suppressor gene WT1. *Cancer Res.* **55**, 5386–5389.
18. Buckler, A. J., Pelletier, J., Haber, D. A., Glaser, T., and Housman, D. E. (1991) Isolation, characterization, and expression of the murine Wilms' tumor gene (WT1) during kidney development. *Mol. Cell. Biol.* **11**, 1707–1712.
19. Park, S., Schalling, M., Bernard, A., Maheswaran, S., Shipley, G. C., Roberts, D., et al. (1993) The Wilms tumor gene WT1 is expressed in murine mesoderm-derived tissues and mutated in a human mesothelioma. *Nat. Genet.* **4**, 415–420.
20. Davies, R., Moore, A., Schedl, A., Bratt, E., Miyahawa, K., Ladomery, M., et al. (1999) Multiple roles for the Wilms' tumor suppressor, WT1. *Cancer Res.* **59(Suppl. 7)**, 1747s–1750s (*see also* discussion on 1751s).

Wilms Tumor Gene WT1 in Leukemia

21. Moore, A. W., McInnes, L., Kreidberg, J., Hastie, N. D., and Schedl, A. (1999) YAC complementation shows a requirement for Wt1 in the development of epicardium, adrenal gland and throughout nephrogenesis. *Development* **126,** 1845–1857.

22. Miwa, H., Beran, M., and Saunders, G. F., (1992) Expression of the Wilms tumor gene (WT1) in human leukemias. *Leukemia* **6,** 405–409.

23. Miyagi, T., Ahuja, H., Kubota, T., Kubonishi, I., Koeffler, H. P., and Miyoshi, I. (1993) Expression of the Candidate Wilms' tumor gene, WT1, in human leukemia cells. *Leukemia* **7,** 970–977.

24. Inoue, K., Sugiyama, H., Ogawa, H., Nakagawa, M., Yamagami, T., Miwa, H., et al. (1994) WT1 as new prognostic factor and a new marker for the detection of minimal residual disease in acute leukemia. *Blood* **84,** 3071–3079.

25. Bergmann, L., Miething, C., Maurer, U., Brieger, J., Karakas, T., Weidmann, E., and Hoelzer, D. (1997) High levels of Wilms' tumor gene (wt1) mRNA in acute myeloid leukmias are associated with a worse long-term outcome. *Blood* **90,** 1217–1225.

26. Brieger, J., Weidmann, E., Fenchel, K., Mitrou, P. S., Hoelzer, D., and Bergmann, L. (1994) The expression of the Wilms' tumor gene in acute myelocytic leukemias as a possible marker for leukemic blast cells. *Leukemia* **8,** 2138–2143.

27. Menssen, H. D., Renkl, H.-J., Rodeck, U., Maurer, J., Notter, M., Schwartz, S., Reinhardt, R., and Thiel, E. (1995) Presence of Wilms' tumor gene (wt1) transcripts and the WT1 nuclear protein in the majority of human acute leukemias. *Leukemia* **9,** 1060–1067.

28. Menssen, H. D., Renkl, H. J., Rodeck, U., Kari, C., Schwartz, S., and Thiel, E. (1997) Detection by monoclonal antibodies of the Wilms' tumor (WT1) nuclear protein in patients with acute leukemia. *Intl. J. Cancer* **70,** 518–523.

29. Patmasiriwat, P., Fraizer, G. C., Claxton, D., Kantarjian, H., and Saunders, G. F. (1996) Expression pattern of WT1 and GATA-1 in AML with chromosome 16q22 abnormalities. *Leukemia* **10,** 1127–1133.

30. Im, H. J., Kong, G., and Lee, H. (1999) Expression of Wilms tumor gene (WT1) in children with acute leukemia. *Pediatr. Hematol. Oncol.* **16,** 109–118.

31. Tamaki, H., Ogawa, H., Inoue, K., Soma, T., Yamagami, T., Miyake, S., et al. (1996) Increased expression of the Wilms tumor gene (WT1) at relapse in acute leukemia. *Blood* **88,** 4396–4399.

32. Inoue, K., Ogawa, H., Yamagami, T., Soma, T., Tani, Y., Tatekawa, T., et al. (1996) Long-term follow-up of minimal residual disease in leukemia patients by monitoring WT1 (Wilms tumor gene) expression levels. *Blood* **88,** 2267–2278.

33. Bergmann, L., Maurer, U., and Weidmann, E. (1997) Wilms tumor gene expression in acute myeloid leukemias. *Leuk. Lymph.* **25,** 435–443.

34. Ogawa, H., Tsuboi, A., Oji, Y., Tamaki, H., Soma, T., Inoue, K., and Sugiyama, H. (1998) Successful donor leukocyte transfusion at molecular rlapse for a patient with acute myeloid leukemia who was treated with allogeneic bone marrow transplantation: importance of the monitoring of minimal residual disease by WT1 assay. *Bone Marrow Transplant.* **21,** 525–527.

35. Tamaki, H., Ogawa, H., Ohyashiki, K., Ohyashiki, J.-H., Iwama, H., Inoue, K., et al. (1999) The Wilms' tumor gene WT1 is a good marker for diagnosis of disease progression of myelodysplastic syndromes. *Leukemia* **13**, 393–399.
36. Sako, M., Ogawa, H., Okamura, J., Tamaki, H., Nakahata, T., Kishimoto, T., and Sugiyama, H. (1998) Abnormal expression of the Wilms' tumor gene WT1 in juvenile chronic myeloid leukemia and infantile monosomy 7 syndrome. *Leuk. Res.* **22**, 965–967.
37. Menssen, H. D., Renkl, H.-J., Reider, H., Bartelt, S., Schmidt, A., Notter, M., and Thiel, E. (1998) Distinction of eosinophilic leukaemia from idiopathic hypereosinophilic syndrome by analysis of Wilms' tumor gene expression. *Br. J. Haematol.* **101**, 325–334.
38. Oji, Y., Ogawa, H., Tamaki, H., Oka, Y., Tsuboi, A., Kim, E. H., et al. (1999) Expression of the Wilms' tumor gene WT1 in solid tumors and its involvement in tumor cell growth. *Jpn. J. Cancer Res.* **90**, 194–204.
39. Inoue, K., Ogawa, H., Sonoda, Y., Kimura, T., Sakabe, H., Oka, Y., et al. (1997) Aberrant overexpression of the Wilms tumor gene (WT1) in human leukemia. *Blood* **89**, 1405–1412.
40. Yamagami, T., Sugiyama, H., Inoue, K., Ogawa, H., Tatekawa, T., Hirata, M., et al. (1996) Growth inhibition of human leukemic cells by WT1 (Wilmt tumor gene) antisense oligodeoxynucleotides: Implications for the involvement of WT1 in leukemogenesis. *Blood* **87**, 2878–2884.
41. Inoue, K., Tamaki, H., Ogawa, H., Oka, Y., Soma, T., Tatekawa, T., et al. (1998) Wilms' tumor gene (WT1) competes with differentiation-inducing signal in hematopoietic progenitor cells. *Blood* **91**, 2969–2976.
42. Tsuboi, A., Oka, Y., Ogawa, H., Elisseeva, O. A., Tamaki, H., Oji, Y., et al. (1999) Constitutive expression of the Wilms' tumor gene WT1 inhibits the differentiation of myeloid progenitor cells but promotes their proliferation in response to granulocyte-colony stimulating factor (G-CSF). *Leuk. Res.* **23**, 499–505.
43. Osaka, M., Koami, K., and Sugiyama, T. (1997) WT1 contributes to leukemogenesis: expression patterns in 7, 12-dimethylbenz [a] anthracence (DMBA)-induced leukemia. *Intl. J. Cancer* **72**, 696–699.
44. Maheswaran, S., Park, S., Bernard, A., Morris, J. F., Rausher, F. J. III, Hill, D. E. and Haber, D. A. (1993) Physical and functional interaction between WT1 and p53 proteins. *Proc. Natl. Acad. Sci. USA* **90**, 5100–5104.
45. Johnstone, R. W., See, R. H., Sells, S. F., Wang, J., Muthukkumar, S., Englert, C., et al. (1996) A novel repressor, par-4, modulates transcription and growth suppression functions of the Wilms' tumor suppressor WT1. *Mol. Cell. Biol.* **16**, 6945–6956.
46. Johnstone, R. W., Wang, J., Tommerup, N., Vissing, H., Roberts, T., and Shi, Y. (1998) Ciao 1 is a novel WD40 protein that interacs with the tumor suppressor protein WT1. *J. Biol. Chem.* **273**, 10,880–10,887.
47. Algar, E., Blackburn, D., Kromykh, T., Taylor, G., and Smith, P. (1997) Mutation analysis of the W gene in sporadic childhood leukaemia. *Leukemia* **11**, 110–113.

Wilms Tumor Gene WT1 in Leukemia

48. Carapeti, M., Goldman, J. M., and Cross, N. C. (1997) Dominant-negative mutations of the Wilms' tumour predisposing gene (WT1) are infrequent in CML blast crisis and de novo acute leukaemia. *Eur. J. Haematol.* **58,** 346–349.
49. King-Underwood, L., Renshow, J., and Pritchard-Jones, K. (1996) Mutations in the Wilms' tumor gene WT1 in leukemias. *Blood* **87,** 2171–2179.
50. King-Underwood, L. and Pritchard-Jones, K. (1998) Wilms' tumor (WT1) gene mutations occur mainly in acute myeloid leukemia and may confer drug resistance. *Blood* **91,** 2961–2968.
51. Miyagawa, K., Hayashi, Y., Fukuda, T., Mitani, K., Hirai, H. and Kamiya, K. (1999) Mutations of the *WT1* gene in childhood nonlymphoid hematological malignancies. *Genes Chrom. Cancer* **25,** 176–183.
52. Oka, Y., Udaka, K., Tsuboi, A., Elisseeva, O. A., Ogawa, H., Aozasa, K., et al. (2000) Cancer immunotherapy targeting Wilms' tumor gene WT1 product. *J. Immunol.* **164,** 1873–1880.
53. Oka, Y., Elisseeva, O. A., Tsuboi, A., Ogawa, H., Tamaki, H., Li, H., et al. (2000) Human cytotoxic T lymphocyte responses specific for peptides of wild-type Wilms' tumor gene WT1 product. *Immunogenetics*, **51,** 99–107.

18

Detection of Aberrant Methylation of the $p15^{INK4B}$ Gene Promoter

Toshiki Uchida

1. Introduction

The 5' promoter regions of some genes contain CpG-rich areas, known as CpG islands. Methylation of the cytosines in these CpG dinucleotides by DNA methyltransferase generating 5-methylcytosine has important regulatory effects on gene expression *(1)*. Almost all gene-associated CpG islands are protected from methylation on autosomal chromosomes *(2)*. by contrast, DNA methylation of CpG islands normally occurs in selected imprinted genes *(3)* and genes on the inactive X-chromosome of females *(4)*, and may play an important role during normal embryonic development.

Since the functional significance of promoter hypermethylation would be the same as point mutation or allelic loss, it is suggested that DNA methylation also plays an important role in carcinogenesis *(5)*. We have demonstrated $p15^{INK4B}$ gene inactivation by promoter hypermethylation in myelodysplastic syndromes (MDSs), in which no genetic alterations of the $p15^{INK4B}$ gene have been detected *(6)*. Recent studies have also shown that aberrant DNA methylation occurs frequently in several tumor suppressor genes and may be an important event during multistep carcinogenesis *(7)*. To clarify the roles of tumor suppressor genes in carcinogenesis, it is necessary to analyze the methylation status of the promoter region in addition to performing genetic analyses, i.e., searching for deletions and point mutations.

Various methods to detect DNA methylation have been developed. These can be divided into two groups: those using methylation-sensitive restriction endonucleases, and those using bisulfite modification of cytosine. The former is based on the principle that methylation-sensitive restriction endonucleases cannot cut methylated DNA. Southern blotting *(8)* and methylation-based polymerase chain reaction (PCR) assays *(9)* are included in this group. The latter is

From: *Methods in Molecular Medicine, vol. 68: Molecular Analysis of Cancer*
Edited by: J. Boultwood and C. Fidler © Humana Press Inc., Totowa, NJ

240   Uchida

based on the principle that unmethylated cytosines are modified by bisulfite and changed to uracil, whereas methylated cytosines escape from bisulfite modification and remain as cytosine *(10)*. Although direct sequence analysis of modified DNA can detect DNA methylation, new, simple, and highly sensitive methods using this modification have been developed recently; such as methylation-specific PCR *(11)* and methylation-sensitive single nucleotide primer extension *(12)*.

This chapter discusses methylation analyses of the $p15^{INK4B}$ gene using Southern blotting and methylation-specific PCR.

2. Materials

2.1. Southern Blotting

1. Five micrograms of DNA to be analyzed.
2. Bovine serum albumin (BSA) (1 mg/mL). Store at –20°C.
3. Sterile distilled water.
4. Restriction endonuclease: methylation-insensitive restriction endonucleases, *Hind*III, methylation-sensitive restriction endonucleases, and *Eco*52I (or the isoschizomer *Eag*I). Store at –20°C.
5. 10X Stock of the appropriate restriction enzyme buffer. Store at –20°C.
6. TE buffer: 10 m*M* Tris-HCl, pH 7.4, 0.1 m*M* EDTA, pH 8.0. Store at room temperature.
7. Vacuum centrifuge.
8. Reagents for gel electrophoresis: molecular biology grade agarose, gel-loading solution, ethidium bromide, DNA size markers, Tris-acetate (TAE).
9. Heating plate or microwave oven.
10. Suitable gel apparatus and power pack.
11. Ultraviolet (UV) light transilluminator.
12. Nylon membrane (Hybond N+; Amersham).
13. Nylon mesh sheet.
14. Whatmann 3MM paper.
15. Paper towel.
16. 20X Saline sodium citrate (SSC): 3 *M* NaCl, 0.3 *M* Na₃ citrate. Store at room temperature.
17. Hybridization buffer (Rapid-hyb buffer; Amersham). Store at room temperature.
18. 10% Sodium dodecyl sulfate (SDS): Store at room temperature.
19. Salmon sperm DNA (10 mg/mL). Store at –20°C.
20. Labeled probe for the $p15^{INK4B}$ gene (**Fig. 1**). Store at –20°C.
21. Hybridization oven and tubes.
22. Suitable autoradiographic film.

2.2. Methylation-Specific PCR

1. One microgram of DNA to be analyzed.
2. Sterile distilled water.

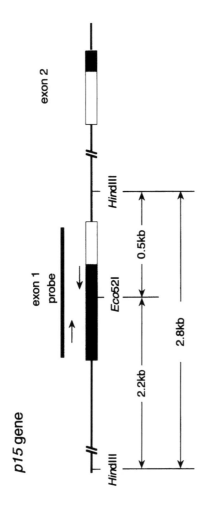

Fig. 1. Schematic representation of the *p15^INK4B* gene. Exons are depicted as boxes in which noncoding regions are shaded gray. The CpG islands extend from the 5' flanking region of exon 1 through the entire region of exon 1, i.e., the region around the transcriptional start site. The bold line in exon 1 indicates the region used as the probe for Southern blotting. The restriction sites for *Hin*dIII and methylation-sensitive *Eco*52I, and the predicted sizes of restriction fragments are also shown. The arrows show the sites of sense and antisense primers used in methylation-specific PCR.

3. NaOH pellets.
4. 10 mM Hydroquinone.
5. 3 M Sodium bisulfite.
6. 5 M NH$_4$OAc.
7. Ethanol (70 and 100%).
8. TE buffer.
9. pH Meter and pH indicator paper.
10. Desalting column (Wizard DNA purification resin; Promega, Madison, WI).
11. Vacuum centrifuge.
12. 10X PCR buffer: 65 mM MgCl$_2$, 100 mM Tris-HCl, pH 9.0, 500 mM KCl, 1% Triton X-100, 2 mg/mL of BSA. Store at –20°C.
13. Deoxynucleotide triphosphates (dNTPs): each at 2.5 mM. Store at –20°C.
14. PCR primers specific for methylated (M), unmethylated (U), and wild-type (W) DNAs (10 μmol/L) (**Figs. 1** and **2**). Store at –20°C.
15. Dimethylsulfoxide (DMSO). Store at room temperature.
16. *Taq* polymerase (5 U/μL). Store at –20°C.
17. Thermal cycler.
18. Reagents for gel electrophoresis: agarose or acrylamide, gel-loading solution, ethidium bromide, DNA size markers, TAE.
19. Heating plate or microwave oven.
20. Suitable gel apparatus and power pack.
21. UV light transilluminator.

3. Methods

3.1. Southern Blotting (see Note 1)

3.1.1. Restriction Endonuclease Digestion of Sample DNA

1. After deciding on the final volume, prepare 5 μg of sample DNA, 1/10 vol of reaction buffer (*see* **Note 2**), and 1/10 vol of BSA, then mix into sterile Eppendorf tubes.
2. Add sterile distilled water to the final volume.
3. Add 2 μL of *Hind*III (10 U/μL) to the reaction mixture, and incubate at 37°C overnight.
4. Confirm sufficient digestion of sample DNA by gel electrophoresis, and add 2 μL of *Eco*52I (5 U/μL).
5. After incubation at 37°C for 12 h, again add 2 μL of *Eco*52I to reaction mixture and incubate at 37°C for a further 12 h (*see* **Note 3**).
6. Resuspend the digested DNA in 16 μL of TE after ethanol precipitation.

3.1.2. Agarose Gel Electrophoresis

1. Melt the mixture of powdered agarose and TAE on a hot plate or in a microwave, and make a 0.7% agarose gel in the gel apparatus.

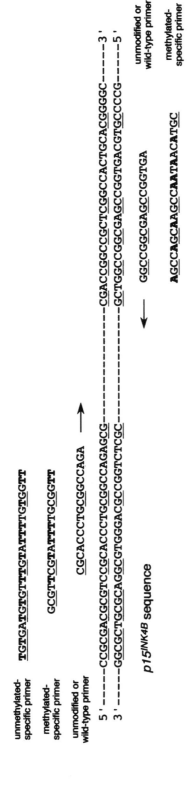

Fig. 2. Primer design for methylation-specific PCR. Genome sequences of the *p15INK4B* gene are shown with those of wild-type, methylated-specific, and unmethylated-specific primers. Bisulfite changes unmethylated cytosines to uracil, whereas methylated cytosines escape from bisulfite modification. Since the primers are designed to discriminate between methylated and unmethylated alleles, some CpG dinucleotides (underlined) must be contained near the 3' end of the primer sequences. Also, the primer sequences must contain frequent cytosines to distinguish unmodified from modified DNA. Sequence changes caused by bisulfite modification are shown in bold. Wild-type primer set, methylated-specific primer set, and unmethylated-specfic primer set produced 137-, 147-, and 154-bp products by methylation-specific PCR, respectively.

244   *Uchida*

2. Place the gel into the running apparatus and fill with 1X TAE to just cover the wells.
3. Mix the digested DNA with 4 μL of 5X loading solution and load into the wells of the gel. Size marker should be loaded in one of the lanes.
4. Add ethidium bromide to TAE in the running apparatus and run the gel for an appropriate time. After electrophoresis, confirm the digested DNA products on a UV transilluminator.

3.1.3. Blotting and Hybridization

1. Shake the gel gently in alkaline solution (0.5 M NaOH, 1.5 M NaCl) for 30 min at room temperature.
2. Neutralize the gel with 1 M Tris-HCl, pH 7.4, and 1.5 M NaCl for 30 min at room temperature and rinse with ddH$_2$O.
3. Cut the nylon membrane to fit the size of the gel and float it in transfer buffer (10X SSC) to wet completely.
4. Transfer the denatured DNA from the gel to the membrane by capillary action.
5. Expose the side of the membrane carrying the DNA to a source of UV irradiation to fix the DNA to the membrane.
6. Rinse the blotted nylon membrane and nylon mesh sheet in ddH$_2$O, place them into a hybridization tube, and gently add 10 mL of hybridization buffer (*see* **Note 4**). The mesh sheet should be placed on the inside of the membrane. Prehybridize the membrane by incubating at 65°C for 15 min in a hybridization oven.
7. Remove the prehybridization buffer from the hybridization tube and add the ^{32}P-labeled probe (*see* **Note 5**) and 100 μL of salmon sperm DNA (*see* **Note 6**) denatured by boiling for 5–10 min to the buffer.
8. Mix gently and return to the hybridization tube. Incubate with rotation at 65°C for 2 h.
9. After removing the mesh sheet, place the membrane in 500 mL of 2X SSC and 0.1% SDS, and wash twice with gentle shaking at room temperature for 5 min each time to wash off unbound probe.
10. Wash the membrane twice in 500 mL of preheated 0.5X SSC and 0.1% SDS at 65°C for 5 min each time.
11. Wash the membrane in 500 mL of preheated 0.1X SSC and 0.1% SDS at 65°C. Occasionally monitor the radioisotope count and stop the wash at an appropriate time.
12. Remove the membrane from the wash solution and wrap it with polyethylene film (*see* **Note 7**).
13. Expose the membrane to X-ray film at –70°C (*see* **Note 8**).

3.1.4. Evaluation

The *Hind*III and *Eco*52I double-digested DNA fragments give bands of 2.8, 2.2, and 0.5 kb with the *p15^{INK4B}* probe (**Fig. 1**). Evaluate the methylation status of the *p15^{INK4B}* gene according to the band pattern as shown in **Fig. 3**.

Aberrant Methylation of p15[INK4B] Promoter

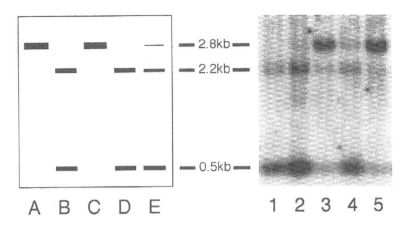

Fig. 3. Southern blotting of the *p15[INK4B]* gene. *Lanes A–E* are a schematic representation of typical examples. Lane A, control unmethylated DNA digested with *Hin*dIII alone; *lane B*, control unmethylated DNA digested with both *Hin*dIII and *Eco*521; *lane C*, completely methylated sample digested with *Hin*dIII and *Eco*521; *lane D*, unmethylated sample digested with *Hin*dIII and *Eco*521; *lane E*, partially methylated sample or contamination of methylated sample into unmethylated sample digested with *Hin*dIII and *Eco*521. There was also the possibility of incomplete digestion of unmethylated samples. *Lanes 1–5* are the results from patients with MDS. DNAs in *lanes 1* and *2* were almost completely digested by *Eco*521, implying the unmethylated status of the *p15[INK4B]* gene. By contrast, DNAs in *lanes 3* and *5* were slightly digested by *Eco*521, indicating densely methylated status. The weak band at 2.8 kb in *lane 4* indicates slightly methylated status or contamination of methylated DNA into unmethylated DNA.

3.2. Methylation-Specific PCR (see Note 9)

3.2.1. DNA Modification (see **Note 10**, **Fig. 4**)

1. Denature 1 µg of DNA in a volume of 50 µL by adding 3.5 µL of freshly prepared 3 *M* NaOH (final concentration of 0.2 *M*) followed by incubating for 10 min at 37°C (*see* **Note 11**).
2. Add 30 µL of 10 m*M* hydroquinone and 520 µL of 3 *M* sodium bisulfite, pH 5.0 (pH adjustment with 10 *M* NaOH), both freshly prepared, to the denatured DNA.
3. Incubate this mixture under mineral oil at 50°C for 16–24 h.
4. Purify the modified DNA using a desalting column and elute into 50 µL of TE (*see* **Note 12**).
5. Add 5.5 µL of freshly prepared 3 *M* NaOH (final concentration of 0.3 *M*) to the modified DNA and incubate for 5 min at room temperature.
6. Neutralize this solution by adding 10 µL of 5 *M* NH$_4$OAc, and resuspend the DNA in 20 µL of TE after ethanol precipitation.

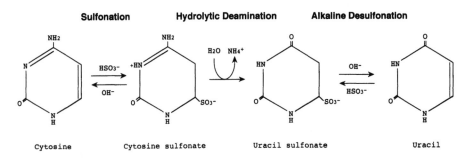

Fig. 4. Conversion from cytosine to uracil by bisulfite. Chemical modification progresses through three steps: sulfonation, hydrolytic deamination, and alkaline desulfonation. This conversion is highly single-strand specific.

3.2.2. PCR Amplification

1. Prepare three primer sets (M, U, W), PCR buffers, dNTPs, and DMSO, and make the following master mixes: 2 µL of 10X PCR buffer, 2 µL of 2.5 m*M* dNTP mix (*see* **Note 13**), 0.8 µL of PCR primer set (M, U, or W), 1 µL of DMSO, 10.2 µL of ddH$_2$O for a subtotal of 16µL.
2. Aliquot 16 µL of each master mix (M, U, or W) into corresponding PCR tubes.
3. Centrifuge these PCR tubes after adding mineral oil.
4. Add 2 µL of modified DNA into the mixture under the mineral oil in each tube.
5. After denaturation at 95°C for 5 min, pipet 2 µL of *Taq* polymerase (diluted to 0.5 U/mL with ddH$_2$O) directly into the mixture under mineral oil (*see* **Notes 14 and 15**).
6. Perform 35 cycles of PCR under the following conditions: denaturation at 95°C for 45 s, annealing at 60°C for 45 s, extension at 72°C for 60 s.

3.2.3. Gel Electrophoresis

1. Run 5 µL of PCR product with an appropriate amount of loading dye on a 2% agarose or 10% polyacrylamide gel. Use DNA markers to determine the size of the PCR products.
2. After electrophoresis, stain the gel with ethidium bromide for 20–30 min. The products can be viewed on a UV transilluminator.

3.2.4. Evaluation

Evaluate the methylation status of the *p15^{INK4B}* gene according to the band pattern as shown in **Fig. 5** (*see* **Note 16**).

4. Notes

1. Refer to the comprehensive review of Southern blotting in **ref. 3**.
2. Methylation analysis using Southern blotting requires methylation-sensitive restriction endonuclease and methylation-insensitive restriction endonuclease.

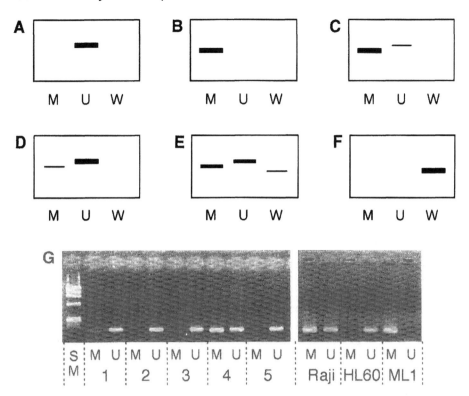

Fig. 5. Methylation-specific PCR of the *p15^INK4B* gene. (**A–F**) Schematic representation of typical examples. (**A**) Unmethylated sample; (**B**) completely methylated sample; (**C** and **D**) partially methylated sample or contamination of unmethylated DNA in methylated DNA, (**E**) incomplete chemical modification (*see* **Note 16**); (**F**) failure of chemical modification. (**G**) Examples of methylation-specific PCR analysis for patients with MDS and cell lines. DNA from patients 2 and 5 were not amplified with methylated-specific (M) primer, indicating unmethylated status of the *p15^INK4B* gene. By contrast, PCR products amplified with M primer were visible in patients 1, 3, and 4, indicating that the *p15^INK4B* gene was methylated to various degrees. In the analysis of clinical samples, the U products were usually visible because contamination by the normal component was inevitable. Methylation-specific PCR showed partially methylated, unmethylated, and methylated status of the *p15^INK4B* gene in Raji, HL60 and ML1 cell lines, respectively. Results of PCR amplification with wild-type primers are not shown. M, Product amplified with methylated-specific primer; U, Product amplified with unmethylated-specific primer; W, Product amplified with wild-type specific primer; SM, DNA size marker (øX174*Hae*III).

Usually, each enzyme has an optimal reaction buffer. We performed all reactions in a buffer specific for *Eco*52I in this study because *Hin*dIII has sufficient activity in this buffer.

3. To avoid partial digestion, we usually add an excess of methylation-sensitive restriction endonuclease to the sample DNA twice.
4. There are several commercially available hybridization buffers. We usually use Rapid-hyb buffer because it requires only 2 h for hybridization.
5. The probe should be designed to exclude exon 2 of the *p15^{INK4B}* gene because it has 93% similarity with exon 2 of the *p16^{INK4A}* gene. We used a cDNA probe produced by RT-PCR using the following primers.
   a. Sense primer: TCCCAGAAGCAATCCAGGCG.
   b. Antisense primer: GCCTCCCGAAACGGTTGACT.
6. To block nonspecific attachment of the probe to the surface of the membrane, we usually add denatured salmon sperm DNA to the labeled probe.
7. Wrapped membranes are stable for at least 3 mo when stored at room temperature. If the membrane is allowed to dry out, it will be extremely difficult to remove the probe for further washing or reprobing.
8. Instead of X-ray film, Phosphor imaging plates (Imaging plate BAS III, Fuji) can be used. These require a shorter exposure than the X-ray film and enable examination with a laser image analyzer (Fujix BAS2000; Fuji).
9. During methylation-specific PCR analysis, we always use aerosol-resistant pipet tips to avoid contamination.
10. Commercial DNA modification kits (CpGenome™ DNA Modification Kit, Oncor) are available.
11. For samples with nanogram quantities of human DNA, add 1μL of salmon sperm DNA as a carrier.
12. For cleaning up DNA after chemical modification, Glass Milk™ (BIO 101) may also be used instead of a desalting column.
13. If PCR amplification with the U primer set is insufficient, double the amount of dNTP mix (from 2 to 4 μL).
14. Sequences closely related to each primer introduce the possibility of mispriming. To avoid this and other PCR-related artifacts, "hot-start" PCR is recommended in methylation-specific PCR.
15. Alternatives to hot-start PCR are also available:
    a. Use of AmpliTaq Gold™ (Perkin-Elmer). This enzyme becomes active only after heating at 94 to 95°C for 9–12 min.
    b. Physical separation of *Taq* polymerase and PCR mixture with wax beads. *Taq* polymerase combines with the PCR mixture only after the wax melts.
    c. Use of an anti-*Taq* antibody. After antibody denaturation during the 95°C incubation, *Taq* polymerase becomes active.
16. Amplification of the sample DNA with the W primer set is an indication of incomplete chemical modification. However, this will not affect the validity of the assay because unmodified DNA is not recognized by primers specific for methylated and unmethylated DNA.

References

1. Bird, A. (1992) The essentials of DNA methylation. *Cell* **70,** 5–8.
2. Bird, A. (1986) CpG-rich islands and the function of DNA methylation. *Nature* **321,** 209–213.

3. Li, E., Beard, C., and Jaenisch, R. (1993) Role for DNA methylation in genomic imprinting. *Nature* **366,** 362–365.
4. Pfeifer, G. P., Steigerwald, S. D., Mueller, P. R., Wold, B., and Riggs, A. D. (1989) Genomic sequencing and methylation analysis by ligation mediated PCR *Science* **246,** 810–813.
5. Counts, J. L. and Goodman, J. I. (1995) Alterations in DNA methylation may play a variety of roles in carcinogenesis. *Cell* **83,** 13–15.
6. Uchida, T., Kinoshita, T., Nagai, H., Nakahara, Y., Saito, H., Hotta, T., and Murate, T. (1997) Hypermethylation of the p15INK4B gene in myelodysplastic syndromes. *Blood* **90,** 1403–1409.
7. Baylin, S. B., Herman, J. G., Graff, J. R., Vertino, P. M., and Issa, J. P. (1998) Alterations in DNA methylation: a fundamental aspect of neoplasia. *Adv. Cancer Res.* **72,** 141–196.
8. Herman, J. G., Jen, J., Merlo, A., and Baylin, S. B. (1996) Hypermethylation-associated inactivation indicates a tumor suppressor role for *p15INK4B. Cancer Res.* **56,** 722–727.
9. Singer-Sam, J., Grant, M., LeBon, J. M., Okuyama, K., Chapman, V., Monk, M., and Riggs, A. D. (1990) Use of a HpaII-polymerase chain reaction assay to study DNA methylation in the Pgk-1 CpG island of mouse embryos at the time of X-chromosome inactivation. *Mol. Cell. Biol.* **10,** 4987–4989.
10. Clark, S. J., Harrison, J., Paul, C. L., and Frommer, M. (1994) High sensitivity mapping of methylated cytosines. *Nucleic Acids Res.* **22,** 2990–2997.
11. Herman, J. G., Graff, J. R., Myöhänsen, S., Nelkin, B. D., and Baylin, S. B. (1996) Methylation-specific PCR: a novel PCR assay for methylation status of CpG islands. *Proc. Natl. Acad. Sci. USA* **93,** 9821–9826.
12. Gonzalgo, M. L. and Jones, P. A. (1997) Rapid quantitation of methylation differences at specific sites using methylation-sensitive single nucleotide primer extension (Ms-SNuPE). *Nucleic Acids Res.* **25,** 2529–2531.
13. Harwood, A. J. (1996) *Basic DNA and RNA Protocols, vol. 58: Methods in Molecular Biology.* Humana, Totowa, NJ.

19

Clonality Studies in Cancer Based on X Chromosome Inactivation Phenomenon

John T. Phelan II and Josef T. Prchal

1. Introduction

The understanding that human neoplasms are clonal cell proliferations ultimately derived from a single transformed somatic cell represents a major advance in cancer biology. A cell population is designated as clonal if it can be demonstrated to have arisen from a single parent or progenitor cell. The clonality of select human neoplastic cell populations can be determined in several ways. One way is by detection of stable, unique somatic chromosome abnormalities (Philadelphia chromosome; 8, 21 translocation); somatic gene mutations (*H-ras*); or immunoglobulin heavy/light chain rearrangements. The drawbacks of these are that they either are rare, are fortuitous, or require labor-intensive techniques. Another way to assess clonality in human cell populations is to exploit the unique position of the X chromosome in human female development.

1.1. X-Chromosome Inactivation Phenomena

The chromosomes in eukaryotic organisms are derived from two parental organisms, male and female or paternal and maternal. One half of the chromosomes are maternally derived, the other half are paternally derived. All of the chromosomes are transcriptionally active except one of the two X chromosomes of cells found in mature females. Early in development, one of the two X chromosomes (most but not all of its genes) in the cells constituting a human female embryo becomes transcriptionally inactivated *(1–3)*. This appears to be a random process in that some of the cells of the early human female embryo express only paternal X chromosome genes whereas other cells from the same embryo express only maternal X chromosome genes. This phenomenon of X

From: *Methods in Molecular Medicine, vol. 68: Molecular Analysis of Cancer*
Edited by: J. Boultwood and C. Fidler © Humana Press Inc., Totowa, NJ

251

chromosome maternal/paternal molecular mosaicism persists throughout the life of the human female and represents a gene dosage compensation mechanism whereby comparable X chromosome gene expression in males and females is ensured.

One protein whose gene is X chromosome linked is glucose-6-phosphate dehydrogenase (*G6PD*). G6PD is a rate-controlling enzyme for the hexose monophosphate shunt, which produces NADPH and pentose sugars. Deficiency of G6PD is the most common and most polymorphic red cell enzymopathy in the world known so far. The typical clinical manifestation of the common deficient variants is an acute, short-lasting nonspherocytic hemolysis in affected males and in affected heterozygous females. The study of the biology of *G6PD* mosaicism in females by Beutler et al. *(3)* in the late 1950s to early 1960s inspired some of the initial research on tumor clonality. They demonstrated biphenotypic erythrocytes in females known to be heterozygous for G6PD deficiency *(3)*. Erythrocyte mosaicism was first demonstrated by showing that erythrocytes from heterozygous females exhibited a glutathione consumption curve identical to that of a 50:50 mixture of cells from an affected and unaffected male, respectively. In later work, erythrocytes from two adult females heterozygous for sickle cell trait and G6PD deficiency, separated based on oxidant-induced generation of sickle cells, were either G6PD deficient or had normal G6PD activity *(4)*. Davidson et al. *(5)* further showed that skin cells obtained from G6PD heterozygous females, when cultured and later subjected to single-cell platings, produced clonal populations with either normal or absent G6PD activity. These results, in addition to Lyon's *(1)* animal experiments and Ohno and Hauschka's *(2)* observations, provided some early experimental confirmation of the Lyon hypothesis of X chromosome inactivation.

Not all *G6PD* mutations produce a hemolytic phenotype. Some exhibit differences in qualitative electrophoretic mobility relative to the wild-type molecule (designated "B" by convention). For example, G6PD A is a mutation characterized by rapid mobility on electrophoresis relative to G6PD B *(6)*. G6PD A hemizygosity is associated with almost normal in vitro enzyme activity and no hemolytic phenotype. By contrast, while the G6PD A-isoenzyme has the same rapid mobility on electrophoresis as G6PD A, it has reduced red cell enzymatic activity as a result of intrinsic protein instability. This instability results in shortened red cell survival time (hemolysis) on oxidant exposure of the older erythrocytes that have very low G6PD activity since erythrocytes do not possess protein synthesis machinery.

X Chromosome Inactivation Phenomenon

1.2. Review of Methods Used to Study X-Chromosome Inactivation

1.2.1. Protein-Based Methods

In 1965, Linder and Gartler (7) exploited the electrophoretic mobility differences of these three isoenzymes. They studied leimyomas obtained from females who were known G6PD A/B heterozygotes undergoing hysterectomies for multiple uterine leimyomas. Electrophoresis was performed on crude extracts of individual leimyomas. Individual leimyomas were either exclusively A or exclusively B. Electrophoresis was also performed on the surrounding uninvolved myometria; both A and B bands were observed. Finally, Beutler et al. (8) subjected cell extracts of antemortem and postmortem neoplastic and nonneoplastic tissue obtained from two known G6PD A/B heterozygotes. One had chronic lymphocytic leukemia (CLL), and the other had metastatic colon cancer. The individual with CLL demonstrated exclusively A clonal lymph node tissue; the individual with colon cancer showed some neoplastic tissue specimens with exclusively A bands, others with exclusively B bands, and still others with both A and B bands. These studies emphasized the potential problem of contaminating supporting/stromal tissue cells (monocytes, fibroblasts, and so on) when evaluating fresh, unprocessed neoplastic tissue. In addition, the finding of both clonal A and B neoplastic tissue in the colon cancer patient was suggestive of more than one initial transformed cell. In summary, the first studies of tumor cell clonality exploiting the hypothesis of random X chromosome inactivation derived initially from pioneering work by Beutler et al. (8) and his studies of G6PD mosaicism. More widespread applicability was restricted primarily by the limited ethnic distribution of the of the qualitative G6PD mutation in question (women of African descent).

1.2.2. DNA-RNA-Based Methods

The next phase in the study of tumor cell clonality harnessed technologic advances drawn from the detailed study of DNA and the discovery of bacterial enzymes (restriction endonucleases) that cleave DNA at specific (restricted) sites determined by DNA nucleotide sequence. The frequency of genomic DNA polymorphisms vastly exceeds the frequency of protein polymorphisms. Interindividual DNA sequence differences that may be exploited for clonality studies may occur between X chromosome-linked genes and also occur in exons or introns of the X chromosome-linked genes themselves. By convention, these differences in DNA sequence are referred to as polymorphisms rather than mutations if they are not associated with a disease state and if they are observed in sufficiently high frequencies. A particular gene displays a characteristic pattern on Southern blot gel electrophoresis when genomic DNA is digested with a given restriction endonuclease. If a polymorphism occurs at the restriction site of that enzyme, that pattern will be altered and this particular polymorphism would be conveniently detectable by Southern blot; this phenomenon is referred to as a restriction fragment length polymorphism. Studies of the transcriptional activity of genomic DNA also demonstrated that differential cytosine residue methylation marks some genes (X and non-X chromosome linked) as transcriptionally inactive *(9)*. Not all cytosine residues in all genes are methylated when transcriptionally inactivated. However, cytosine residue methylation (typically but not always indicating transcriptional inactivation) occurs consistently at some sites in some genes. These methylated and unmethylated nucleotide sequences can be distinguished by methylation-sensitive restriction endonucleases. Thus, an ubiquitously expressed X-linked gene with a common restriction site polymorphism and differentially methylated cytosine residues (reflecting transcriptional activation/inactivation status), which constitute a separate, methylation-sensitive restriction endonuclease site, could potentially serve as a clonality marker in a very large population of females.

In the mid 1980s, Vogelstein et al. *(10)* pioneered a novel clonality assay based on detection of X-linked gene restriction site polymorphisms and differential methylation as a marker for X chromosome transcriptional activation/inactivation. The hypoxanthine phosphoribosyltransferase (*HPRT*) gene is an X chromosome gene encoding an essential enzyme for the purine/pyrimidine salvage pathway. The *HPRT* gene has a readily identifiable *Bam*HI restriction site polymorphism for which approximately one-third of females are heterozygous *(11)*. In addition, the *HPRT* gene is hypermethylated at cytosine residues distant from the *Bam*HI site when transcriptionally active *(12)*. Some of the methylation-prone cytosine residues also make up a methylation-sensitive restriction endonuclease site. DNA isolated from solid tumors obtained from females known to be heterozygous for the *HPRT Bam*HI restriction site polymorphism subjected to *Bam*HI digestion followed by methylation-sensitive endonuclease digestion, Southern blotting, and autoradiography shows only one of the two polymorphic loci. By contrast, DNA obtained from nontumor tissue close to the excised tumors showed an autoradiographic pattern consistent with hypermethylation of both polymorphic loci, indicating that this population of cells is polyclonal (i.e., composed of a mixture of cells using either the maternally derived or the paternally derived X chromosome). Other X-linked loci with restriction endonuclease site polymorphisms and cytosine residues located in methylation-sensitive restriction endonuclease sites whose methylation status coincided with transcriptional activation were found (monoamine oxidase and phosphoglycerate kinase) *(13,14)*. Another, the human androgen receptor (*HUMARA*) locus, was unique in four ways: The restriction site polymorphism consisted of a variable number of tandem repeats of a CAG

X Chromosome Inactivation Phenomenon

trinucleotide sequence, the restriction site polymorphism was located in the coding region (exon 1), the restriction site polymorphism was very closely linked to a methylation-sensitive restriction site, and more than 90% of human females were potentially heterozygous for the restriction site polymorphism *(15)*. Exploiting these properties, Busque et al. *(16)* confirmed the correlation between methylation and transcriptional activation at the *HUMARA* locus.

In summary, the development of differential methylation-based clonality assays represented a significant technologic step forward. Their development expanded the potential number of females available for clonality studies. The restriction site polymorphisms discovered to date are not limited to a specific demographic grouping, as is the G6PD isoenzyme assay. However, reliance on differential DNA methylation as a marker for transcriptional activation has some limitations. The functional significance and mechanisms of regulation of DNA methylation are poorly understood *(17)*. The relationship of DNA methylation to transcriptional activation is far from well understood. Some genes have methylated cytosine residues when transcriptionally inactivated *(16)*; other genes have methylated cytosine residues when transcriptionally active *(18)*. Furthermore, the DNA extracted from tumor cells is somewhat hypomethylated relative to nontumor DNA; this may impact interpretation of tumor clonality data derived from differential methylation assays *(17)*. Finally, the differential methylation clonality assays are only applicable to nucleated cells and require large numbers of such cells for sufficient DNA. Nonnucleated cells such as erythrocytes and platelets are not suitable for differential methylation clonality assays. Reliance on differential DNA methylation as a marker for transcriptional activation may not represent an optimal method for studying clonality. As X chromosome-based clonality assays have evolved, the following has become clear. First, the assay must be applicable to large numbers of females. Second, the assay must be based on a biologically sound method of discriminating between the transcriptionally active and inactive X chromosome. Third, the X chromosome gene transcription product must be ubiquitously expressed and not tumor or tissue specific. Finally, it would be desirable for the assay to be applicable to nucleated and nonnucleated cells.

Recent sequencing of a number of X chromosome-linked genes has resulted in the discovery of polymorphisms in the coding regions of a number of ubiquitously expressed housekeeping genes. In three of these X chromosome-linked gene exonic polymorphic sequences, the polymorphism is conservative (i.e., the nucleotide substitutions in the polymorphic codon codes for the same amino acid as the wild-type sequence). These exonic X chromosome polymorphisms are present in the *G6PD*, palmitoylated erythrocyte membrane antigen (*p55*), and the iduronate-2-sulfatase (*IDS*) genes *(19–21)*. These polymorphisms do not appear to affect mRNA stability, posttranscriptional processing, or translation.

Expression-based clonality assays have been developed that can detect and quantitate the expression of coding region polymorphisms in both nucleated and nonnucleated cells and use this as a marker for clonality.

The first clonality assay based on the discrimination of the active X chromosome by its transcript was developed independently by two groups. Their work was based on observations by Vulliamy et al. *(22)*, who found that some individuals possessed a C-to-T transposition at nucleotide (nt) 1311 (exon 11) of the *G6PD* gene. Beutler et al. *(19,23)* demonstrated that this transposition actually represented a very common polymorphism. One of these groups *(24)* utilized this polymorphism *(22)* in a study of a woman with X-linked chronic granulomatous disease. Family studies revealed that the propositus was heterozygous for the C1311T G6PD polymorphism; her mother was homozygous for the C allele and her father was hemizygous for the T allele. These investigators extracted total RNA from the propositus's granulocytes and polymerase chain reaction (PCR) amplified the resulting cDNA with primers complementary to the region flanking G6PD nt 1311. The products were then separated on a denaturing polyacrylamide gel, dot-blotted, and probed with radiolabeled allele-specific oligomers *(25)*. The oligomers were allele specific in that they were 19–20-mers complementary to the nucleotide sequences flanking the C1311T site, differing only at the site complementary to nt 1311. A single mismatched base pair between such duplexes results in significant duplex instability; only perfect complementarity between the probe and its binding partner results in a high degree of target molecule/oligomer hybridization stability. The granulocytes of the propositus were found to express only the paternal X chromosome, demonstrating a spontaneous chronic granulomatous disease mutation in the patient's paternal X chromosome.

Prchal et al. *(28)*, working simultaneously to exploit the G6PD C1311T polymorphism for a transcription-based clonality assay, built on the foundation and the work of Barany *(26)* and Landegren et al. *(27)*, who developed a method of detecting nucleotide differences using thermostable DNA ligase. DNA ligase is a nuclear enzyme that ligates juxtaposed oligonucleotides complementary to a denatured DNA target strand. The DNA ligase-based assays can distinguish single nucleotide substitutions in otherwise identical DNA target sequences with high fidelity. These thermostable ligase properties were utilized for a clonality assay that detects the *G6PD* C1311T polymorphism by a ligase detection reaction (LDR) assay. Since this particular polymorphism is not recognizable by any known restriction enzymes, LDR detects both alleles at this locus *(26)*. In this procedure, a thermostable DNA ligase covalently binds two adjacent DNA oligonucleotides provided they are perfectly complementary to the target DNA region of interest. Thus, allele-specific oligonucleotides (of different size) can be constructed to detect the presence of either, or both, allelic transcripts. Experimental conditions were developed that allow detection of both alleles in the same tube using either PCR-amplified genomic DNA or cDNA as templates. In addition, since the ligase utilized was also thermostable, the reaction could be subjected to multiple thermal cycles to linearly amplify product.

This particular quantitative transcription technique was used for the study of clonality in a female with long-standing polycythemia vera who was heterozygous for the *G6PD* C1311T exonic polymorphism *(28)*. Using 5–10 cc of peripheral blood, RNA was extracted from separated reticulocytes, granulocytes, platelets, and mononuclear cells. Total RNA from each separated cell population was reverse transcribed to cDNA and amplified using *G6PD* C1311T flanking region-specific primers. These reverse transcriptase (RT)-PCR products were then utilized in an LDR assay *(26)* using variant oligomers with 3' termini specific for either the C or T allele at the *G6PD* nt 1311 polymorphism. Although heterozygous at the *G6PD* C1311T polymorphism, this individual's reticulocytes, platelets, and granulocytes displayed only one band on autoradiography. This suggested to the investigators that these cells all derived from a single stem cell (i.e., were clonal). The mononuclear cells (mostly T-lymphocytes) exhibited two bands on autoradiography, suggesting cells derived from more than one stem cell (i.e., were polyclonal), as were the cells from her nonhematopoietic tissues (oral mucosal epithelial cells, urinary epithelial cells, and hair follicle cells). In normal females heterozygous for the G6PD C1311T polymorphism, all peripheral blood cells, as well as the cells from nonhematopoietic tissues, were found to be polyclonal *(29)*. These two original studies demonstrated that a common, single nucleotide polymorphism in the coding region of an X-linked housekeeping gene could be exploited in a clonality assay based on differentiation of the active X chromosome by its transcript.

The differentiation of the active from the inactive X chromosome by their transcripts was also exploited for the studies of normal hematopoiesis. In these studies using RT-PCR/LDR *(28,30)*, the conditions for RT-PCR/LDR were developed that allowed quantitation of the X chromosome allelic transcript ratio. This methodology was shown to be reproducible with <5% interassay variability, sensitive for analysis of as few as 100 cells, and permitting studies of rare populations of cells isolated by fluorescence activated cell sorting (FACS) sorting. Among normal *G6PD* C1311T heterozygous females, the relative autoradiographic intensities of the two bands, in the single individual, was noted to vary from one tissue to the other, while this ratio was constant in all hematopoietic cells (platelets; reticulocytes; granulocytes; monocytes; B-, T-, and NK-lymphocytes). By contrast, the X chromosome allelic transcript ratio of hematopoietic cells varies from one individual to another individual *(29)*.

This interindividual variation in X chromosome allelic transcript ratio was subjected to computer analyses and, assuming that no preferential selection occurred *(31,32)*, suggested that eight progenitor cells for all of the blood cells were present in the embryo at the time of X chromosome inactivation *(30)*. Thus, "skewing" of the X chromosome allelic transcript ratio is a normal phenomenon. Longitudinal evaluation by this method of peripheral blood cells from these same normal *G6PD* C131T heterozygous females over time showed that this pattern of individual variation remained constant in all lineages for a period of 3 yr of observation *(30)*. This observation provided no support for "clonal succession theory of hematopoiesis," although it could not formally exclude it.

The clonality assay based on a transcriptional polymorphism of the X chromosome using the *G6PD* C1311T polymorphism is limited by its applicability to less than one-fourth of females *(30,33)*. A similar RT-PCR/LDR assay was developed to detect expression from a common single-nucleotide exonic polymorphism found on the X-linked gene p55 (T358G) *(34)*. About 60% of females are heterozygous for either the G6PD or p55 exonic polymorphisms *(33)*. Of note, while the G6PD and p55 genes are adjacent to each other on the X chromosome (<100 kb), frequent crossovers between these loci were encountered, suggesting an ancient origin of these polymorphisms in evolution *(33)*.

A third exonic conservative polymorphism of the single-nucleotide X chromosome gene has been reported in the *IDS* gene (C146T) *(21)*. El-Kassar et al. *(35)* have utilized the *IDS* exonic polymorphism for clonality study of nonnucleated platelets in essential thrombocythemia and found discrepancies between the clonality results from the methylation-based *HUMARA* assay *(15)* and the transcription-based *IDS* assay when granulocytes from these subjects were used for analysis. This work suggested the superiority of the transcription-based clonality assays. When large numbers of normal females were genotyped for polymorphisms in the X-linked G6PD p55 and IDS genes, 60–70% of Caucasian and African American females were heterozygous for at least one of these three polymorphisms *(33,36)*. Unfortunately, while the IDS polymorphism was most informative in Caucasian and African American females, it was not informative among Asian females *(36)*. A fourth X chromosome-linked gene exonic polymorphism exists at the *HUMARA* locus and has been used for a transcription-based clonality assay *(16)*. We had difficulty standardizing this assay, perhaps because of different efficacy of PCR when HUMARA cDNA templates of different lengths, owing to a variable number of tandem CAG trinucleotide repeats, are used. This suggests that large numbers of women are potentially informative for expression-based clonality studies utilizing one or more of these genes.

These assays have several potential advantages over the *G6PD* isoenzyme detection or differential DNA methylation assays. They are not limited by racial

X Chromosome Inactivation Phenomenon 259

specificity and are applicable to nucleated and nonnucleated cells. In addition, they can be quantitative and only a small amount of tissue is needed for analysis. In the presence of appropriate controls, these assays can also quantify the relative percentages of clonal and nonclonal cells in a particular tissue sample.

The RT-PCR/LDR assay is already providing insight and improving our understanding of a number of clinical syndromes and diseases. To date, these have been almost exclusively hematologic/immunologic diseases primarily because of the ease of accessibility of the affected tissue (blood and marrow) and the availability of established methods to separate nearly pure populations of affected cells uncontaminated by stromal/supportive cells. These have included studies of myeloproliferative disorders (MPD) *(35,37,38)*, juvenile chronic myelogenous leukemia *(39)*, X-linked hyper IgM syndrome *(40)*, and common variable immunodeficiency *(41)*.

These assays still entail potential exposure to radioactivity and are somewhat labor-intensive. More rapid, less hazardous assays have been developed that are broadly based on principles similar to those of the RT-PCR/LDR assays. Allele-specific PCR (ASPCR) refers to a PCR-based technique that can accurately identify single-nucleotide base differences between two otherwise identical genomic DNA or cDNA strands *(33,36)*. The technique requires two PCR rounds. The first round utilizes primers specific for sequences flanking the polymorphic nucleotide of interest and generates a high concentration of "template" products containing the polymorphic nucleotide of interest. In the second PCR round, an aliquot of first-round products is added to two PCR reaction tubes each containing buffer, nucleotides, $MgCl_2$, and a common 3' primer. The 5' primer in each second-round reaction tube is allele specific; its 3' terminus is designed to be complementary to the polymorphic nucleotide or the wild-type allele. The second PCR round is very brief, usually only four to six cycles. If there is a lack of complementarity between the polymorphic locus on the template strand and the 3'-terminal nucleotide of the second-round 5' primer, *Taq* polymerase-mediated amplification cannot proceed efficiently, and a sufficient amount of visible product of agarose gel does not accumulate. Thus, only the template-round products are visible on agarose gel electrophoresis.

A modification of these assays was introduced by El-Kassar et al. *(35)* and Harrison et al. *(42)* whereby they utilized a PCR mismatch system instead of ASPCR. In their respective techniques, the target molecule (DNA or cDNA) is subjected to a single round of PCR using primers that hybridize to sequences flanking the X-linked exonic polymorphic site in question. The primers do not hybridize to the polymorphic site itself, as in ASPCR. One of the primers contains a nucleotide mismatch two or four nucleotides upstream from the primer 3' terminus (four or five nucleotides from the polymorphic site on the target molecule). PCR products generated under such conditions will substitute a new, complementary nucleotide at the site of primer/target molecule mismatch. In the presence of one polymorphism (but not the other), this reconstitutes a cryptic restriction endonuclease site. When a target DNA or cDNA molecule containing the other polymorphism is amplified under these conditions, no such cryptic restriction site is generated. The PCR reaction products are then subjected to restriction endonuclease digestion and gel electrophoresis; the relative expression of each allele in the cell population under study can then be determined by the band pattern generated. Since the primers do not hybridize directly to the polymorphic site in question, equal amplification of both polymorphisms is ensured. In addition, many rounds of PCR are eliminated. Both Harrison et al. *(42)* and El-Kassar et al. *(35)* also demonstrated a high degree of correlation between the DNA-based differential methylation *HUMARA* assay and their primer mismatch RT-PCR assays (utilizing the aforementioned *G6PD*, *p55*, and *IDS* exonic polymorphisms) in their studies of clonality in essential thrombocythemia.

1.3. Interpreting Data from DNA–RNA-Based Clonality Methods

X chromosome inactivation occurs early in development and has been hypothesized to be a gene dosage equalizing mechanism in the XX eukaryotic female *(43)*. X inactivation appears to be regulated by an X inactivation–specific transcript (Xist), an RNA transcript originating from the X inactivating center (Xic) of the X chromosome *(44)*. Deletion of Xist or the Xic abolishes random X inactivation *(43)*. By mechanisms yet to be elucidated, the Xist transcript induces apparently random transcriptional inactivation in one of the two X chromosomes at a specific developmental stage in the female embryo. In addition, studies in murine embryos show that X inactivation is tissue specific; different embryonic tissues sequentially undergo X inactivation *(45)*. The number of adult tissue progenitor cells present at the time of X inactivation in a particular embryonic tissue would thus be expected to influence the relative proportion of mature cells ultimately expressing either the maternally derived or paternally derived X chromosome. For example, if only two progenitor cells are present in the embryo at the time of tissue-specific X inactivation, it is highly likely that those two progenitor will express only the paternal or only the paternal X chromosome. If all the organism's blood cells derive from these two progenitors, then that organism would appear to have clonal hematopoiesis on X chromosome-based clonality analysis. However, if 8, 16, or 32 progenitors are present at the time of random X chromosome inactivation, it is highly likely that close to one half of the progenitor cells will express only the maternal and the other half only the

X Chromosome Inactivation Phenomenon

paternal X chromosome, and the tissue would appear to be nonclonal on X chromosome-based clonality analysis.

The tissue specificity of embryonic X chromosome inactivation and the possibility of X chromosome allelic skewing resulting from a relatively small number of adult tissue progenitor cells present at the time of X inactivation dictates that X chromosome-based clonality data may exhibit significant interindividual variation. Such data should therefore be interpreted with caution and in the presence of appropriate tissue-specific positive controls. Clonality studies performed on peripheral blood cells from normal women show that approx 20–35% exhibit allelic skewing *(46–48)*. Skewing of the X chromosome allelic usage ratio in peripheral blood cells becomes more pronounced as individuals age *(47)*; whether this is owing to exhaustion of the hematopoietic stem cell pool or a progressive effect of cell selection owing to expression of X chromosome alleles that are detrimental to proliferation/survival ("pseudoclonality") *(31,32)* has not yet been established. It is also possible that this phenomenon may reflect the methylation differences of DNA among the cells rather than true clonal selection; since it has been observed only when methylation-based clonality assay was used and not in X-chromosome inactivation-based transcription clonality assay.

1.4. Conclusions

Overall, advances made in the understanding of the regulation of gene transcription and the biology of the X chromosome have contributed substantially to the development of widely applicable X chromosome-based clonality assays. Those assays, which rely on detection of exonic polymorphisms, require very pure study cell populations. Contaminating lymphocytes, fibroblasts, and monocytes may inadvertently contribute nonclonal RNA, and substantially alter results in small tissue specimens, thereby possibly limiting their applicability to solid tumors. Even in very uniform cell populations, the possibility of differential DNA methylation (as seen in malignant tissue *[17]* when methylation-based clonality assays are used), potential interindividual variability in the number of progenitor cells present at the time of X chromosome inactivation, age-related allelic skewing, and "pseudoclonality" observed in females heterozygous for X-linked inherited diseases *(31,32)* all necessitate thoughtful use of appropriate controls and, possibly, use of more than one clonality assay for proper conclusions to be reached.

There are clearly many clonality assays available to the researcher. Here we describe a rapid, reproducible, and nonradioactive clonality assay based on detection of exonic polymorphisms of the X chromosome genes p55 and G6PD using ASPCR *(33)*.

2. Materials

2.1. Isolation of Blood Cells: Preparation of Granulocyte and T-Lymphocyte Fractions from Peripheral Blood

2.1.1. Separation of Granulocytes and Mononuclear Cells by Density Gradient Centrifugation

1. Density gradient: Histopaque-1077 (Sigma, St. Louis, MO).
2. Phosphate-buffered saline (PBS) (Sigma).

2.1.2. Separation of T-Lymphocytes by Rosetting with Sheep Red Blood Cells

1. Neuraminidase-treated sheep red blood cells (RBCs) (TCS Biologicals, UK).
2. Fetal calf serum (Sigma).
3. 1% Stock solution of polybrene (Sigma).

2.2. Preparation of RNA

1. TRIzol™ reagent (Gibco-BRL, Gaithersburg, MD).
2. Chloroform.
3. Isopropanol.
4. 75% Ethanol in RNase-free water.
5. RNase-free water: Add 0.01% diethylpyrocarbonate to distilled water in glass bottles, allow to stand overnight, and autoclave).

2.3. First-Strand cDNA Synthesis

1. SuperScript™ II RNase H- Reverse Transcriptase (200 U/mL) (Gibco-BRL).
2. 5X First-strand buffer: 250 mM Tris-HCl, pH 8.3, 375 mM KCl, 15 mM MgCl$_2$, supplied with enzyme.
3. 0.1 M Dithiothreitol (DTT) (supplied with enzyme).
4. 25 mM dNTPs (25 mM each of dATP, dCTP, dGTP, and dTTP) (Gibco-BRL).
5. RNasin (40 U/mL) (Promega, Madison, WI).
6. Random hexamer pd(N)$_6$ (1 mg/mL) (Pharmacia, Washington, DC).
7. Single-strand DNA-binding protein (US Biochemical, Cleveland, OH).
8. RNase-free water.

2.4. Analysis of Genomic DNA for Genotype Determination by ASPCR

2.4.1. Polymerase Chain Reaction

1. 10X PCR buffer II (Perkin-Elmer, Foster City, CA).
2. 25 mM MgCl$_2$ (supplied with buffer).
3. 10 mM dNTPs (10 mM each of dATP, dCTP, dGTP, and dTTP).
4. AmpliTaq™ DNA polymerase (5 U/mL) (Perkin-Elmer).
5. Single-strand DNA-binding protein (US Biochemical).
6. Oligonucleotide primers. Refer to **ref. 33** for details of sequences.

X Chromosome Inactivation Phenomenon 263

7. Mineral oil (Sigma).
8. Sterile distilled water.
9. Perkin-Elmer 9600 thermocycling machine.

2.4.2. Agarose Gel Electrophoresis

1. 1X TAE buffer: 50X TAE buffer contains 242 g of Tris base, 57.1 mL of glacial acetic acid, and 100 mL of 0.5 M EDTA, pH 8.0, adjusted to 1 L total volume with distilled water.
2. Ethidium bromide (10 mg/mL stock solution).
3. DNA-grade agarose.
4. 10X Gel-loading dye: 0.25% bromophenol blue, 0.25% xylene cyanol, 15% Ficoll-400 (Pharmacia).
5. λ*Hind*III DNA molecular marker (Gibco-BRL).
6. Distilled water.

3. Methods

3.1. Isolation of Blood Cells: Preparation of Granulocyte and T-Lymphocyte Fractions from Peripheral Blood

Peripheral blood samples anticoagulated with EDTA can be used for genotyping and for determination of clonality in females known to have a clonal hematopoietic disorder. The method described here is for the separation of granulocytes and T-lymphocytes from 20 mL of peripheral blood. Further separation of the myeliod lineage may be required for some clonality studies.

3.1.1. Separation of Granulocytes and Mononuclear Cells by Density Gradient Centrifugation

1. Collect 20 mL of peripheral blood into trisodium EDTA tubes.
2. Gently layer the blood onto 25 mL of Histopaque-1077 in a 50-mL polypropylene conical tube and centrifuge at 400*g* (Sorvall RT6000B benchtop centrifuge) for 30 min at room temperature.
3. Transfer the interface (the mononuclear cell layer) to a sterile 50-mL conical tube, using a Pasteur pipet, and process as described in **Subheading 3.1.2.**
4. Aspirate the layers using a Pasteur pipet and discard to leave the RBC/granulocyte layer.
5. Add PBS to the RBC/granulocyte layer to give a total volume of 50 mL and mix by gentle inversion.
6. Centrifuge at 400*g* at room temperature for 10 min.
7. Remove the supernatant using a Pasteur pipet and discard.
8. Repeat **steps 5–7**.
9. To lyse the red cells, distribute the packed RBC/granulocyte layer into conical tubes containing freshly prepared red cell lysis buffer (approx 1 mL of RBCs/50 mL of red cell lysis buffer), and leave at room temperature for 15 min, with occasional mixing.

10. Centrifuge at 400g for 10 min at room temperature and pour off the supernatant.
11. Pool each granulocyte pellet into two conical tubes.
12. Fill the tubes to 50 mL with PBS and centrifuge at 400g for 10 min at room temperature. Pour off the supernatant.
13. Repeat **step 12**.
14. Pool the pellets into one conical tube and resuspend in PBS to a total volume of 10 mL.
15. Take an aliquot and obtain a cell count using an automated counter.

3.1.2. Separation of T-Lymphocytes by Rosetting with Sheep RBCs

This protocol is based on the erythrocyte rosetting method of Kaplan and Clark *(49)*.

1. Dilute the mononuclear cell fraction from **step 3** to obtain a concentration of 2–6×10^6/mL white blood cells.
2. Add 1–2 vol of neuraminidase-treated sheep RBCs (TCS Biologicals), 0.5–1 vol of FCS, and 100–300 μL of a fresh 1:30 dilution of a 1% stock solution of polybrene to the cell suspension.
3. Centrifuge the suspension at 750 rpm for 5 min at 4°C, and then incubate at 4°C for a minimum of 5 h or maximum overnight.
4. Remove the supernatant from the packed cell pellet (sheep RBCs and rosetted T-lymphocytes) and add 1 vol of PBS.
5. Resuspend the cells by rotating the meniscus through the cell pellet.
6. Layer the cell suspension onto an equal volume of Histopaque and centrifuge at 400g for 30 min at room temperature.
7. Aspirate and discard the upper layer, interface (non-T-cell), and Histopaque layer leaving the sheep RBC/T-lymphocyte layer.
8. Add PBS to 50 mL and centrifuge at 400g for 10 min at room temperature.
9. Remove the supernatant using a Pasteur pipet and discard.
10. Repeat **steps 8** and **9**.
11. To lyse the sheep RBCs, distribute the cell pellet into conical tubes containing freshly prepared red cell lysis buffer (approx 1 mL of cells/50 mL of lysis buffer), and incubate at room temperature for 15 min with occasional mixing.
12. Centrifuge at 400g for 10 min and pour off the supernatant.
13. Treat the T-cell pellets exactly as the granulocyte pellets from **step 11** of **Subheading 3.1.1.**

3.2. Preparation of RNA

RNA preparation is perfomed using TRIzol reagent according to the manufacturer's instructions, with minor modifications.

1. After counting, pellet the cells by centrifugation. Aspirate off the supernatant.
2. Add 1 ml of TRIzol reagent per 1×10^7 cells in a polypropylene tube. Using a syringe and a 25-gage needle, aspirate the cells and TRIzol repeatedly in order to lyse the cells (seven or eight times is usually sufficient). At this point the sample

X Chromosome Inactivation Phenomenon

may be transferred to a 1.5-mL microcentrifuge tube if the required volume of TRIzol is 1 mL or less.

3. Incubate the lysed cells in TRIzol for 5 min at room temperature (15–30°C).
4. Add 0.2 mL of chloroform/mL of TRIzol and shake the tubes in order to mix the contents thoroughly. Incubate at room temperature for 2 to 3 min. Centrifuge at 4000 rpm for 30 min at 4°C.
5. Aspirate off the upper aqueous phase and transfer to a clean tube. Avoid disturbing the interface because this may result in contamination of the RNA preparation by DNA.
6. Add isopropanol to the aqueous phase (use 0.5 mL of isopropanol/mL of TRIzol used in **step 2**). Mix and incubate at room temperature for 10 min. Centrifuge at 4000 rpm for 30 min at 4°C. The precipitated RNA should form a clear pellet at the bottom of the tube.
7. Aspirate off the supernatant and wash with 75% ethanol (use 1 mL of ethanol/1 mL of TRIzol used in **step 2**). Briefly vortex to expose the pellet to ethanol, and centrifuge at 4000 rpm for 10 min.
8. Remove the supernatant and air-dry the RNA pellet for 10 min to allow any remaining ethanol to evaporate. Dissolve the pellet in an appropriate volume of RNase-free water; incubating the solution in a 55°C water bath for 10 min will facilitate this.
9. Determine the concentration of RNA in solution using a spectrophotometer at A_{260}. One A_{260} unit of single-stranded RNA corresponds to a concentration of 40 mg/mL. Pure RNA preparations should have an $A_{260}:A_{280}$ ratio of 2.0. RNA should be stored at –70°C to prevent degradation.

3.3. First-Strand cDNA Synthesis

1. Add 1 mL random hexamers 1 mg/mL of $(pd(N)_6$ to an RNase-free 500-mL microcentrifuge tube together with a volume of RNA constituting between 3 and 5 mg (to a maximum volume of 11.5 mL). Add RNase-free water to bring the total volume to 12.5 mL (*see* **Note 1**).
2. Incubate at 70°C for 10 min. Quench the reaction on ice for 2 min. Briefly spin and set back on ice.
3. To each tube, add 5 mL first-strand buffer, 2 mL of 0.1 M DTT, 1 mL of 25 mM dNTPs, 0.5 mL of RNasin (40 U/mL), 1 mL of single-strand DNA-binding protein (0.5 mg/mL), and 1.5 mL of RNase-free water.
4. Add 1.5 mL of SuperScript II RNase H-Reverse Transcriptase (200 U/mL) to each tube, and incubate at 37°C for 1 h. The total reaction volume should equal 25 mL.
5. Inactivate the enzymes by heating to 65°C for 10 min.
6. Store synthesized cDNA at –20°C.

3.4. Analysis of Genomic DNA for Genotype Determination by ASPCR

ASPCR for G6PD and p55 genotyping consists of two rounds of PCR (*see* **Note 1**).

1. In the first round, aliquot the following into a sterile 200-mL tube for each PCR reaction (total volume of 50 µL) 1–10 µL of genomic DNA (extracted from the fractionated blood cells using standard conditions), 5 µL of 10X PCR buffer II, 2 mM MgCl$_2$, 0.2 mM dNTPs, 25 pmol of forward primer (6J-p55 or 7g-G6PD), 25 pmol of reverse primer (8gR-p55 or 9gR-G6PD) *(33)*, 1 U of *Taq* polymerase, and sterile distilled water to give a final volume of 50 µL.
2. Pipet 50 µL of mineral oil taking care not to puncture the layer. Cap the tube.
3. Perform PCR amplification in a Perkin-Elmer 9600 thermocycling machine using the following conditions: initial denaturation step at 95°C for 1 min, followed by 35 cycles of PCR at 94°C for 40 s, 62°C for 1 min, and 72°C for 1 min.
4. Visualize amplified PCR product in all reactions by agarose gel electrophoresis. Use a 1% agarose gel and 1X TAE running buffer. Load 5 mL of PCR product plus 1 mL of 10X gel-loading dye and include a lane containing a λ*Hind*III marker in order to assess the size of the product. Run at 90 V until the dark blue dye front is approximately two-thirds down the gel.
5. Stain the gel with ethidium bromide. Visualize the DNA on an ultraviolet (UV) transilluminator and photograph the gel.
6. In the second round (a sample from the first round is used as a template), aliquot the following into a sterile 200-mL tube for each PCR reaction (total volume of 50 µL) 5 µL of first-round products, 5 µL of 10X PCR buffer II, 1.5 mM MgCl$_2$, 0.2 mM dNTPs, 10 pmol of allele-specific primer as forward primer (e.g., 1gT or 3gG for p55/3C, or T4 for G6PD) and the same reverse primer as that used in the first round of PCR (8gR-p55 or 9gR-G6PD) *(33)*, 1 U of *Taq* polymerase, and sterile distilled water to give a final volume of 50 µL.
7. Pipet 50 µL of mineral oil taking care not to puncture the layer. Cap the tube.
8. Perform PCR amplification in a Perkin-Elmer 9600 thermocycling machine using the following conditions: initial denaturation step at 95°C for 1 min, followed by five cycles of PCR at 94°C for 30 s, 64°C for 1 min, and 72°C for 1 min.
9. Visualize 15 µL of amplified PCR products (from each second-round PCR) in all reactions on 1% agarose gels. Genomic DNA from homozygote individuals will generate second-round allele-specific products in only one well. Genomic DNA from heterozygote individuals will generate second-round allele-specific products in both wells *(see* **Note 2**).

3.5. Analysis of cDNA for Determination of Clonality by ASPCR

For rapid determination of clonality, the template for the first round of PCR is cDNA synthesized from total RNA by reverse transcription. Second-round PCR is conducted in an identical fashion as with genomic DNA. Clonal samples (using cDNA from heterozygous patients) will generate second-round allele-specific products in only one well. Nonclonal samples (using cDNA from heterozygous patients) will generate second-round allele-specific products in both wells.

4. Notes

1. A limitation of G6PD, p55, and recently introduced IDS assay *(50)* is that only 76% of Caucasian females, 62% of African-American females, and even lower

X Chromosome Inactivation Phenomenon

proportion of Asian females are heterozygous for at least one of these assays and thus suitable for clonality analysis. However, these limitations are now being overcome by assays currently under development.

2. The first-round products always should be visualized under UV light as the same high molecular weight band on first- and second-round agarose gels, and thus serve as an internal control.

References

1. Lyon, M. F. (1961) Gene action in the X-chromosome in the mouse (Mus musculus L.). *Nature* **190,** 372,373.
2. Ohno, S. and Hauschka, T. S. (1960) Allocycly of the X-chromosome in tumors and normal tissue. *Cancer Res.* **20,** 541–545.
3. Beutler, E., Yeh, M., and Fairbanks, V. F. (1962) The normal human female as a mosaic of X chromosome activity: studies using the gene for G6PD deficiency as a marker. *Proc. Natl. Acad. Sci. USA* **48,** 9–16.
4. Beutler, E. and Baluda, M. C. (1964) The separation of glucose-6-phosphate-dehydrogenase-deficient erythrocytes from the blood of heterozygotes for glucose-6-phosphate-dehydrogenase deficiency. *Lancet* **1,** 189–192.
5. Davidson, R. G., Nitowsky, H. M., and Childs, B. (1963) Demonstration of two populations of cells in the human female for glucose 6 phosphate dehydrogenase variants. *Proc. Natl. Acad. Sci. USA* **50,** 481–485.
6. Boyer, S. H., Porter, I. H., and Weilbacher, R. G. (1962) Electrophoretic heterogeneity of glucose 6 phosphate dehydrogenase and its relationship to enzyme deficiency in man. *Proc. Natl. Acad. Sci. USA* **48,** 1868–1876.
7. Linder, D. and Gartler, S. M. (1965) Glucose-6-phosphate dehydrogenase mosaicism: utilization as a cell marker in the study of leiomyomas. *Science* **150,** 67–69.
8. Beutler, E., Collins, Z., and Irwin, L. E. (1967) Value of genetic variants of glucose-6-phosphate dehydrogenase in tracing the origin of malignant tumors. *N. Engl. J. Med.* **276(7),** 389–391.
9. Razin, A. and Riggs, A. D. (1980) DNA methylation and gene function. *Science* **210,** 604–610.
10. Vogelstein, B., Fearon, E. R., Hamilton, S., and Feinberg, A. P. (1985) Use of restriction fragment length polymorphisms to determine the clonal origin of human tumors. *Science* **227,** 642–645.
11. Nussbaum, R. L., Crowder, W., Nyhan, W. L., and Caskey, C. T. (1983) A three-allele restriction-fragment-length polymorphism at the hypoxanthine phosphoribosyltransferase locus in man. *Proc. Natl. Acad. Sci. USA* **80,** 4035–4039.
12. Wolf, S. F., Jolly, D. J., Lunnen, K. D., Friedmann, T., and Migeon, B. R. (1984) Methylation of the hypoxanthine phosphoribosyltransferase locus on the human X-chromosome: implications for X-chromosome inactivation. *Proc. Natl. Acad. Sci. USA* **81,** 2806–2810.
13. Hendriks, R. W., Chen, Z. Y., Hinds, H., Schuurman, R. K. B., and Craig, I. W. (1992) An X chromosome inactivation assay based on differential methylation of a CpG island coupled to a VNTR polymorphism at the 5' end of the monoamine oxidase A gene. *Hum. Mol. Genet.* **1(3),** 187–194.

14. Keith, D. H., Singer-Sam, J., and Riggs, A. D. (1986) Active X chromosome DNA is unmethylated at eight CCGG sites clustered in a guanine-plus-cytosine-rich island at the 5' end of the gene for phosphoglycerate kinase. *Mol. Cell. Biol.* **6,** 4122–4125.

15. Allen, R. C., Zoghbi, H. Y., Moseley, A. B., Rosenblatt, H. M., and Belmont, J. W. (1992) Methylation of HpaII and HhaI sites near the polymorphic CAG repeat in the human androgen-receptor gene correlates with X chromosome inactivation. *Am. J. Hum. Genet.* **51,** 1229–1239.

16. Busque, L., Zhu, J., DeHart, D., Griffith, B., Willman, C., Carroll, R., Black, P. M., and Gilliland, D. G. (1994) An expression based clonality assay at the human androgen receptor locus (HUMARA) on chromosome X. *Nucleic Acids Res.* **22,** 697,698.

17. Goelz, S. E., Vogelstein, B., Hamilton, S. R., and Feinberg, A. P. (1985) Hypomethylation of DNA from benign and malignant human colon neoplasms. *Science* **228,** 187–190.

18. Boyd, Y. and Fraser, N. J. (1990) Methylation patterns at the hypervariable X-chromosome locus DXS255 (M27B): correlation with X-inactivation status. *Genomics* **7,** 182–187.

19. Beutler, E. and Kuhl, W. (1990) The NT 1311 polymorphism of the G6PD gene: G6PD Mediterranean mutation may have originated independently in Europe and Asia. *Am. J. Hum. Genet.* **47,** 1008–1012.

20. Metzenberg, A. B. and Gitschier, J. (1992) The gene encoding the palmitoylated erythrocyte membrane protein, p55, originates at the CpG island 3' to the Factor VIII gene. *Hum. Mol. Genet.* **1(2),** 97–101.

21. Bunge, S., Cordula, S., Beck, M., Rosenkranz, W., Schwinger, E., Hopwood, J. J., and Gal, A. (1992) Mutation analysis of the iduronate-2-sulfatase gene in patients with mucopolysaccharidosis type II (Hunter syndrome). *Hum. Mol. Genet.* **1(5),** 335–339.

22. Vulliamy, T. J., D'Urso, M., Battistuzzi, G., Estrada, M., Foulkes. N. S., Martini, G., Calabro, V., et al. (1988) Diverse point mutations in the human glucose-6-phosphate dehydrogenasegene cause enzyme deficiency and mild or severe hemolytic anemia. *Proc. Natl. Acad. Sci. USA* **85,** 5171–5175.

23. Kay, A. C., Kuhl, W., Prchal, J. T., and Beutler, E. (1992) The origin of glucose-6-phosphate dehydrogenase (G6PD) polymorphisms in African-Americans. *Am. J. Hum. Genet.* **50,** 394–398.

24. Curnutte, J. T., Hopkins, P. J., Kuhl, W., and Beutler, E. (1992) Studying X inactivation. *Lancet* **339,** 749.

25. Conner, B. J., Reyes, A. A., Morin, C., Itakura, K., Teplitz, R. L., and Wallace, R. B. (1983) Detection of sickle beta globin allele by hybridization with synthetic oligonucleotides. *Proc. Natl. Acad. Sci. USA* **80,** 278–282.

26. Barany, F. (1991) Genetic disease detection and DNA amplification using cloned thermostable ligase. *Proc. Natl. Acad. Sci. USA* **88,** 189–193.

27. Landegren, U., Kaiser, R., Sanders, J., and Hood, L. (1988) A ligase-mediated gene detection technique. *Science* **241,** 1077–1080.

X Chromosome Inactivation Phenomenon 269

28. Prchal, J. T., Guan, Y. L., Prchal, J. F., and Barany, F. (1993) Transcriptional analysis of the active X-chromosome in normal and clonal hematopoiesis. *Blood* **81,** 269–271.
29. Prchal, J. T. and Guan, Y. L. (1993) A novel clonality assay based on transcriptional analysis of the active X chromosome. *Stem Cells* **11,** 62–65.
30. Prchal, J. T., Prchal, J. F., Belickova, M., Chen, S., Guan, Y. L., Gartland, G. L., and Cooper, M. D. (1996) Clonal stability of blood cell lineages indicated by X-chromosomal transcriptional polymorphism. *J. Exp. Med.* **183,** 561–567.
31. Nyhan, W. L., Bakay, B., Connor, J. D., Marks, J. F., and Keele, D. K. (1970) Hemizygous expression of glucose-6-phosphate dehydrogenase in erythrocytes of heterozygotes for the Lesch-Nyhan syndrome. *Proc. Natl. Acad. Sci. USA* **65,** 214–218.
32. Prchal, J. T., Carroll, A. J., Prchal, J. F., Crist, W. M., Skalka, H. W., Gealy, W. J., Harley, J., and Malluh, A. (1980) Wiskott-Aldrich syndrome: cellular impairments and their implications for carrier detection. *Blood* **56,** 1048–1054.
33. Liu, Y., Phelan, J., Go, R. C. P., Prchal, J. F., and Prchal, J. T. (1997) Rapid determination of clonality by detection of two closely-linked X chromosome exonic polymorphisms using allele specific PCR. *J. Clin. Invest.* **99(8),** 1984–1990.
34. Luhovy, M., Liu, Y., Belickova, M., Prchal J. F., and Prchal, J. T. (1995) A novel clonality assay based on transcriptional polymorphism of X chromosome gene p55. *Biol. Blood Marrow Transplant.* **1,** 81–87.
35. El-Kassar, N., Hetet, G., Briere, J., and Grandchamp, B. (1997) Clonality analysis of hematopoiesis in essential thrombocythemia: advantages of studying T lymphocytes and platelets. *Blood* **89(1),** 128–134.
36. Gregg, X. T., Liu, Y., and Prchal, J. T. (1996) Development of a new clonality assay based on a transcriptional polymorphism of the iduronate-2-sulfatase gene. *Blood* **88(10 Suppl. 1),** 370a.
37. Prchal, J. T., Liu, Y., Prchal, J. F., Hoffman, R., and Tushinski, R. (1994) Are normal stem cells present in myeloproliferative syndrome? *Blood* **84(Suppl. 1),** 55a.
38. Gregg, X. T., Liu, Y., Prchal, J. T., Gartland, G. L., Cooper, M. D., and Prchal, J. F. (1996) Clonality in myeloproliferative disorders. *Blood* **88(Suppl. 1),** 479a.
39. Busque, L., Gilliland, D. G., Prchal, J. T., Sief, C. A., Weinstein, H. J., Sokol, J. M., Belickova, M., Sokol, L., and Emmanuel, P. D. (1995) Clonality in juvenile chronic myelogenous leukemia. *Blood* **85,** 21–30.
40. Atkinson, T., Smith, C. A., Garber, E., Hsu, Y. M., Howard, T. T., Prchal, J. T., and Cooper, M. D., (1998) Leukocyte transfusion-asociated granulocyte responses in a patient with X-linked hyper-IgM syndrome. *J. Clin. Immunol.* **18,** 430–439.
41. Belickova, M., Schroeder, H. W., Guan, Y. L., Cooper, M. D., and Prchal. J. T. (1995) Clonal hematopoiesis and acquired thalassemia in common variable immunodeficiency. *Mol. Med.* **1,** 56.
42. Harrison, C. N., Gale, R. E., and Linch, D. C. (1998) Quantification of X-chromosome inactivation patterns using rtPCR of the polymorphic iduronate-2-sulphatase gene and correlation of the results obtained with DNA-based techniques. *Leukemia* **12,** 1834–1839.

43. Kay, G. F. (1998) Xist and X chromosome inactivation. *Mol. Cell. Endocrinol.* **140,** 71–76.
44. Penny, G. D., Kay, G. F., Sheardown, S. A., Rastan, S., and Brockdorf, N. (1996) Requirement for Xist in X chromosome inactivation. *Nature* **379,** 131–137.
45. Tan, S. S., Williams, E. A., and Tam, P. P. L. (1993) X-chromosome inactivation occurs at different times in different tissues of the post-implantation mouse embryo. *Nat. Genet.* **3,** 170–174.
46. Busque, L., Mio, R., Mattioli, J., Brais, E., Blais, N., Lalonde, Y., et al (1996) Nonrandom X-inactivation patterns in normal females: Lyonization ratios vary with age. Blood **88(1),** 59–65.
47. Champion, K. M., Gilbert, J. G. R., Asimakopoulos, F. A., Hinshelwood, S., and Green, A. R. (1997) Clonal haematopoiesis in normal elderly women: implications for the myeloproliferative disorders and myelodysplastic syndromes. *Br. J. Haematol.* **97,** 920–926.
48. Gale, R. E., Fielding, A. K., Harrison, C. N., and Linch, D. C. (1997) Acquired skewing of X-chromosome inactivation patterns in myeloid cells of the elderly suggests stochastic clonal loss with age. *Br. J. Haematol.* **98,** 512–519.
49. Kaplan, M. E. and Clark, C. An improved rosetting assay for detection of human T lymphocytes. *J. Immunol. Methods* **5(2),** 131–135.
50. Gregg, X. T., Kralovics, R., and Prchal, J. T. (2000) A polymorphism of the X-linked gene IDS increases the number of females informative for transcriptional clonality assays. *Am. J. Hemat.* **63,** 184–191.

20

Telomere Length Changes in Human Cancer

Dominique Broccoli and Andrew K. Godwin

1. Introduction

Telomere length is now known to be directly responsible for limiting the capacity of cellular division in a number of human cell types *(1,2)*. Comparison of telomere length in tumors and matched normal tissue from the same individual has indicated that the telomere repeat array is often shorter in tumors than in adjacent untransformed tissue *(3–5)* (**Fig. 1**). Changes in telomere length during human tumorigenesis are believed to reflect loss of terminal sequences resulting from the end replication problem during the cell divisions required for tumor formation. Although telomeres are often shorter in tumors than in matched normal tissue from the same individual, these telomeres are usually stabilized at a new length setting by the activation of the telomere maintenance enzyme, telomerase *(6,7)*.

Telomere length is usually determined by Southern analysis of terminal restriction fragments (TRFs). This is technically the most simple protocol for visualizing telomere arrays. However, difficulties in interpreting the telomere length data generated from this technique arise owing to the heterogeneity in the number of telomeric repeats present at individual chromosome ends. In contrast to the discrete bands usually resulting from Southern analysis, telomeric signals appear as a smear of hybridization. The intensity of the signal is biased toward the larger telomeric fragments because these fragments contain a greater number of target sequences for hybridization. In addition, the TRFs being visualized via this method represent not only the canonical TTAGGG repeats but a variable amount of subtelomeric sequences (**Fig. 2**).

Recently, two additional methods for ascertaining telomere length have been developed. First, hybridization of TRFs can be done in solution with an oligonucleotide probe complementary to the single-stranded protrusion present at

From: *Methods in Molecular Medicine, vol. 68: Molecular Analysis of Cancer*
Edited by: J. Boultwood and C. Fidler © Humana Press Inc., Totowa, NJ

271

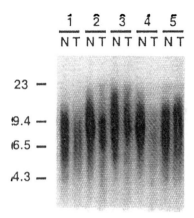

Fig. 1. Analysis of telomere length changes in breast tumors. TRFs are from normal (N) and tumor (T) tissue from five individuals. Genomic DNA was digested with *Hinf*I and visualized following Southern hybridization with the telomeric oligonucleotides (TTAGGG)$_4$ and (CCCTAA)$_4$. Note that TRFs are usually shorter in tumors than in adjacent normal tissue from the same individual.

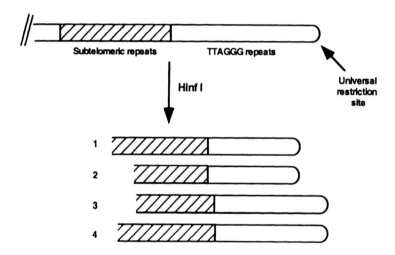

Fig. 2. Telomeric arrays appear as a smear rather than as discrete bands following Southern analysis owing to heterogeneity in the amount of subtelomeric sequences (1 vs 2 and 3 vs 4) and in the number of TTAGGG repeats present at each chromosome end (1 vs 4 and 2 vs 3).

the 3' ends of chromosomes *(8,9)*. This method reduces heterogeneity in signal intensity owing to variable amounts of target sequence, allowing quantitation of telomere length to be somewhat simplified. However, there are several of problems associated with this technique, including the necessity of running hot

Telomere Length and Change in Human Cancer 273

gels and the care to determine that one's DNA samples do not become denatured. Second, telomere length can be determined by *in situ* hybridization using peptide nucleic acid–based probes *(10)*. This technique permits accurate determination of telomere length based on signal intensity and allows investigation of telomere length on an individual chromosome basis. However, this technique requires the generation of metaphase spreads from actively growing cultures, and data collection is onerous. Thus, peptide nucleic acid-based *in situ* hybridization is not yet suitable for analysis of telomere length in large numbers of human tumor samples.

This chapter describes the analysis of human telomere length in human tumors using Southern hybridization of TRFs. This is the technique that is most widely used in the field of telomere dynamics, and where possible, we have optimized the use of commercially available reagents and kits to minimize interlaboratory variation.

2. Materials
2.1. Preparation of Genomic DNA

1. Matched samples from tumor and normal tissue.
2. 10X PBSA: 1.37 M NaCl, 26.8 mM KCl, 106 mM Na$_2$HPO$_4$, 14.7 mM K$_2$H$_2$PO$_4$.
3. TNE lysis Buffer: 0.5 M Tris-HCl, pH 8.9, 10 mM NaCl , 15 mM EDTA.
4. Proteinase K (10 mg/mL).
5. Phenol (saturated with 0.1 M Tris/0.2% β-mercaptoethanol, pH 8.0).
6. 3 M Sodium acetate, pH 5.7.
7. Absolute and 70% ethanol.
8. T$_{10}$E$_{20}$: 10 mM Tris-HCl/20 mM EDTA, pH 7.5.
9. RnaseA (10 mg/mL).
10. 10% Sodium dodecyl sulfate (SDS).
11. Phenol/chloroform/isoamyl alcohol (25:24:1) (Fisher).
12. T$_{10}$E$_1$: 10 mM Tris-HCl/1 mM EDTA, pH 8.0.
13. Centrifuge.
14. Polypropylene tubes (15 and 50 mL).
15. Rotator.

2.2. Digestion and Quantitation of DNA Samples

1. *Hinf*I restriction endonuclease and reaction buffer (New England Biolabs).
2. Incubator.
3. Flurometer (Bio-Rad, Hercules, CA).
4. DNA quantitation kit (Bio-Rad) containing 10X TEN (100 mM Tris-HCl, 2 M NaCl, 10 mM EDTA, pH7.4), 1 mg/mL of calf thymus DNA, and 10 mg/mL of Hoechst 33258 (bisbenzamide). Alternatively, components for quantitation can be purchased separately.
5. Cuvets.
6. Eppendorf tubes.

2.3. Southern Blotting

1. Agarose.
2. Ethidium bromide (10 mg/mL).
3. 5X Tris-borate EDTA (TBE) buffer.
4. DNA molecular weight standards (New England Biolabs).
5. Agarose gel electrophoresis chamber and power supply.
6. 0.25 N HCl.
7. Denaturing solution: 0.5 M NaOH, 1.5 M NaCl.
8. Neutralizing solution: 1 M Tris-HCl, pH 7.5, 1.5 M NaCl.
9. Hybond N (Amersham).
10. Stratalinker (Stratagene).
11. Transfer apparatus (capillary or electroblot).

2.4. Probe Preparation and Hybridization

1. Hybridization mix: 0.5 M NaH$_2$PO$_4$, 10% BSA, 7% SDS.
2. Filter unit (500-mL, 0.45-μm) (Nalgene).
3. Hybridization setup (water bath, oven, and so on).
4. ProbeQuant G-50 microcolumns (Pharmacia).
5. T4 kinase and 5X Forward Reaction Buffer (Gibco-BRL).
6. γ^{32}P-ATP (3000 Ci/mmol).
7. (TTAGGG)$_4$ and (CCCTAA)$_4$ oligonucleotides (100 ng/μL).
8. TES: 10 mM Tris-HCl, pH 7.4, 1 mM EDTA, pH 8.0, 0.1% SDS.
9. Pyrex dish or tupperware.
10. 4X Saline sodium citrate (SSC), 0.1% SDS.
11. Autoradiographic film or Phosphorimager cassette.

3. Methods
3.1. Preparation of Genomic DNA (see Note 1)

It is essential that tissue samples are pathologically evaluated to minimize cross contamination of tumor tissue with normal tissue. Tissues should be flash frozen and stored at –70°C until use.

1. Rinse approx 1 g (1 cm^3) of frozen tissue with 1X PBSA.
2. Decant the wash and finely mince the specimen (~1 g or 1 cm^3) with a razor or scalpel blade.
3. Place the minced tissue into a 50-mL polypropylene tube and add 10 mL of TNE lysis buffer supplemented with 500 μg/mL of proteinase K and 1% SDS.
4. Parafilm the cap and incubate overnight at 37°C with constant rocking.
5. Add an equal volume of phenol saturated with 0.1 M Tris/0.2% β-mercaptoethanol (pH 8.0), and mix gently at room temperature for 10–15 min.
6. Centrifuge at 1400g for 10 min.
7. Remove the aqueous phase (upper layer) with a wide-bored pipet (e.g., 25-mL disposable pipet), and transfer to a fresh 50-mL polypropylene tube. Repeat the

Telomere Length and Change in Human Cancer

phenol extraction as described previously until the interphase between the aqueous and organic layers is clear.

8. Transfer the final aqueous phase to a fresh tube. This solution will be very viscous, and care should be taken to slowly and gently remove the aqueous phase to limit the contamination with the phenol solution.
9. Add 0.1 vol of 3 M sodium acetate (pH 5.7) and 2 vol of cold absolute ethanol.
10. Precipitate the DNA by rotating gently for 5–10 min. The genomic DNA will precipitate into a white stringy clump. Loosely spool strands of DNA around a glass pipet or a yellow pipet tip and transfer to a fresh 50-mL tube.
11. Wash the spooled DNA by rotating the DNA in 25–35 mL of 70% EtOH for 5–10 min at room temperature.
12. Air-dry the DNA and place in a 15-mL polypropylene tube (Falcon 2059). Resuspend the DNA in 3 mL of $T_{10}E_{20}$ by rotating overnight at 4°C.
13. Add 100 µg/mLof RNase A (10 mg/mL stock) and incubate at 37°C for 30 min.
14. Add proteinase K and SDS to final concentrations of 200 µg/mL and 1%, respectively. Incubate for 1 h at 48°C.
15. Extract twice with equal volumes of phenol/chloroform/isoamyl alcohol (25:24:1) as described in **steps 5–8**.
16. Add 0.1 vol of 3 M sodium acetate, 2 vol of cold absolute EtOH to the aqueous phase, and spool the DNA as before.
17. Wash the DNA with 70% ethanol.
18. Air-dry the DNA and then vacuum dry the pellet.
19. Resuspend the dried DNA in 1 to 2 mL of $T_{10}E_1$ by rotating overnight at 4°C.
20. Store the DNA samples at 4°C. The concentration of the sample may be determined using a spectrophotometer at this time, but because the viscosity of the solution makes accurate pipetting difficult, these measurements are not very reliable.

3.2. Digestion and Quantitation of DNA Samples

1. Digest 5–10 µL of the DNA sample (no more than 5 µg) in a 50-µL reaction overnight at 37°C with 25U of *Hinf*I. The DNA should be pipeted using sawed-off tips to minimize shearing and facilitate pipetting. Incubation should be carried out in an incubator rather than a water bath to minimize condensation of the reaction on the lid of the Eppendorf tube.
2. Briefly spin the tubes to collect the reaction volumes at the bottom of the tube.
3. Quantitate the amount of DNA in each reaction using the Bio-Rad fluorometer (or similar equipment) and the DNA quantitation kit (Bio-Rad).
4. Prepare sufficient 1X TEN (2 mL/sample to be quantitated).
5. Add Hoechst 33258 to a final concentration of 1 µg/mL.
6. Zero the fluorometer using 2 mL of the TEN/dye solution.
7. Calibrate the fluorometer by adding 5 µL of 100 µg/mL calf thymus DNA (equivalent to a total of 500 ng of DNA).
8. Check the calibration by adding 10 µL of 10 µg/mL calf thymus DNA to 2 mL of TEN/dye solution.

276

Broccoli and Godwin

9. Determine the concentration of DNA in each digest by adding 2 μL of the reaction to 2 mL of TEN/dye solution.
10. Calculate the volumes required to load 1 μg to 2.5 μg of DNA/lane on an agarose gel.

3.3. Southern Blotting

1. Pour a $20 \times 20 \text{ cm}^2$ agarose gel. The agarose mix is composed of 0.7% agarose in 0.5X TBE buffer supplemented with 1 μg/mL of ethidium bromide.
2. Load equal amounts of each DNA sample on the gel. We add 0.1 vol of loading dye to each sample. Also include molecular weight markers (*see* **Note 2**).
3. Run the gel at 30 V until the dye front has entered the gel. The gel can then be turned up to 80 V or continued running at 30 V. The gel should be run for a total of 700–1000 Vh.
4. Check the gel by observing on an ultraviolet light box. The gel should run until the 2-kb molecular weight marker is at the bottom. The majority of the genomic DNA should have run off the gel since *Hinf*I is a frequent cutter in bulk genomic DNA with resulting average sized fragments <2 kb. The intensity of ethidium bromide staining should appear equal for all lanes.
5. Take a picture of the gel with a ruler next to the molecular weight markers.
6. Incubate the gel for 15 min at room temperature with 0.25 N HCl on a rotator. The volume should be sufficient to cover the gel completely.
7. Treat the gel twice for 20 min each in denaturing solution on a rotator.
8. Treat the gel twice for 30 min each in neutralizing solution on a rotator.
9. Rinse the gel with ddH$_2$O.
10. Transfer the DNA to a Hybond N membrane by capillary transfer or using an electroblot apparatus. After transfer is complete, mark the location of the wells.
11. Crosslink the DNA to the membrane by treating in a Statalinker (Stratagene) at 1200 mJ (the "autocrosslink" setting). The membrane can be stored for an unlimited time or immediately be hybridized to detect the TRFs.

3.4. Probe Preparation and Hybridization

The hybridization mix is made in 500-mL aliquots and will last for months at room temperature. The solution should be incubated at 50°C overnight to ensure complete dissolution of the SDS and BSA. The following morning, the hybridization mix is filtered through a 0.45-μm filter unit. This step eliminates "speckling" appearing on the films. Where possible, the procedures below utilize commercially available reagents to eliminate variation from experiment to experiment.

1. Prehybridize the filter at 55°C in 10 mL hybridization mix for at least 30 min at 55°C.
2. While the filter is prehybridizing, label the oligonucleotides. We use a 1:1 mixture of the two oligonucleotides (a total of 200 ng of oligonucleotide) (*see* **Note 3**).
3. End label the oligonucleotides using T4 kinase and 20 pmol (12 μL of 3000 Ci/mmol) of γ^{32}PATP for 45 min to 1 h at 37°C in a final volume of 20 μL (4 μL of 5X forward reaction buffer, 1 μL of each oligonucleotide [100 ng/μL], 2 μL of T4 kinase, 12 μL of γ^{32}P-ATP).

Telomere Length and Change in Human Cancer

4. Stop the reaction by adding 30 μL of TES to the reaction to achieve a final volume of 50 μL.
5. Remove the unincorporated radionuclotide from the reaction using ProbeQuant G-50 microcolumns (Pharmacia).
6. Determine the efficiency of labeling in a crude manner using a Geiger counter. The probe should be labeled such that the counter is saturated on the most sensitive setting when the monitor is held approx 1 in. from the tube.
7. Add the probe to 7 mL of hybridization mix. Replace the prehybridization solution with the hybridization solution and incubate at 55°C overnight.
8. Wash the filter twice for 20 min each in 4X SSC/0.1% SDS at room temperature. Use a Geiger counter to monitor the filter. There should be very few counts remaining in the center of the filter and background levels of radiation at the top and bottom of the filter. If necessary, wash the filter an additional time in 4X SSC/0.1% SDS at 55°C.
9. Wrap the filter in plastic wrap and expose to autoradiographic film or a Phosphorimager cassette. The exposure time and use of intensifying screens varies with experiments and efficiency of hybridization and can range from 2 h with two screens at –70°C to 3 d with two screens at –70°C.

4. Notes

1. Genomic DNA can be prepared using a number of commercially available kits. We have had mixed results using kits and recommend determining the quality of DNA prepared in this manner by running 1 μL of the sample on a gel prior to digestion. Up to 50% of the genomic DNA isolated using kits may be degraded and therefore unsuitable for this type of analysis.
2. Internal telomeric fragments of approx 2 and 2.3 kb act as internal controls for loading and the integrity of DNA.
3. Because of the highly repetitive nature of telomeres, hybridization to these sequences is occasionally uneven. This is owing to insufficient quantities of probe sequence relative to target sequence, i.e., unsaturated conditions. The amount of oligonucleotide suggested in the protocol is usually sufficient to prevent this problem. However, in the event of uneven hybridization patterns, 100–200 ng of unlabeled oligonucleotides should be added to the hybridization mix.

References

1. Vaziri, H. and Benchimol, S. (1998) Reconstitution of telomerase activity in normal human cells leads to elongation of telomeres and extended replicative life span. *Curr. Biol.* **8,** 279–282.
2. Bodnar, A. G., Ouellette, M., Frolkis, M., Holt, S. E., Chiu, C. P., Morin, G. B., et al. (1998) Extension of life-span by introduction of telomerase into normal human cells. *Science* **279,** 349–352.
3. de Lange, T. (1998) Telomeres and senescence: ending the debate. *Science* **279,** 334,335.

4. de Lange, T., Shiue, L., Myers, R. M., Cox, D. R., Naylor, S. L., Killery, A. M., and Varmus, H. E. (1990) Structure and variability of human chromosome ends. *Mol. Cell. Biol.* **10,** 518–527.
5. Hastie, N. D., Dempster, M., Dunlop, M. G., Thompson, A. M., Green, D. K., and Allshire, R. C. (1990) Telomere reduction in human colorectal carcinoma and with ageing. *Nature* **346,** 866–868.
6. Shay, J. W. and Wright, W. E. (1996) The reactivation of telomerase activity in cancer progression. *Trends Genet.* **12,** 129–131.
7. Shay, J. W. and Bacchetti, S. (1997) A survey of telomerase activity in human cancer. *Eur. J. Cancer* **33,** 787–791.
8. Makarov, V., Hirose, Y., and Langmore, J. P. (1997) Long G tails at both ends of human chromosomes suggest a C strand degradation mechanism for telomere shortening. *Cell* **88,** 657–666.
9. McElligott, R. and Wellinger, R. J. (1997) The terminal DNA structure of mammalian chromosomes. *EMBO J.* **16,** 3705–3714.
10. Lansdorp, P. M., Verwoerd, N. P., van de Rijke, F. M., Dragowska, V., Little, M.-T., Dirks, R. W., et al. (1996) Heterogeneity in telomere length of human chromosomes. *Hum. Mol. Genet.* **5,** 685–691.

21

Measurement of Telomerase Activity in Human Hematopoietic Cells and Neoplastic Disorders

Kazuma Ohyashiki and Junko H. Ohyashiki

1. Introduction

Human chromosomal termini, called telomeres, consist of tandem repeat (TTAGGG) sequences *(1)* and the length of this portion progressively shortens with each cell division *(2–8)*. The terminal portions of chromosomes lose the 5' end, and, thus, since the formation of the Okazaki fragment is not accomplished, DNA does not extend toward 3'. This phenomenon was proposed by Watson *(9)* in 1972 and has been designated as the end-replication problem *(9–11)*. Telomeres in dividing cells become shortened and in somatic cells the proliferative capability ceases by decrement of telomere length at a critical level, approx 2.5 kb *(5,7)*. Telomere shortening is observed in peripheral blood cells at a rate of 40 bp/yr and in cultured cells at 40–60 bp/cell division *(12–14)*. This is why telomeres are referred to as mitotic clocks or mitotic bombs *(15)*. Although telomere erosion occurs by division of actively proliferative cells, immortal cells, including cancer cells, become able to express telomerase activity synthesizing a *de novo* telomere DNA sequence that maintains cellular proliferative capability and, thus, avoids proliferative crisis.

Telomerase is a ribonucleoprotein *(16,17)* that is detected in >90% of primary cancer tissues using a telomeric repeat amplification protocol (TRAP) assay *(18)*. Recently, it has been demonstrated that peripheral blood cells and some normal hematopoietic stem cells have telomerase activity *(14,19–21)*. This indicates that active proliferative cells in the component of stem cells have telomerase activity to prevent progressive shortening of telomeres resulting in cell death. However, the telomere dynamics of the most primitive stem cells, which may be quiescent, have not been clarified. Telomerase activity is not detectable in somatic cells, except hematopoietic cells and cryptic cells in

From: *Methods in Molecular Medicine, vol. 68: Molecular Analysis of Cancer*
Edited by: J. Boultwood and C. Fidler © Humana Press Inc., Totowa, NJ

279

the intestine *(22)* and hair follicles *(23)*; thus, the definition of telomerase activity in cancer cells, except for hematologic neoplasias, is easy to determine. In hematologic neoplasias, the determination of telomerase-positive cells derived from neoplastic clone can be difficult, because normal hematopoietic cells have detectable telomerase activity *(24,25)*. This clearly indicates that caution should be exerted in the determination of telomerase-positive leukemia cells, and one should determine the telomerase activity quantitatively.

1.1. Telomere Length in Hematologic Neoplasias

Telomere structures protect chromosomal ends from illegitimate recombination *(4,26)*. Thus, reduction of telomere length associated with cell division may induce telomeric association, e.g., the presence of dicentric chromosomes and chromosome instability *(26)*. Telomere length is measurable using Southern blot analysis of *Hinf*I-digested DNA *(1)*. The telomeres are detected as smearlike bands, the most dense portion of which is measured and represented as a terminal restriction fragment (TRF). Thus, telomere length may vary among cell types and chromosomes even within a single cell, but at this time one can only define TRF as a representative telomere length *(28)*. Based on this study, the reduction of TRF correlated with the number of division of cells in in vitro and in vivo conditions *(15)* (**Fig. 1**). When cultured cells became immortal and telomere length shortened, telomeric association became evident, however, in clinical samples telomeric association is uncommon. Since detectable cytogenetic changes in clinical samples result from clonal selection of neoplastic cells, one might not show an exact association between telomere shortening and the presence of certain chromosome abnormalities. TRFs in peripheral mononuclear cells, possibly reflecting the TRFs of the major part of normal resting lymphocytes, reduced in size with aging *(13,14)*. As reported previously, however, the TRFs in bone marrow cells are not particularly different from those in peripheral mononuclear cells *(27,28)*. We and other researchers have identified the formula for the reduction rate of TRF in peripheral mononuclear cells *(27,28)*; thus, in this review the term reduced TRF means reduction in telomere length compared to this formula obtained from normal peripheral mononuclear cells. Reduction in telomere length, therefore, should be determined based on the age of each individual.

1.2. Detection of Telomerase Activity in Leukemia Cells

1.2.1. Detection of Telomerase Activity

The introduction of the TRAP assay based on a polymerase chain reaction (PCR) by Kim *(see **refs.** 18, 29, and 30)* has made it possible to detect telomerase with a much greater sensitivity than previously *(31)*. With this

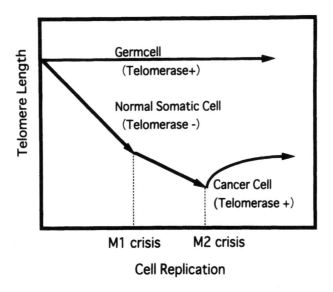

Fig. 1. Reduction in telomere length depends on cell division. Without the presence of telomerase activity, likely in normal somatic cells, telomere length reduces its size owing to the end-replication problem. At the M1 crisis, most cells cease cell division. DNA virus transformed somatic cells can overcome the M1 crisis without upregulation of telomerase activity. At the M2 crisis, cells without telomerase activity stop dividing and senesce. In cancer cells, even though they have reduced telomere length, they maintain cell replication owing to upregulation of telomerase activity (i.e., the telomere-telomerase hypothesis originally proposed by Harley *[15]*).

method, telomerase activity was demonstrated in >90% of primary tumors and almost all established cancer cell lines *(18)*. TRAP assay uses a certain protein content, and dilution experiments permit the determination of inhibitor(s) for PCR. It is easy to count blood mononuclear cells, including leukemia cells; therefore, we counted the number of cells and used them for the TRAP assay. This allows us to calculate the telomerase activity easily. Moreover, as reported previously, hematopoietic stem cells and peripheral mononuclear cells in younger individuals have detectable telomerase activity *(14,20)*; thus, we modified the TRAP assay to detect telomerase activity semiquantitatively, called fluorescence-based TRAP assay. On the other hand, Tatematsu et al. *(21)* developed a "stretch PCR assay" also to detect telomerase activity semiquantitatively.

1.2.2. Fluorescence-Based TRAP Assay

To semiquantitate telomerase activity, we use fluorescence end-labeled CX and TS primers, an internal control, and an automated laser fluorescence DNA sequencer *(32,33)*. This technique allows us to determine telomerase activity in real time and to calculate relative telomerase activity without using a photocapture system. We first calculate 2000 blood mononuclear cells and extract protein from the sample using a previously reported method (18). Telomerase activity was assessed according to the method of Kim et al. (18) and Piatyszek et al. (29) with modifications using the TRAP-eze detection kit (Oncor), and an automated laser fluorescence DNA sequencer. The TRAP assay procedure was performed according to the supplier's instruction and the report by Holt et al. (34). The frozen cell pellets were dissolved in 10–30 µL of 1X CHAPS lysis buffer, incubated on ice for 30 min, and then centrifuged at 10,000g for 30 min at 4°C. The supernatants were collected, and the protein content was determined using standard procedures (BCA protein assay). Briefly, 2 µL of the cell extract (equivalent to 3 µg of protein) was added to a 48-µL reaction solution consisting of 10X TRAP buffer (Oncor), 50X deoxynucleotide triphosphates (dNTPs) mix (Oncor), 10 pmol of fluorescein isothiocyanate–labeled TS primer 5'-AAT CCG TCG AGC AGA GTT-3' (5'-end labeling using FluorePrime™; Pharmacia Biotech, Uppsala, Sweden), TRAP primer mix already including a 36-bp internal standard (Oncor), 2 U of *Taq* polymerase (Takara Shuzo, Shiga, Japan), and distilled H_2O. The mixture was incubated at 30°C for 10 min and then was heated at 90°C for 90 s. The PCR conditions were 30 cycles of 94°C for 30 s, 55°C for 30 s, and 72°C for 1.5 min. The PCR products (1.5 µL) were subjected to 12% denaturing electrophoresis in an automated laser fluorescence DNA sequencer II (Pharmacia Biotech) and analyzed by the Fragment Manager program (Pharmacia Biotech). To compare the relative amount of telomerase activity between samples, a ratio of the 36-bp internal standard to the telomerase peak was calculated (**Fig. 2**). To confirm that the sample contained telomerase activity, multiple periodic 6-bp peaks of telomerase signal had to be detected, and preincubation of the extract with heat (95°C, 1.5 min) or RNase eliminated the periodic peak.

1.3. Telomerase Activity in Normal Hematopoietic Cells

1.3.1. Telomerase Activity in Hematopoietic Stem Cells

Human hematopoietic stem cells are considered to be enriched in CD34+ cells' population, although in the mouse most primitive stem cells exist in the CD34− fraction, and it is still controversial whether or not human hematopoietic stem cells exist in the CD34− fraction. In the CD34+ cell fraction, cells with CD38 antigen have more committed characteristics with elevated telomerase activity compared with the CD34+/CD38+ population (20). Engelhardt et al. (35) confirmed this evidence that telomerase activity in CD34+/CD38+ cells exceeds levels in CD34+/CD38− and CD34− cells. They also demonstrated that telomerase activity is highest in bone marrow CD34+

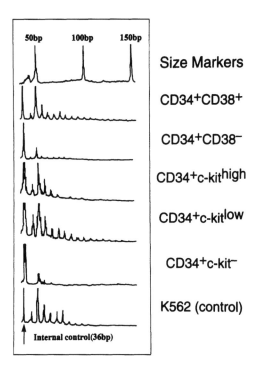

Fig. 2. Fluorocurve of the fluorescence-based TRAP assay. Each 6-bp peak corresponds to telomerase activity. In comparison with the area of the 36-bp internal control signal, telomerase signals could be calculated and determined as relative telomerase activity *(39)*.

cells followed by peripheral blood and umbilical cord blood. It is noteworthy, that they did not observe any particular difference in telomere length between bone marrow CD34+ cells and peripheral blood (7.6 kb vs 7.4 kb), but that cord blood cells had long telomeres (10.4 kb) *(35)*. Moreover, they found a correlation between telomerase activity, cell cycle status, and the expression of cyclin D1 and cyclin A *(35)*. Other investigators also confirmed these observations *(36,37)*. Chiu et al. *(38)* demonstrated that early progenitors (CD34+/CD71+) expressed telomerase activity at a higher level, which was subsequently downregulated in response to cytokines, and that primitive hematopoietic stem cells (CD34+/CD71^{low}/CD45RA^{low}) had low levels of telomerase activity *(38)*. Moreover, c-kit negative cells in the CD34+ fraction are considered to contain the most primitive stem cells within the CD34+ fraction.

Regarding telomerase activity, CD34+/c-kit− cells carry very low telomerase activity, whereas those with CD34+/c-kit− apparently have telomerase activity (**Fig. 3**) *(39)*. This clearly indicates that most primitive hematopoietic stem

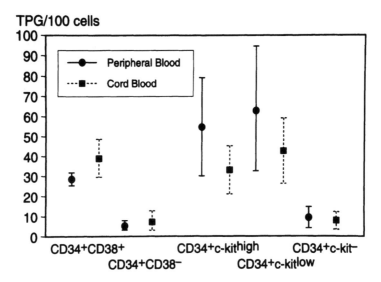

Fig. 3. Telomerase activity in hematopoietic stem cells sorted. Both cord blood cells and granulocyte colony-stimulating factor induced peripheral blood cells expressing CD34$^+$/c-kit$^-$ cells with much higher telomerase activity compared with those with CD34$^+$/c-kit^{high} and CD34$^+$/c-kit^{low}. These results indicate that CD34$^+$/c-kit$^-$ cells may be the most primitive hematopoietic stem cells. TPG, total product generation.

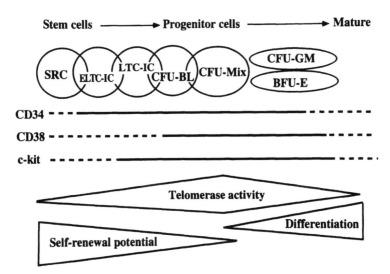

Fig. 4. Schematic presentation of differential level and expression of telomerase activity in hematopoietic stem cells.

cells might be low or negative for telomerase activity, and after they enter the cell cycle they become telomerase positive (**Fig. 4**). Thus, most primitive stem

Telomerase in Human Leukemias

cells may not have telomerase activity since they are quiescent, and it is currently demonstrated that cells in the G0 phase do not express telomerase activity. When a part of them enters a proliferative population, telomere erosion starts and telomerase activity may be upregulated.

The telomere-telomerase relationship allows us to speculate that there is a certain controlling mechanism or mechanisms that upregulate telomerase activity. Therefore, all these results supported the concept that purified hematopoietic stem cells show dramatic functional differences in turnover time and the ability to produce cells with stem cell properties *(40)*.

1.3.2. Telomerase Activity in Normal Peripheral Blood Cells

Peripheral blood mononuclear cells obtained from normal individuals show detectable telomerase activity *(14,20,21)*. As Tatematsu et al. *(21)* demonstrated, peripheral leukocytes from younger individuals show detectable telomerase activity, whereas those in older individuals do not. The exact mechanism of downregulation of telomerase activity with aging is obscure. Our study demonstrated that about half of the samples of peripheral mononuclear cells obtained from subjects older than 40 yr did not have detectable telomerase activity and the remaining samples had very low telomerase activity *(14)*. By contrast, all samples obtained from subjects younger than 20 yr have detectable telomerase activity and show relatively high telomerase activity when compared with those age 20 yr *(14)*. Thus, telomerase activity in normal individuals younger than 40 yr progressively declined with increased age, whereas those age 40 yr or older had a very low level or no detectable telomerase activity that was stably maintained (**Fig. 5**). In peripheral granulocytes, however, no telomerase activity was detectable *(41)*.

1.3.3. Upregulation of Telomerase Activity After Cytokine or Mitogen Exposure

Most primitive bone marrow progenitors expressing telomerase activity showed downregulation of activity after cytokine exposure *(35,36)*; Yui et al. *(36)* demonstrated that telomerase activity was up-regulated after culturing purified hematopoietic stem cells (CD34$^+$/CD71^{low}/CD45RA^{low}) with stem cell factors, interleukin-3 and Flt3-ligand, but not with a combination of stem cell factor and Flt3-ligand, indicating that IL-3 is a key cytokine in the differentiation of hematopoietic stem cells. Engelhardt et al. *(35)* also found that telomerase activity was upregulated within 48–72 h after culturing with IL-3, IL-6, erythropoietin, and granulocyte colony-stimulating factor, decreasing to baseline after 3 to 4 wk.

It is well known that mitogen-stimulated lymphocytes show upregulation of telomerase activity *(20)*: circulating T-lymphocytes *(20,42)* and B-lymphocytes

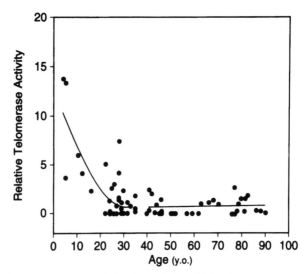

Fig. 5. Relative telomerase activity in peripheral blood mononuclear cells obtained from normal individuals of various ages. Most individuals younger than 20 yr had detectable telomerase activity. However, about 50% of individuals older than 40 yr had no telomerase activity in the peripheral blood cells *(14)*.

(19,43) in peripheral blood have telomerase activity. In T-lymphocytes, telomerase upregulation was noted by stimulation of not only anti-CD3 monoclonal antibody but also Ca ionophore and phorbol myristate acetate, which were considered to be the stimulants that bypass T-cell receptor signaling *(44,45)*. It was also demonstrated that telomerase activity is induced in the B-lymphocyte activation of the antigen-specific immune response *(46–49)*.

1.4. Telomerase Activity in Acute Leukemia

1.4.1. Telomerase Activity in Freshly Obtained Acute Leukemia Cells

Most acute leukemia cases have reduced telomere length, and this may represent active cell division. It has been demonstrated that leukemia cells have a short telomere length at the time of diagnosis and that their length returns to within the normal range during the complete remission state *(27,28)*. This trend is particularly common in acute myelogenous leukemia (AML) *(27,28,50)* and acute lymphoid leukemia *(51)*. Although Takeuchi et al. *(50)* reported that t(8;21) acute leukemia had a significant short telomere length at the time of diagnosis, other investigators did not confirm this change *(27,28)*. In acute leukemia, a significant overlapping of telomerase activity between acute leukemia cells and normal peripheral mononuclear cells has been reported *(52,53)*. In some patients with acute leukemia, telomere length decreases, but the short-

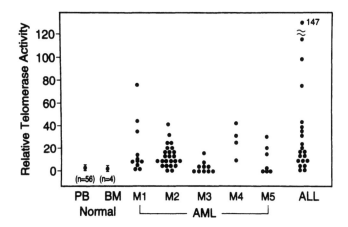

Fig. 6. Relative telomerase activity in acute leukemia patients. Patients with AML-M3 had low but detectable telomerase activity. About 70% of acute leukemia patients had high telomerase activity compared with that of age-matched normal individuals.

ening of telomeres might not reach the critical level for upregulation of telomerase activity, whereas some leukemia patients may have normal TRFs that may result from upregulation of telomerase activity. This is supported by the finding that the length of TRFs and level of telomerase activity in each patient did not show any particular correlation *(52)*.

Thus, we should determine both TRF length and telomerase activity in leukemia patients. In previously reported studies, about 70% of acute leukemia patients had elevated telomerase activity at the time of diagnosis *(52–54)*, and the remaining patients had detectable telomerase activity but within the age-matched normal range (**Fig. 6**). By using a stretch PCR assay, Tatematsu et al. *(21)* demonstrated that most AML patients in their study had telomerase activity. At the time of relapse, higher telomerase activity was noted compared with that at the time of diagnosis *(52,54)*. This may partially support the concept that relapsed leukemia cells have more malignant characteristics. Nevertheless, although most acute leukemia patients have shortened TRFs, some acute leukemia patients hve telomeres that might not reach the critical point for reactivating telomerase activity. It has been demonstrated that telomerase activity in myeloid leukemia cells is downregulated during the process of cellular differentiation *(53)*. AML is categorized into several subtypes based on morphologic and cytologic characteristics (M0–M7), and some of them have cellular differentiation mimicking either normal or catastrophic differentiation. This suggests the possibility that telomerase activity in certain leukemia cells showing differentiation potential may be downregulated. Another key point is that telomerase activity in leukemia cells may be controlled by the cell cycle; quiescent cells (e.g., cells in the G0 phase and most primitive stem cells) have downregulation of the expression of telomerase activity. It is well known that a part of the population of *de novo* leukemia cells enters the G0 phase. These observations may indicate that telomerase activity in leukemia cells may depend on the population of leukemia cells in certain cell-cycle phases and with cellular differentiation, in addition to controlling the mechanism of the telomere-telomerase relationship.

Zhang et al. *(53)* demonstrated that acute leukemia patients with high telomerase activity are significantly frequent among in patients showing –7/7q– and 11q23 anomalies, and high telomerase activity indicates an extremely poor prognosis. As already discussed in a study by Ohyashiki et al. *(52)*, about 30% of acute leukemia patients had telomerase activity within the normal range. About 10% of the acute leukemia pateints had high levels of telomerase activity (equivalent level of telomerase activity in solid tumors), and they had a significantly poorer outcome (**Fig. 7**): all of them expired within 12 mo after the diagnosis of acute leukemia *(52)*. Therefore, high levels of telomerase activity in acute leukemia might be an indicator of unfavorable prognosis. Acute leukemia patients with extremely high telomerase activity consisted of one patient with AML and four with ALL, and they showed t(6;9), t(9;22), and t(17;19) anomalies *(52)*, and these cytogenetic changes were linked to poor outcome. Thus, although acute leukemia patients with high levels of telomerase activity might have an unfavorable prognosis, it is difficult to conclude whether prognosis of those leukemia patients is related to upregulation of telomerase activity or transformation activity related to gene translocation.

1.4.2. Telomerase Activity Downregulate in Differentiated Leukemia Cells

In patients with acute promyelocytic leukemia (FAB-M3), telomerase activity is not elevated compared with other types of leukemia *(52)*. In a differentiation experiment using an AML cell line, HL-60, cells differentiated using all-*trans*-retinoic acid had reduced telomerase activity *(53,55,56,57)*. However, some differentiated cells without proliferative capability maintain elevated telomerase activity, indicating that the signaling pathway that affects cellular differentiation may also reduce telomerase activity independently. Although some solid tumors with differentiation have relatively low telomerase activity compared with those with undifferentiated tumors, the level of telomerase activity is not simply related to differentiation stage of cancer cells.

1.5. Telomere Dynamics in Chronic Leukemia

1.5.1. Telomerase Activity in Chronic Myeloid Leukemia

Chronic myelogenous leukemia (CML) is characterized by a specific t(9;22)(q22;q34) chromosomal translocation that creates $p210^{BCR/ABL}$ chimeric

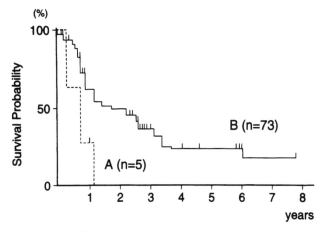

Fig. 7. Survival probability of acute leukemia patients depends on telomerase activity. Acute leukemia patients with high telomerase activity (relative telomerase activity >50, equivalent to solid tumor level) had a significantly poorer outcome compared with those with <50 relative telomerase activity *(52)*.

protein, and this is important in signal transduction, which promotes proliferation of leukemia cells. In CML, most patients in the chronic phase have shortened telomere lengths. The most likely explanation for this observation might be that active cell division of hematopoietic stem cells without apparent elevated telomerase activity resulted in telomere erosion. However, hematopoietic cells possess telomerase activity and CML is one of the stem cell diseases, thus, reduction rates of telomeres in CML patients in the chronic phase overcome the rate of repair of chromosomal ends by telomerase activity. The high replicative capability of CML cells might result in progressive telomere shortening. Telomerase activity in the chronic phase of CML is enhanced. There is no significant difference in telomerase levels between peripheral mononuclear cells from normal subjects (resting lymphocytes) and mononuclear cells (myeloid cells) of CML cells *(58)*. However, granulocytes from normal individuals do not express telomerase activity; upregulation of telomerase activity in CML myeloid cells might represent neoplastic characteristics. Telomerase activity in granulocytes in CML patients might be downregulated during the process of granulocytic differentiation, as reported by Zhang et al. *(53)* using myeloid leukemia cells. Thus, the telomerase activity in the granulocytes of CML patients might not exactly reflect telomerase activity in the stem cells of CML patients. Blast crisis in some CML patients is accompanied by additional cytogenetic anomalies, and blastic transformation is considered to result from genetic alterations and clonal selection.

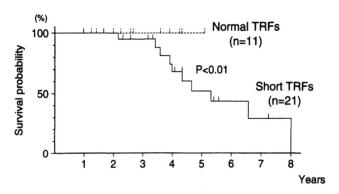

Fig. 8. Survival probability of CML patients depends on telomere length. CML patients with telomere length within the age-matched normal range had a significantly better outcome compared with those with shortened telomere length *(59)*.

1.5.1.1. TELOMERE DYNAMICS IN CML IN THE CHRONIC PHASE

In the chronic phase of CML, low, but detectable, telomerase activity is demonstrated *(21,58,59)*. Telomere length in the chronic phase varies and some patients show normal telomere length (i.e., TRF length within the normal range) *(59)*. We have demonstrated that CML patients with normal TRF lengths at the time of diagnosis responded well to interferon-alpha treatment, and they had a favorable prognosis (**Fig. 8**) *(59)*. This indicates that telomere length in CML patients may reflect disease severity and further suggests that measurement of telomere length might provide an indicator for interferon-alpha treatment. When CML patients were divided into two groups according to TRF length, CML patients with normal TRF length had significantly low levels of telomerase activity compared with those with shortened TRF length at the time of diagnosis *(59)*. It is possible, therefore, that CML patients with short telomere length with elevated telomerase activity might reflect the excess amount of myeloid progenitor cells and be related to disease severity.

1.5.1.2. TELOMERASE ACTIVITY IN CML IN THE BLASTIC PHASE

In blast crisis, telomerase activity is significantly elevated compared with that in the chronic phase (**Fig. 9**) *(21,58)*. It is still controversial whether elevated telomerase activity in the blast phase reflects blast clones in the chronic phase or whether it is owing to reduction in telomeres *(24,25)*. We have reported a relationship between reduction in telomere length and reactivation of telomerase activity during the process of establishing leukemia cell lines *(60)*. In the chronic phase, reduction in telomere length was not remarkable *(61)*, but telomeres became shortened to the critical point, and high telomerase activity was evident when they developed blast crisis. If the short

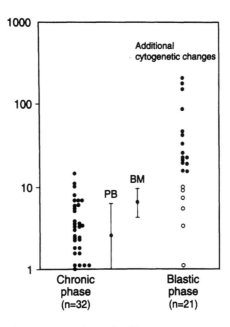

Fig. 9. Relative telomerase activity in CML patients in the chronic and blastic phases. A significant elevation of telomerase activity was noted in the blast phase, and most patients with high telomerase activity showed additional cytogenetic changes. PB, peripheral blood cells; BM, bone marrow cells.

telomeres and high telomerase activity reflect blast cells that exist in the chronic phase (preexisting as a minor clone), how can one explain why they show very short TRFs in the blast phase?

The blast cells in both the chronic and blast phases carry the Ph translocation and they may have transforming potential. Thus, the most plausible explanation for the telomere dynamics in CML might be that Ph chromosome-positive cells, including CML stem cells, have a high proliferative potential in the chronic phase that may overcome telomerase activity, resulting in progressive erosion of telomeres. CML stem cells that can produce blast crisis (actually present in the chronic phase) may be quiescent. Thus, they may keep telomere length without the presence of upregulated telomerase. However, we do not have any evidence that blast cells in the chronic phase are quiescent until blast crisis is clinically detectable. One can speculate that additional genetic changes cause the quiescent blast cells to "wake up," and then the blast cells obtain high proliferative capability resulting in the telomere length becoming shorter and shorter. Furthermore, this process may upregulate telomerase activity. According to this hypothesis, telomere dynamics in the chronic phases and blast phase might not be similar events. This aspect might be clarified by detecting telomerase activity at each cell level in the chronic and blast phases.

1.5.2. Telomerase Activity in Chronic Lymphocytic Leukemia

In chronic lymphocytic leukemia (CLL), Counter et al. *(19)* telomerase activity was reported to be undetectable in the stable phase, whereas in the blast phase telomerase is upregulated. The important evidence for this is that telomerase activity in the CLL-stable phase is undetectable; thus, it is lower than in normal peripheral blood cells. This indicates that telomerase activity is not related to the mass of neoplastic cells but is linked to the population of quiescent cells. In CLL patients, active production of CLL cells is present, but once the cells (CLL cells in the peripheral blood) become quiescent, they lose their telomerase activity, indicating that telomerase activity in neoplastic cells could also be downregulated. When CLL cells actively proliferate (terminal phase), they restore or show upregulation of telomerase activity. Therefore, it is easy to consider that upregulation and downregulation of telomerase activity can be coexistent not only in the same patient but also in the same tumor.

1.6. Telomere Dynamics in Myelodysplastic Syndromes

Myelodysplastic syndrome (MDS) encompasses a heterogeneous category of diseases showing cytopenia in the peripheral blood and characteristic dysplastic morphologic features *(62)*. Approximately 30% of MDSs develop into leukemia, but some of them suffer from "bone marrow failure." We reported an association between the disease progression pattern and reduction of telomeres in the developmental process of disease in MDS patients *(63)*. The likely explanation of the genetic change during the process of disease progression is the genetic instability that was demonstrated by microsatellite alteration. Although the question of any correlation among cytogenetic changes, microsatellite alteration, and telomere reduction in MDS patients is obscure, this may be partially owing to the heterogeneous category of this disease entity. Chromosomal changes related to telomere reduction are also rarely seen in MDS with disease progression. Therefore, we focused on the disease progression pattern in MDS and cytogenetic changes or telomere length. Some MDS patients showed telomere reduction and karyotypic progression with disease progression, whereas some had telomere shortening before disease progression with multiple chromosomal changes. Telomere shortening was evident in all subtypes of MDS; thus, the replication history in each MDS patient that depends on telomere erosion is not related to the percentage of blast cells. There have been no reports regarding telomerase activity in MDS patients. Further studies in this field might disclose a possible association between telomere dynamics and the outcome of MDS patients.

1.6.1. Telomere Length in Myelodysplastic Syndromes

As mentioned below, telomerase activity in MDS patients is detectable but not as elevated as in those with *de novo* acute leukemia, and telomere length is

Telomerase in Human Leukemias

correlated with disease severity *(64)*. About 70% of MDS patients had shortened TRF length. This might be owing to the insufficient upregulation mechanism of telomerase. MDS patients with shortened TRF length had a significantly high incidence of cytogenetic abnormalities, multiple cytopenias, and marrow blast percentage. Patients with shortened TRF length were frequently seen in the International Prognostic Scoring System (IPSS) *(65)* high-risk group ($p < 0.01$) *(66)*. MDS patients with shortened TRF length had a very poor prognosis ($p < 0.01$), suggesting that telomere dynamics may be linked to clinical outcome in MDS patients *(66)*. Thus, an abnormal mechanism of telomere maintenance mechanism in subgroups of MDS patients may be an early indication of genomic instability. This study demonstrates that telomere stability is frequently impaired in a high-risk group of MDS patients and suggests that in combination with the IPSS classification system, measurement of TRFs may be useful for risk stratification and, in the future, management of the care of MDS patients *(66)*.

1.7. Conclusion

Telomeres are very important structures that protect chromosomal ends from recombination, but the structure itself induces irreversible reduction without the presence of telomerase activity. Researchers are now collecting evidence of telomere dynamics in clinical samples, but we are still far from being able to discuss telomere dynamics and chromosomal changes in such materials. Although there is a growing body of evidence that telomerase might be a very important key enzyme to obtain immortality, and possibly oncogenesis, other pathways for immortal characteristics are currently being reported. Moreover, we do not have any evidence at hand to indicate whether quiescent cells, especially most primitive stem cells, have telomerase activity or not *(67–73)*.

2. Materials
2.1. Preparation of Cell Lysate

1. Wash buffer: 10 mM HEPES, pH 7.5, 1.5 mM MgCl$_2$, 10 mM KCl, 1 mM dithiothreitol.
2. Lysis buffer: 10 mM Tris-HCl, pH 7.5, 1 mM MgCl$_2$, 1 mM EGTA, 0.1 M phenlymethylsulfonyl fluoride, 5 mM β-mercaptoethanol, 0.5% CHAPS (Pierce), 10% glycerol.

2.2. Amplification

1. Fluorescence-labeled CX reverse primer: 5' CCC TTA CCC TTA CCC TTA CCC TTA 3'.
2. Ampliwax (Perkin-Elmer).
3. 1 M Tris-HCl, pH 8.3.

4. 50 mM MgCl$_2$.
5. KCl.
6. Tween-20.
7. 0.1 M EGTA.
8. Deoxynucleoside triphosphates: 2.5 mM each.
9. Fluorescent-labeled TS forward primer: 5' AAT CCG TCG AGC AGA GTT 3'.
10. T4 gene 32 protein (Boehringer Mannheim).
11. Bovine serum albumin (BSA).
12. *Taq* DNA polyerase.
13. RNase.
14. Thermal cycler.

2.3. Analysis

1. Long Ranger polyacrylamide gel mix (AT Biochem).
2. 1X Tris-borate EDTA (TBE): 45 mM Tris-borate, 1 mM EDTA.
3. Loading buffer: 90% formamide, 10% blue dextran.
4. Fluorescent size markers (100, 150, and 200 bp).
5. ALF automated DNA sequencer II (Pharmacia Biotech).
6. ALF Fragment Manager Program (Pharmacia Biotech).

3. Methods
3.1. Preparation of Cell Lysate

1. Resuspend 1×10^7 cells from either fresh samples or dimethylsulfoxide-free samples stored at –80°C in 1 mL of ice-cold wash buffer, and centrifuge at 16,000g at 4°C for 1 min.
2. Resuspend the cell pellets in 100 µL of ice-cold lysis buffer.

3.2. Amplification

1. Lyophilize 0.1 µg of fluorescence labeled CX reverse primer in a microtube, and seal with Ampliwax.
2. Add 50 µL of TRAP reactions above the wax barrier containing 20 mM Tris-HCl, pH 8.3, 1.5 mM MgCl$_2$, 63 mM KCl, 0.005% Tween-20, 1 mM EGTA, 50 µM deoxynucleoside triphosphates, 0.1 µg of fluorescence labeled TS forward primer, 1 µg of T4 gene 32 protein, 0.1 mg/mL of BSA, 2 U of *Taq* DNA polymerase, and 5 µg of the CHAPS cell extract. For RNase treatment, incubate 5 µg of extract 1 µg of RNase for 20 min at 37°C before PCR amplification. For standardization of telomerase activity, we used internal telomerase assay standard (provided by Prof. Jerry W. Shay, Department of Cell Biology and Neuroscience, The University of Texas, Southwestern Medical Center, Dallas, TX) generating the 150-bp product or internal standard (TRAP-eze kit; Oncor) generating the 36-bp product.
3. Place the prepared microtube at 22°C for 10 min for telomerase-mediated extension of the TS primer. Heat-inactivate the reaction mixture at 90°C for 90 s.
4. Perform the PCR in a thermal cycler under the following conditions: 27 cycles of 94°C for 30 s, 50°C for 30 s, and 72°C for 90 s.

Telomerase in Human Leukemias

3.3. Analysis

1. Prepare an 8% denaturing gel (Long Ranger) containing 6 M urea according to the supplier's instructions. Use glass plates for the ALF DNA sequencer II.
2. Add 1X TBE running buffer to the gel apparatus of the sequencer.
3. Mix 1 µL of the PCR product with 1 µL of loading buffer.
4. Denature for 1 min at 95°C, and then chill quickly on ice. Load the samples on the 8% denaturing gel. Use 100-, 150-, and 200-bp fluorescent size markers.
5. Run the DNA sequencer.
6. The fluorescent gel data obtained by the ALF DNA sequencer II are collected and analyzed automatically by the Fragment Manager Program. Each fluorescent peak is quantitated in terms of size (base pair), peak height, and peak area.

References

1. Moyzis, R. K., Buckingham, J. M., Cram, L. S., Dani, M., Deaven, L. L., Jones, M. D., et al. (1988) A highly conserved repetitive DNA sequence, (TTAGGG)$_n$, present at the telomeres of human chromosomes. *Proc. Natl. Acad. Sci. USA* **85,** 6622–6626.
2. Zakian, V. A. (1989) Structure and function of telomeres. *Annu. Rev. Genet.* **23,** 579–604.
3. Blackburn, E. H. (1991) Structure and function of telomeres. *Nature* **350,** 569–573.
4. de Lange, T., Shiue, L., Myers, R. M., Cox, D. R., Naylor, S. L., Killery, A. M., and Varmus, H. E. (1990) Structure and variability of human chromosome ends. *Mol. Cell. Biol.* **10,** 518–527.
5. de Lange, T. (1995) Telomere dynamics and genome instability in human cancer, in *Telomeres* (Blackburn, E. H. and Greider, C. W., eds.), Cold Spring Harbor Laboratory Press, Plainview, NY, pp. 265–293.
6. Harley, C. B., Futcher, A. B., and Greider, C. W. (1990) Telomeres shorten during ageing of human fibroblasts. *Nature* **345,** 458–460.
7. Hastie, N. D., Dempster, M., Dunlop, M. G., Thompson, A. M., Green, D. K., and Allshire, R. C. (1990) Telomere reduction in human colorectal carcinoma and with ageing. *Nature* **346,** 866–868.
8. Allsopp, R. C., Vaziri, H., Patterson, C., Goldstein, S., Younglai, E. V., Futcher, A. B., et al. (1992) Telomere length predicts replicative capacity of human fibroblasts. *Proc. Natl. Acad. Sci. USA* **89,** 10.114–10.118.
9. Watson, J. D. (1972) Origin of concatemeric T7 DNA. *Nature* **239,** 197–201.
10. Olovnikov, A. M. (1973) A theory of marginotomy. The incomplete copying of template margin in enzymic synthesis of polynucleotides and biological significance of the phenomenon. *J. Theor. Biol.* **41,** 181–190.
11. Levy, M. Z., Allsopp, R. C., Futcher, A. B., Greider, C. W., and Harley, C. B. (1992) Telomere end-replication problem and cell aging. *J. Mol. Biol.* **225,** 951–960.
12. Lindsey, J., Mcgill, N. I., Lindsey, L. A., Green, D. K., Cooke, H. J. (1991) In vivo loss of telomeric repeats with age in humans. *Mut. Res.* **256,** 45–48.
13. Satoh, H., Hiyama, K., Takeda, M., Awaya, Y., Watanabe, K., Ihara, Y., et al. (1996) Telomere shortening in peripheral blood cells was related with aging but not with white blood cell count. *Jpn. J. Hum. Genet.* **41,** 413–417.

14. Iwama, H., Ohyashiki, K., Ohyashiki, J. H., Hayashi, S., Yahata, N., Ando, K., et al. (1998) Telomeric length and telomerase activity vary with age in peripheral blood cells obtained from normal individuals. *Hum. Genet.* **102,** 397–402.
15. Harley, C. B. (1991) Telomere loss, Mitotic clock or genetic time bomb? *Mut. Res.* **256,** 271–282.
16. Morin, G. B. (1989) The human telomere terminal transferase enzyme is a ribonucleoprotein that synthesizes TTAGGG repeats. *Cell* **59,** 521–529.
17. Blackburn, E. H. (1982) Telomerases. *Annu. Rev. Biochem.* **61,** 113–129.
18. Kim, N. W., Piatyszek, M. A., Prowse, K. R., Harley, C. B., West, M. D., Ho, P. L. C., et al. (1994) Specific association of human telomerase activity with immortal cells and cancer. *Science* **266,** 2011–2015.
19. Counter, C. M., Gupta, J., Harley, C. B., Leber, B., Bacchetti, S. (1995) Telomerase activity in normal leukocytes and in hematologic malignancies. *Blood* **85,** 2315–2320.
20. Hiyama, K., Hirai, Y., Koizumi, S., Akiyama, M., Hiyama, E., Piatyszek, M. A., et al. (1995) Activation of telomerase in human lymphocytes and hematopoietic progenitor cells. *J. Immunol.* **155,** 3711–3715.
21. Tatematsu, K., Nakayama, J., Danbara, M., Shionoya, S., Sato, H., Omine, M., and Ishikawa, F. (1996) A novel quantitative "stretch PCR assay" that detects a dramatic increase in telomerase activity during the progression of myeloid leukemias. *Oncogene* **13,** 2265–2274.
22. Hiyama, E., Hiyama, K., Tatsumoto, N., Kodama, T., Shay, J. W., and Yokoyama, T. (1996) Telomerase activity in human intestine. *Intl. J. Oncol.* **9,** 453–458.
23. Ramirez, R. D., Wright, W. E., Shay, J. W., and Taylor, R. S. (1997) Telomerase activity concentrates in the mitotically active segments of human hair follicles. *J. Invest. Dermatol.* **108,** 113–117.
24. Shay, J. W. and Wright, W. E. (1996) The reactivation of telomerase activity in cancer progression. *Trends Genet.* **12,** 129–131.
25. Greaves, M. F. (1996) Is telomerase activity in cancer due to selection of stem cells and differentiation arrest? *Trends Genet.* **12,** 127,128.
26. Counter, C. M., Avilion, A. A., LeFeuvre, C. E., Stewart, N. G., Greider, C. W., Harley, C. B., and Bacchetti, S. (1992) Telomere shortening associated with chromosome instability is arrested in immortal cells which express telomerase activity. *EMBO J.* **11,** 1921–1929.
27. Yamada, O., Oshimi, K., Motoji, T., and Mizoguchi, H. (1995) Telomeric DNA in normal and leukemic blood cells. *J. Clin. Invest.* **95,** 1117–1123.
28. Fujimura, T. (1995) Telomere shortening in hematopoietic neoplasias and its clinical implications. *J. Tokyo Med. Coll.* **53,** 652–663 (in Japanese).
29. Piatyszek, M. A., Kim, N. W., Weinrich, S. L., Hiyama, K., Hiyama, E., Wright, W. E., and Shay, J. W. (1995) Detection of telomerase activity in human cells and tumors by a telomeric repeat amplification protocol (TRAP). *Meth. Cell Sci.* **17,** 1–15.
30. Wright, W. E., Shay, J. W., and Piatyszek, M. A. (1995) Modifications of a telomeric repeat amplification protocol (TRAP) result in increased reliability, linearity and sensitivity. *Nucleic Acids Res.* **23,** 3794,3795.

Telomerase in Human Leukemias

31. Nilsson, P., Mehle, C., Remes, K., and Roos, G. (1994) Telomerase activity in vivo in human malignant hematopoietic cells. *Oncogene* **9,** 3043–3048.
32. Ohyashiki, J. H., Ohyashiki, K., Sano, T., and Toyama, K. (1996) Non-radioisotopic and semi-quantiative procedure for terminal repeat amplification protocol. *Jpn. J. Cancer Res.* **87,** 329–331.
33. Ohyashiki, J. H., Ohyashiki, K., Toyama, K., and Shay, J. W. (1996) A nonradioactive, fluorescence-based telomeric repeat amplification protocol to detect and quantitate telomerase activity. *Trends Genet.* **12,** 395–396.
34. Holt, S. E., Norton, J. C., Wright, W. E., and Shay, J. W. (1996) Comparison of the telomeric repeat amplification protocol (TRAP) to the new TRAP-eze telomerase detection kit. *Methods Cell Sci.* **18,** 237–248.
35. Engelhardt, M., Kumar, R., Albanell, J., Pettengell, R., Han, W., and Moore, M. A. (1997) Telomerase regulation, cell cycle, and telomere stability in primitive hematopoietic cells. *Blood* **90,** 182–193.
36. Yui, J., Chiu, C. P., and Lansdorp, P. M. (1998) Telomerase activity in candidate stem cells from fetal liver and adult bone marrow. *Blood* **91,** 3255–3262.
37. Hohaus, S., Voso, M. T., Orta-La Barbera, E., Cavallo, S., Bellacosa, A., et al. (1997) Telomerase activity in human hematopoietic progenitor cells. *Haematologica* **82,** 262–268.
38. Chiu, C. P., Dragowska, W., Kim, N. M., Vaziri, H., Yui, J., Thomas, Y. E., et al. (1996) Differential expression of telomerase activity in hematopoietic progenitors from adult human bone marrow. *Stem Cell* **14,** 239–248.
39. Sakabe, H., Yahata, N., Kimura, T., Zeng, Z. Z., Minamiguchi, H., Kaneko, H., et al. (1998) Human cord blood-derived primitive progenitors are enriched in CD34+c-kit⁻ cells, correlation between long-term culture-initiating cells and telomerase expression. *Leukemia* **12,** 728–734.
40. Lansdorp, P. M., Poon, S., Chavez, E., Dragowska, V., Zijlmans, M., Bryan, T., et al. (1997) Telomeres in haematopoietic system. *Ciba Found. Symp.* **211,** 209–218.
41. Engelhardt, M., Ozkaynak, M. F., Drullinsky, P., Sandoval, C., Tugal, O., Jayabose, S., and Moore, M. A. (1998) Telomerase activity and telomere length in pediatric patients with malignancies undergoing chemotherapy. *Leukemia* **12,** 13–24.
42. Pan, C, Xue, B-H., Ellis, T. M., Peace, D. J., and Diaz, M. O. (1997) Changes in telomerase activity and telomere length during human T lymphocyte senescence. *Exp. Cell Res.* **231,** 346–353.
43. Broccolli, D., Young, J. W., de Lange, T. (1995) Telomerase activity in normal and malignant hematopoietic cells. *Proc. Natl. Acad. Sci. USA* **92,** 9082–9086.
44. Igarashi, H. and Sakaguchi, N. (1996) Telomerase activity is induced by the stimulation to antigen receptor in human peripheral lymphocytes. *Biochem. Biophys. Res. Commun.* **219,** 649–655.
45. Weng, N. P., Levine, B. L., June, C. H., and Hodes, R. J. (1996) Regulated expression of telomerase activity in human T lymphocyte development and activation. *J. Exp. Med.* **183,** 2471–2479.
46. Igarashi, H. and Sakaguchi, N. (1997) Telomerase activity is induced in human peripheral B lymphocytes by the stimulation to antigen receptor. *Blood* **89,** 1299–1307.

47. Weng, N. P., Granger, L., and Hodes, R. J. (1997) Telomere lengthening and telomerase activaion during human B cell differentiation. *Proc. Natl. Acad. Sci. USA* **94,** 10,827–10,832.
48. Weng, N. P., Palmer, L. D., Levine, B. L., Lane, H. C., June, C. H., and Hodes, R. J. (1997) Tales of tails, regulation of telomere length and telomerase activity during lymphocyte development, differentiation, activation, and aging. *Immunol. Rev.* **160,** 43–54.
49. Yamada, O., Motoji, T., Mizoguchi, H. (1996) Up-regulation of telomerase activity in human lymphocytes. *Biochem. Biophy. Acta* **1314,** 260–266.
50. Takauchi, K., Tashiro, S., Ohtaki, M., Kamada, N. (1994) Telomere reduction of specific chromosome translocation in acute myelocytic leukemia. *Jpn. J. Cancer Res.* **85,** 127–130.
51. Adamson, D. J. A., King, D. J., Haites, N. E. (1992) Significant telomere shortening in childhood leukemia. *Cancer Genet. Cytogenet.* **61,** 204–206.
52. Ohyashiki, J. H., Ohyashiki, K., Iwama, H., Hayashi, S., Toyama, K., and Shay, J. W. (1997) Clinical implications of telomerase activity levels in acute leukemia. *Clin. Cancer Res.* **3,** 619–625.
53. Zhang, W., Piatyszek, M. A., Kobayashi, T., Estey, E., Andreeff, M., Deisseroth, A. B., et al. (1996) Telomerase activity in human acute myelogenous leukemia, inhibition of telomerase activity by differentiation-inducing agents. *Clin. Cancer Res.* **2,** 799–803.
54. Yamada, O. (1996) Telomeres and telomerase in human hematologic neoplasia. *Intl. J. Hematol.* **64,** 87–99.
55. Albanell, J., Han, W., Mellado, B., Gunawardane, R., Scher, H. I., Dmitrovsky, E., and Moore, M. A. (1996) Telomerase activity is repressed during differentiation of maturation-sensitive but nor resistant human tumor cell lines. *Cancer Res.* **56,** 1503–1508.
56. Xu, D., Gruber, A., Peterson, C., Pisa, P (1996) Suppression of telomerase activity in HL60 cells after treatment with differentiating agents. *Leukemia* **10,** 1354–1357.
57. Yamada, O., Takanashi, M., Ujihara, M., Mizoguchi, H. (1998) Down-regulation of telomerase activity is an early event of cellular differentiation without apparent telomeric DNA change. *Leukemia Res.* **22,** 711–717.
58. Ohyashiki, K., Ohyashiki, J. H., Iwama, H., Hayashi, S., Kawakubo, K., Shay, J. W., and Toyama, K. (1997) Telomerase activity and cytogenetic changes in chronic myeloid leukemia with disease progression. *Leukemia* **11,** 190–194.
59. Iwama, H., Ohyashiki, K., Ohyashiki, J. H., Hayashi, S., Kawakubo, K., Shay, J. W., and Toyama, K. (1997) The relationship between telomere length and therapy-related cytogenetic responses in patients with chronic myeloid leukemia. *Cancer* **79,** 1552–1560.
60. Ohyashiki, K., Ohyashiki, J. H., Iwama, H., Shay, J. W., and Toyama, K. (1996) Telomerase reactivation in leukemia cells. *Intl. J. Oncol.* **8,** 417–421.
61. Ohyashiki, K., Ohyashiki, J. H., Fujimura, T., Kawakubo, K., Shimamoto, T., Saito, M., et al. (1994) Telomere shortening in leukemic cells is related to their genetic alterations but not replicative capability. *Cancer Genet. Cytogenet.* **78,** 64–67.

62. Ohyashiki, K., Ohyashiki, J. H., Iwabuchi, A., and Toyama, K. (1996) Clinical aspects, cytogenetics and disease evolution in myelodysplastic syndromes. *Leuk. Lymphoma* **23,** 409–415.
63. Ohyashiki, J. H., Ohyashiki, K., Fujimura, T., Kawakubo, K., Shimamoto, T., Iwabuchi, A., and Toyama, K. (1994) Telomere shortening associated with disease evolution patterns in myelodysplastic syndromes. *Cancer Res.* **54,** 3557–3560.
64. Boultwood, J., Fidler, C., Kusec, R., Rack, K., Elliott, P. J. W., Atoyebi, O., Chapman, R., Oscier, D. G., and Wainscoat, J. S. (1997) Telomere length in myelodysplastic syndromes. *Am. J. Hematol.* **56,** 266–271.
65. Greenberg, P., Cox, C., LeBeau, M. M., Fenaux, P., Morel, P., Sanz, G., et al. (1997) International scoring system for evaluating prognosis in myelodysplastic syndromes. *Blood* **89,** 2079–2088.
66. Ohyashiki, J. H., Iwama, H., Yahata, N., Ando, K., Heyoshi, S., Shay, J. W., and Ohyashiki, K. (1999) Telomere stability is frequently impaired in high-risk groups of patients with myelodysplastic syndromes. *Clin. Cancer Res.* **5,** 1150–1160.
67. Shay, J. W. and Bacchetti, S. (1997) A survey of telomerase activity in human cancer. *Eur. J. Cancer* **33,** 787–791.
68. Holt, S. E., Shay, J. W., and Wright, W. E. (1996) Refining the telomere-telomerase hypothesis of aging and cancer. *Nat. Biotechnol.* **14,** 836–839.
69. Ohyashiki, K., Ohyashiki, J. H., Nishimaki, J., Toyama, K., Ebihara, Y., Kato, H., et al. (1997) Cytological detection of telomerase activity using an in situ telomeric repeat amplification protocol assay. *Cancer Res.* **57,** 2100–2103.
70. Shay, J. W. (1995) Aging and cancer: are telomeres and telomerase the connection? *Mol. Med. Today* **1,** 378–384.
71. Shay, J. W. and Wright, W. E. (1996) Telomerase activity in human cancer. *Curr. Opin. Oncol.* **8,** 66–71.
72. Shay. J. W., Werbin, H., and Wright, W. E. (1996) Telomeres and telomerase in human leukemias. *Leukemia* **10,** 1255–1261.
73. Ishikawa, F. (1997) Telomere crisis, the driving force in cancer cell evolution. *Biochem. Biophys. Res. Commun.* **230,** 1–6.

Index

A

ATM gene, 115–124

C

cDNA microarray analysis, 195–204, 205–222,
    hybidization, 200–202, 216–217
    image acquisition and analysis, 201–202, 217–219
    slide preparation, 198–199, 211–215
cDNA synthesis, 85, 165, 198, 215, 265
Cell separation, 164, 263–264
Chronic myeloid leukemia (CML), 67–68, 288–292
Clonality studies, 251–270,
    allele-specific PCR (ASPCR), *see* Polymerase chain reaction
    DNA-RNA-based methods, 253–261
    protein-based methods, 253
    X-chromosome inactivation, 251–252
Cloning into plasmid vector, 167, 188
Comparative genomic hybridization (CGH), 45–57

D

Differential display, 179–193
DNA (genomic) preparation, 100, 274–275
DNA fingerprinting, 107–114,
    arbitrarily primed PCR, 108–109, 112
    interspersed repetitive element PCR (Alu-PCR), 110–111, 112–113
DNA hybridization, 50–51, 102, 244, 276–277

DNA methylation, *see* Clonality studies

F

Fluorescent *in situ* hybridization (FISH), 7–27, 70–71,
    interphase FISH, 21
    metaphase FISH, 20–21
    microscopy, 19–20
    multicolor FISH, 23
    nick-translation, 15–16

L

Loss of heterozygosity (LOH), 59–65

M

Metaphase chromosome preparation, 12–13, 49–50
Methylation analysis of CpG islands, 230–249,
    methylation-specific PCR, 245–246
    Southern analysis, 242–245
Microsatellite analysis, 59–65, 62–63,
    microsatellite selection, 61–62
Minimal residual disease, 75–78, 225–227
Mutational analysis, 115–124, 125–139, 141–155, 157–170, 171–177,
    denaturing gradient gel electrophoresis (DGGE), 125–139
    direct sequencing, 171–177
    nonisotopic RNase cleavage assay (NIRCA), 141–155
    protein truncation assay, 157–170

302 Index

single-strand conformation
polymorphism (SSCP), 115–124
Myelodysplastic syndromes (MDS),
227–228, 292–293

N

NF1 gene, 157–170
Northern blotting, 187–188

P

Polymerase chain reaction (PCR),
117–118, 121–122, 134–135,
147–148, 165–166, 184,
allele-specific PCR (ASPCR), 265–266
degenerate oligonucleotide primed
PCR (DOP-PCR), 36–39
long-range PCR, 97–105, 100–101
quantitative PCR, 78–84, 85–88
reverse transcription PCR (RT-PCR),
74, 75–78, 184, 232–233

R

RNA preparation, 85, 164–165, 182–183,
199, 215, 264–265

S

Sequencing, 102, 167–168, 171–177,
188–189
Southern blotting, 71–72, 102, 242,
276
Spectral karyotyping (SKY), 29–44

T

Telomerase, 279–299,
TRAP assay, 281–282, 293–295
Telomere measurement, 271–278, 280,
hybridization, 276–277
Southern analysis, 276
Translocation, 67–96,
t(9;22), BCR-ABL, 68–70, 74–78
t(2;5), 97–105
Tumor markers, 223–237

W

Western blotting, 74
Wilms tumor gene *WT1*, 223–237
expression, 222–225
solid tumors, 229–230